ANTIOXIDANTS AS NUTRACEUTICALS

AAP Advances in Nutraceuticals

ANTIOXIDANTS AS NUTRACEUTICALS

Nayan A. Gujarathi, PhD
Raj K. Keservani, PhD
Rajesh K. Kesharwani, PhD
Bhushan R. Rane, PhD
Yogeeta Sameer Goyal, PhD
Editors

AAP | APPLE ACADEMIC PRESS

First edition published 2025

Apple Academic Press Inc.
1265 Goldenrod Circle, NE,
Palm Bay, FL 32905 USA

760 Laurentian Drive, Unit 19,
Burlington, ON L7N 0A4, CANADA

CRC Press
2385 NW Executive Center Drive,
Suite 320, Boca Raton FL 33431

4 Park Square, Milton Park,
Abingdon, Oxon, OX14 4RN UK

Library and Archives Canada Cataloguing in Publication

CIP data on file with Canada Library and Archives

Library of Congress Cataloging-in-Publication Data

CIP data on file with US Library of Congress

ISBN: 978-1-77491-738-1 (hbk)
ISBN: 978-1-77491-739-8 (pbk)
ISBN: 978-1-00353-487-7 (ebk)

ABOUT THE BOOK SERIES: AAP ADVANCES IN NUTRACEUTICALS

Series Editor:
Raj K. Keservani, PhD, MPharm
Faculty of B. Pharmacy, CSM Group of Institutions, Allahabad, India

Rajesh K. Kesharwani, PhD
Nehru Gram Bharati (Deemed to be University), Prayagraj, India

Anil K. Sharma, PhD, MPharm
Department of Pharmacy, School of Medical and Allied Sciences, GD Goenka University, Gurugram, India

In the modern era, mankind has witnessed a paradigm shift with respect to fundamental eating behavior. The lack of physical workouts and busy schedules at offices and in households have promoted the consumption of junk foods, which eventually results in numerous diseases and disorders since the nutritional content from fast food is inadequate. Plumpness and obesity have become a global health threat. The leading causes of death from most developing nations are noncommunicable diseases such as cardiovascular diseases, cancer, arthritis, osteoporosis, and liver toxicity. Patients suffering from such lifestyle ailments are a bit apprehensive towards prolonged use of costly modern therapeutics, which encourages instead the use of alternative approaches for management of such diseases and disorders.

The emerging sector of the nutraceutical industry encompasses products derived from nature, dietary supplements, and functional foods. Nutraceuticals are used for treatment and prevention of a broad range of diseases, such as the common cold, arthritis, sleep-related disorders, cancers, cardiovascular complications, metabolic disorders, and others.

The research on nutraceuticals is increasing day by day, considering the beneficial effects of food or food supplements in the management of diverse diseases. The issue of paramount concern is standardization and establishment of clinical efficacy of nutraceuticals, which is in fact a challenge for researchers around the globe.

This book series aims at realizing the significance of the variety of nutraceuticals for human well-being. The books in the series also emphasize the role of dieticians and nutritionists for the prescription of judicious eating habits. The key food components such as carbohydrates, proteins, and lipids as well as micronutrients (vitamins, minerals) are demonstrated to maintain good health, obviating the need for medicines. Thus, nutraceuticals that are indeed derived from food ingredients are believed to be potential alternative therapeutics.

Asymptomatic diseases/disorders necessitate proper diagnosis. Stressed circumstances have been reported to cause weight loss. Workplace stress is a key variable in the genesis and propagation of metabolic disorders. The nuances of the underlying mechanisms are still to be deciphered. Poor lifestyle trends have been attributed along with the consumption of junk foods in several such instances. Sugar-rich carbonated beverages, the use of contraband drugs, and the consumption of liquor in excess are assigned as risk factors. This book series covers advances and applications in addition to providing the basics of nutraceuticals.

The books in this series are valuable resources for industry professionals to design and develop quality products for end users. In addition, the book series is fortified by ideas of innovation, concept building, manufacturing aspects, quality control, and regulatory status of nutraceuticals.

Ostensibly, business has seen a rise in the nutraceutical consumption in recent years. Pure, safe, efficacious products are the need of the hour globally. There are a number of books on nutraceuticals in the market, yet these are only a few books presenting certain aspects of nutraceuticals therein. This book series offers a holistic view of this promising strategy, which is picking up pace with time. This book series is a unique endeavor to bring manufacturing, research and development, and marketing strategies under a single umbrella.

CURRENT BOOKS IN THE SERIES

- **Micronutrients and Macronutrients as Nutraceuticals**
  Editors: Prakash Chandra Gupta, PhD, Sayan Bhattacharyya, MBBS, MD, Nisha Sharma, PhD, MPharm, Rajesh K. Kesharwani, PhD, and Raj K. Keservani, PhD, MPharm
- **Formulations, Regulations, and Challenges of Nutraceuticals**
  Editors: Tingirikari Jagan Mohan Rao, PhD, Rajesh K. Kesharwani, PhD, Raj. K. Keservani, PhD, and Anil K. Sharma, PhD

- **Food Supplements and Dietary Fibers in Health and Disease**
  Editors: Bhushan R. Rane, PhD, MPharm, Raj K. Keservani, PhD, MPharm, Durgesh Singh, DPhil, Nayan A. Gujarathi, PhD, and Ashish S. Jain, PhD
- **Nutraceuticals in Cancer Prevention, Management, and Treatment**
  Editors: Raj K. Keservani, PhD, MPharm Bui Thanh Tung, PhD, Sippy Singh, DPhil, and Rajesh K. Kesharwani, PhD
- **Advances in Flavonoids for Human Health and Prevention of Diseases**
  Editors: Nisha Sharma, PhD, Deepika Saini, PhD, Rajesh K. Kesharwani, PhD, Prakash Chandra Gupta, and Raj. K. Keservani, PhD
- **The Flavonoids: Extraction and Applications**
  Editors: Deepika Saini, PhD, Rajesh K. Kesharwani, PhD, and Raj K. Keservani, PhD, MPharm
- **Immune-Boosting Nutraceuticals for Better Human Health: Novel Applications**
  Editors: Urmila Jarouliya, PhD, Raj K. Keservani, PhD, MPharm Rajesh K. Kesharwani, PhD, Virendra K. Patel, PhD, and Adi D. Bharti
- **Applications of Functional Foods in Disease Prevention**
  Editors: Raj K. Keservani, PhD, MPharm, and Eknath D. Ahire, MSPharm
- **Plant Metabolites and Vegetables as Nutraceuticals**
  Editors: Raj K. Keservani, PhD, MPharm, Bui Thanh Tung, PhD, Rajesh K. Kesharwani, PhD, MPharm, and Eknath D. Ahire
- **Preventive and Therapeutic Role of Vitamins as Nutraceuticals**
  Editors: Khemchand R. Surana, Eknath D. Ahire, Raj K. Keservani, PhD, MPharm, and Rajesh K. Kesharwani, PhD
- **Nutraceuticals and Bone Health**
  Editors: Deepak Sharma, PhD, Madan Mohan Gupta, PhD, Anil K. Sharma, PhD, MPharm, Raj K. Keservani, PhD, MPharm, and Rajesh K. Kesharwani, PhD
- **Flavonoids as Nutraceuticals**
  Editors: Rajesh K. Kesharwani, PhD, MTech, Deepika Saini, PhD, Raj K. Keservani, PhD, MPharm, and Anil Kumar Sharma, PhD
- **Herbals as Nutraceuticals: Their Role in Healthcare**
  Editors: Raj K. Keservani, PhD, MPharm, Rajeshwar Kamal Kant Arya, PhD, and Rajesh K. Kesharwani, PhD
- **Nutraceutical Fruits: Overview and Disease Prevention**
  Editors: Raj K. Keservani, PhD, MPharm

- **Nutrigenomics and Nutraceuticals**
  Editors: Raj K. Keservani, PhD, MPharm, Eknath D. Ahire, Shubham J. Khainar, PhD, Sanjay J. Kshirsagar, PhD, and Rajesh K. Kesharwani, PhD
- **Nutraceuticals in Cardiac Health Management**
  Editors: Raj K. Keservani, PhD, MPharm, Rajesh K. Kesharwani, PhD, Praveen Kumar Jain, PhD, Bhushan R. Rane, PhD, and Nayan A. Gujarathi, PhD
- **Nutraceuticals for the Treatment and Prevention of Sexual Disorders**
  Editors: Raj K. Keservani, PhD, MPharm, Sharangouda J. Patil, PhD, and Ivan Aranha, PhD
- **Nutraceuticals in Obesity Management and Control**
  Editors: Raj K. Keservani, PhD, MPharm, and Alka Lohani, PhD
- **Antioxidants as Nutraceuticals**
  Editors: Nayan A. Gujarathi, PhD, Raj K. Keservani, PhD, MPharm, Rajesh K. Kesharwani, PhD, Bhushan R. Rane, PhD, and Yogeeta Sameer Goyal, PhD
- **The Nature of Nutraceuticals: History, Properties, Sources, and Nanotechnology**
  Editors: Rajesh K. Kesharwani, PhD, Prashant Kumar, PhD, and Raj K. Keservani, PhD, MPharm
- **Nutraceuticals in Insomnia and Sleep Problems**
  Editors: Raj K. Keservani, PhD, MPharm, Sayan Bhattacharyya, PhD, and Rajesh K. Kesharwani, PhD
- **Nutraceuticals in Respiratory and Pulmonary Diseases**
  Editors: Deepika Saini, PhD, Rajesh K. Kesharwani, PhD, and Raj K. Keservani, PhD, MPharm
- **Nutraceuticals in Arthritis and Psoriasis**
  Editors: Meenakshi Jaiswal, PhD, Raj K. Keservani, PhD, MPharm Rajesh K. Kesharwani, PhD, and Swati G. Talele, PhD
- **Nutraceuticals for the Treatment and Prevention of Sexual Disorders**
  Editors: Raj K. Keservani, PhD, Sharangouda J. Patil, PhD, and Ivan Aranha, PhD
- **Antioxidants as Nutraceuticals**
  Editors: Nayan A. Gujaratih, PhD, Raj K. Keservani, PhD, Rajesh K. Kesharwani, PhD, Bhushan R. Rane, PhD, and Yogeeta Sameer Goyal, PhD

- **Nutraceuticals in Management and Prevention of Diabetes**
  Editors: Raj K. Keservani, PhD, Prashant Kumar, PhD, and Dheeraj Chitara, PhD
- **Nutraceuticals in Mental Disorder and Brain Health**
  Editors: Raj K. Keservani, PhD, Eknath D. Ahire, PhD, and Shubham J. Khairnar, PhD

ABOUT THE EDITORS

Nayan A. Gujarathi, PhD, MPharm
Associate Professor, Department of Pharmaceutics, Shri Vile Parle Kelavani Mandal's Institute of Pharmacy, Dhule, India

Nayan A. Gujarathi, PhD, MPharm, is an Associate Professor at the Department of Pharmaceutics, Shri Vile Parle Kelavani Mandal's Institute of Pharmacy, Dhule, India. He has 16 years of academic experience in pharmaceutical science. He has published 24 peer-reviewed papers in the field of pharmaceutical sciences in national and international journals with 12 book chapters in Apple Academic Press/CRC Press books. He has presented his research work at an international conference organized by the Controlled Release Society and delivered four expert talks on the implementation of outcome-based education for the accreditation process. He is an approved postgraduate teacher in Pharmaceutics by North Maharashtra University, Jalgaon, and Savitribai Phule University, Pune, both in India. He successfully guided 24 MPharm students of Pharmaceutics. He has been appointed as a referee (evaluator) at the university level for Avishkar 2013 and Avishkar 2017 by North Maharashtra University, Jalgaon. He completed a minor research project sanctioned by BCUD, North Maharashtra University, Jalgaon. His research interest encompasses novel drug delivery systems, polymer science, nanotechnology, and nutraceuticals. He received a diploma in Pharmacy from the Government Polytechnic, Jalgaon, India, and a bachelor's degree in Pharmacy from the North Maharashtra University. He completed a Master of Pharmacy degree with a specialization in Pharmaceutics at the School of Pharmaceutical Sciences, Rajiv Gandhi Proudyogiki Vishwavidyalaya, Bhopal, India. He was awarded his PhD in Pharmaceutical Sciences by Jodhpur National University, Jodhpur, India.

Raj K. Keservani, PhD, MPharm
Associate Professor, Faculty of B. Pharmacy, CSM Group of Institutions, Prayagraj, India

Raj K. Keservani, PhD, MPharm, is working as Associate Professor in the Faculty of B. Pharmacy at the CSM Group of Institutions, Prayagraj, India. He has more than 12 years of academic (teaching) experience from various institutes of India in pharmaceutical education. He has supervised more than 25 undergraduate students for their research work. He has published over 30 peer-reviewed papers in the field of pharmaceutical sciences in national and international journals, six patents, over 70 book chapters, three co-authored books, and over 40 edited books. He is also active as a reviewer for several international scientific journals. His research interests include nutraceutical and functional foods, novel drug delivery systems (NDDS), transdermal drug delivery/drug delivery, health science, cancer biology, and neurobiology. Dr. Keservani graduated with a pharmacy degree from the Department of Pharmacy, Kumaun University, Nainital, Uttarakhand, India. He received his Master of Pharmacy (MPharm) (specialization in pharmaceutics) from the School of Pharmaceutical Sciences, Rajiv Gandhi Proudyogiki Vishwavidyalaya, Bhopal, India. He earned his PhD degree from IKG Punjab Technical University, Jalandhar, Punjab, India. Dr. Keservani is a life member of the Society of Pharmaceutical Education and Research (SPER).

Rajesh K. Kesharwani, PhD, MTech
Associate Professor, Department of Computer Application, Nehru Gram Bharati (Deemed to be University), Prayagraj, India

Rajesh K. Kesharwani, PhD, is working as Associate Professor in the Department of Computer Application, Nehru Gram Bharati (Deemed to be University), Prayagraj, India. He has more than 11 years of research and nine years of teaching experience at various institutes of India, imparting bioinformatics and biotechnology education. He has received several awards, including the NASI-Swarna Jayanti Puruskar by The National Academy of Sciences of India. He has supervised one PhD and more than 20 undergraduate and graduate students for their research work. Dr. Kesharwani has authored over 49 peer-reviewed articles, 20 book chapters, and 14 edited books with international publishers. He has been a member of many scientific communities as well as a reviewer for many international journals. He has presented many papers at various national and international conferences. He has been a recipient of a Ministry of Human Resource Development (India) Fellowship and a Senior Research Fellowship from the Indian Council of Medical Research, India. His research fields of interest are medical informatics, protein structure and function prediction, computer-aided drug designing, structural biology, drug delivery, cancer biology, nanobiotechnology, and biomedical sciences. Dr. Kesharwani received his PhD from the Indian Institute of Information Technology, Allahabad, and worked at NIT Warangal for two semesters.

Bhushan R. Rane, PhD, MPharm
Shri. D. D. Vispute, College of Pharmacy and Research Center, New Panvel, Navi Mumbai, India

Bhushan R. Rane, PhD, MPharm, is presently Professor and Head of the Department of Pharmaceutics, Shri. D. D. Vispute, College of Pharmacy and Research Center, New Panvel, Navi Mumbai, India, affiliated to Mumbai University, Maharashtra, India. He has over 15 years of teaching experience at undergraduate and postgraduate levels. To date, he has guided more than 50 students for their MPharm degrees. He has published more than 75 peer-reviewed research and review articles in national and international journals. He has co-authored eight books at the national level and more than 15 book chapters at the international level published by Taylor and Francis Group and Bentham Science Worldwide. He is a reviewer for several scientific and international journals. He received grants from various bodies for research, such as All India Council for Technical Education (AICTE), New Delhi. He is a lifetime member of several professional organizations. His research interests are focused on planning, improvement, and the portrayal of vesicular, microparticulate, and nanoparticulate systems, and advancement of different solid dosage forms for oral conveyance.

Yogeeta Sameer Goyal, PhD, MPharm
Associate Professor, Shri Vile Parle Kelavani Mandal's Institute of Pharmacy, Dhule, India

Yogeeta Sameer Goyal, PhD, MPharm, is an Associate Professor and Head of the Department of Pharmaceutics at Shri Vile Parle Kelavani Mandal's Institute of Pharmacy, Dhule, India. She has 17 years of research and academic experience in pharmaceutical science. She has published 29 peer-reviewed papers in national and international journals. Her h-index is 12 and i10-index is 13. She has published patents at the Indian patent office. She is an approved postgraduate teacher and PhD guide in pharmaceutics by North Maharashtra University, Jalgaon, India. She has successfully guided 25 students for their MPharm degrees and is currently guiding six PhD students. She has successfully completed a major research project sanctioned by the Department of Biotechnology, Govt of India. She received several awards for her work, including gold medals for earning the highest marks at both the BPharm and MPharm levels. She received two minor projects from Kavayitri Bahinabai Chaudhari North Maharashtra University for her research work. She also received a complete international travel grant from the Indian Council of Medical Research (ICMR) to present her research work at an international conference in Dubai. She has participated as delegate and resource person in several workshops and conferences. Her research interests encompass novel drug delivery systems, especially formulation, development, optimization, and in-vitro and in-vivo evaluation of nanostructured lipid carrier.

CONTENTS

Contributors .... *xvii*

Preface .... *xxi*

PART I: Basics of Types of Antioxidants as Nutraceuticals **1**

1. Natural Antioxidants as Nutraceuticals **3**
Dattatraya M. Shinkar, Amit B. Page, Prashant S. Malpure, Bhushan Rane, and Prashant L. Pingale

2. Importance of Phytochemical Antioxidants **39**
Yogeeta Goyal, Mrunali Patil, Kamini More, and Kiran Patil

3. Epigallocatechin Gallate: Nutritional and Pharmacological Intervention in the Treatment of Disease **67**
Myrene Roselyn D'souza and Khalid Mohammed Naji

4. Immunomodulation Property of Antioxidants **95**
Kiran Patil, Sopan Nangare, Meghanath Shete, Madhav Shelke, Matin Shaikh, Mrugendra Potdar, Vinit Agnihotri, and Yogeeta Goyal

PART II: Novel Strategies of Antioxidants in the Treatment of Chronic Diseases **125**

5. Antioxidants as Nutraceuticals in the Prevention and Treatment of Cardiovascular Disease **127**
Amey Sukhia, Nayan A. Gujarathi, Tulshidas S. Patil, Abhijeet Aher, Bhushan Rane, and Raj K. Keservani

6. Novel Strategies of Antioxidants in Chronic Inflammatory Diseases **157**
Sumit Rathod, Ujwal Katolkar, Vinit Agnihotri, Mrugendra Potdar, and Yogeeta Goyal

7. Plant-Derived Antioxidant Nutraceuticals for the Treatment of Neurodegenerative Disorders **195**
Prashant Amale, Kushagra Nagori, Hemant Badwaik, Madhuri Baghel, and Kartik Nakhate

8. Nutraceutical Antioxidants in the Prevention and Treatment of Diabetes Mellitus 225
Neha Panchabhai, Harshad Jadhav, Sanjiri Dilip Shelar, Amey Sukhia, Nayan A. Gujarathi, and Raj K. Keservani

PART III: Functional Foods Rich in Antioxidants 263

9. Antioxidants-Rich Food Sources of Nutraceutical and Functional Foods 265
Sujit Arun Desai, Preeti Khulbe, Yuvraj Dilip Dange, Satwashila Kadam, and Meenakshi Jaiswal

10. Anti-Stress Functional Foods 283
Neelesh Kumar Maurya, Latika Yadav, Pratibha Arya, Abhijeet Aher, and Nayan A. Gujarathi

11. An Update on the Role of Antioxidants in Health and Disease Prevention 305
Mrugendra Bhojraj Potdar, Kiran Patil, Md. Rageeb Md. Usman, and Raju Ratan Wadekar

Index 337

CONTRIBUTORS

Vinit Agnihotri
Department of Pharmaceutics, SVKM Institute of Pharmacy, Dhule, India

Abhijeet Aher
Shri Vile Parle Kelavani Mandal's Institute of Pharmacy, Dhule, Maharashtra, India

Prashant Amale
Priyadarshini J. L. College of Pharmacy, Electronic Zone Building, MIDC, Hingna Road, Nagpur, Maharashtra, India

Pratibha Arya
Institute of Home Science, Bundelkhand University, Jhansi, Uttar Pradesh, India

Hemant Badwaik
Shri Shankaracharya Institute of Pharmaceutical Sciences and Research, Junwani, Bhilai, Chhattisgarh, India

Madhuri Baghel
Shri Shankaracharya Institute of Pharmaceutical Sciences and Research, Junwani, Bhilai, Chhattisgarh, India

Yuvraj Dilip Dange
Annasaheb Dange College of D Pharmacy Ashta Sangli, Maharashtra, India

Sujit Arun Desai
Annasaheb Dange College of D Pharmacy Ashta Sangli, Maharashtra, India

Myrene Roselyn D'souza
Department of Biochemistry, Mount Carmel College Autonomous, Karnataka, India

Yogeeta Sameer Goyal
Department of Pharmaceutics, Shri Vile Parle Kelavani Mandal's Institute of Pharmacy, Dhule, Maharashtra, India

Nayan A. Gujarathi
Shri Vile Parle Kelavani Mandal's Institute of Pharmacy, Dhule, Maharashtra, India

Harshad Jadhav
Department of Pharmaceutical Analysis, National Institute of Pharmaceutical Education and Research, S.A.S Nagar, Mohali, Punjab, India

Meenakshi Jaiswal
Department of Pharmacy, Guru Ghasidas Central University, Koni, Bilaspur, India

Satwashila Kadam
Womens College of Pharmacy, Peth-Vadgaon, Maharashtra, India

Ujwal Katolkar
Department of Pharmacology, R. C. Patel Institute of Pharmaceutical Education and Research, Shirpur, India

Raj K. Keservani
Faculty of B. Pharmacy, CSM Group of Institutions, Prayagraj, Uttar Pradesh, India

Preeti Khulbe
Gyan Vihar School of Pharmacy, Suresh Gyan Vihar University Jaipur, Gyan Vihar Marg, Jagatpura, Jaipur, Rajasthan, India

Prashant S. Malpure
KCT's R. G. Sapkal College of Pharmacy, Trimbakeshwar Road, Nashik, India

Neelesh Kumar Maurya
Department of Home Science, PK University, Shivpuri, Madhya Paradesh, India

Kamini More
Department of Pharmaceutics, Shri Vile Parle Kelavani Mandal's Institute of Pharmacy, Dhule, Maharashtra, India

Kushagra Nagori
Rungta College of Pharmaceutical Sciences and Research, Kohka-Kurud Road, Bhilai, Chhattisgarh, India

Khalid Mohammed Naji
Department of Chemistry, Faculty of Science, Sana'a University, Sana'a, Yemen
Department of Chemical Ecology/Biological Chemistry, Konstanz University, Konstanz, Germany

Kartik Nakhate
Shri Vile Parle Kelavani Mandal's Institute of Pharmacy, Mumbai-Agra Highway, Behind Gurudwara, Dhule, Maharashtra, India

Sopan Nangare
Department of Pharmaceutics, H. R. Patel Institute of Pharmaceutical Education and Research, Shirpur, India

Amit B. Page
SVKM's NMIMS School of Pharmacy and Technology Management, Shirpur, India

Neha Panchabhai
N.D.M.V.P. College of Pharmacy, Nashik, Maharashtra, India

Kiran Patil
Department of Pharmaceutics, Shri Vile Parle Kelavani Mandal's Institute of Pharmacy, Dhule, Maharashtra, India

Mrunali Patil
Department of Pharmaceutical Chemistry, Shri Vile Parle Kelavani Mandal's Institute of Pharmacy, Dhule, Maharashtra, India

Tulshidas S. Patil
Shri Vile Parle Kelavani Mandal's Institute of Pharmacy, Dhule, Maharashtra, India

Prashant L. Pingale
Gokhale Education Society's Sir Dr. M. S. Gosavi College of Pharmaceutical Education and Research, Nashik, India

Mrugendra Bhojraj Potdar
Department of Pharmaceutics, Shri Vile Parle Kelavani Mandal's Institute of Pharmacy Dhule, Maharashtra, India

Md. Rageeb Md. Usman
Smt. Sharadchandrika Suresh Patil College of Pharmacy, Chopda, Maharashtra, India

Bhushan Rane
Shri D. D. Vispute College of Pharmacy and Research Center, New Panvel, Maharashtra, India

Sumit Rathod
Department of Pharmacy, SVKM's Institute of Pharmacy, Dhule, India

Matin Shaikh
Department of Pharmaceutical Chemistry, H. R. Patel Institute of Pharmaceutical Education and Research, Shirpur, India

Sanjiri Dilip Shelar
Department of Pharmaceutical Sciences and Technology, Institute of Chemical Technology, Matunga, Mumbai, Maharashtra, India

Madhav Shelke
Department of Pharmaceutical Quality Assurance, SVKM Institute of Pharmacy, Dhule, India

Meghanath Shete
Department of Pharmaceutics, R. C. Patel Institute of Pharmaceutical Education and Research, Shirpur, India

Dattatraya M. Shinkar
Gokhale Education Society's Sir Dr. M. S. Gosavi College of Pharmaceutical Education and Research, Nashik, India

Amey Sukhia
Department of Pharmacy Sciences, Creighton University, Omaha, Nebraska

Raju Ratan Wadekar
Department of Pharmacognosy, Shri Vile Parle Kelavani Mandal's Institute of Pharmacy Dhule, Maharashtra, India

Latika Yadav
Government Degree College, Punwarka, Saharanpur, Uttar Pradesh, India

PREFACE

The book *Antioxidants as Nutraceuticals* explores the exciting and rapidly growing field of natural compounds with health-promoting properties. Antioxidants and nutraceuticals have gained significant attention in recent years due to their potential to protect against various diseases and improve overall health. These compounds are naturally occurring in fruits, vegetables, and other foods, and are also available in supplement form.

This book provides a comprehensive overview of antioxidants and nutraceuticals, including their sources, mechanisms of action, and health benefits. It covers the latest research on a range of antioxidants and nutraceuticals, including vitamins, minerals, and phytochemicals, and provides practical information on their safe and effective use. The book also addresses the challenges and controversies surrounding the use of antioxidants and nutraceuticals, and provides guidance on their selection and use.

It comprises 11 chapters within three parts that discuss the basics of types of antioxidant nutraceuticals, novel strategies of antioxidants in the treatment of several chronic diseases, and functional foods rich in antioxidants.

PART I: BASICS OF TYPES OF ANTIOXIDANTS AS NUTRACEUTICALS

Chapter 1, *Natural Antioxidants as Nutraceuticals,* written by Dattatraya M. Shinkar and colleagues, summarizes the natural origins of antioxidants as well as their classification, mechanism of action, calculation of antioxidant potential of nutraceutical substances, safety, toxicity, and their significant involvement in the prevention of many degenerative and chronic diseases.

Chapter 2, Phytochemical Antioxidants as Nutraceuticals, written by *Yogeeta Sameer Goyal* and colleagues, describes in detail about the importance of phytochemicals as nutraceuticals.

Chapter 3, *Epigallocatechin Gallate: Nutritional and Pharmacological Intervention in the Treatment of Disease,* is written by Myrene Roselyn D'souza and Khalid Mohammed Naji. They explain that EGCG promotes the prevention and treatment of a variety of health issues, including Alzheimer's, Parkinson's, cancer, cardiovascular disorders, and obesity. Recent developments in EGCG nanodelivery systems are highlighted in the chapter, and the authors explain the significance of utilizing technology to enhance the therapeutic advantages of EGCG.

Chapter 4, *Immunomodulation Property of Antioxidant Nutraceuticals,* written by Kiran Patil and colleagues, elaborate on the application of antioxidants as immunomodulators with special emphasis on different antioxidant defenses for immunomodulation. Moreover, an update of antioxidants as immunomodulators is also summarized. Finally, the present problems and future possibilities of antioxidant immunomodulation properties have been explored.

PART II: NOVEL STRATEGIES OF ANTIOXIDANTS IN THE TREATMENT OF CHRONIC DISEASES

Chapter 5, *Antioxidants as Nutraceuticals in the Prevention and Treatment of Cardiovascular Disease,* written by Amey Sukhia and colleagues, discusses the role of reactive species in the etiology of various heart-related. Further, the chapter deliberates on various nutraceuticals with antioxidant properties that can serve as a potential solution to the problem by scavenging and quenching.

Chapter 6, *Novel Strategies of Antioxidants in Chronic Inflammatory Diseases,* written by Sumit Rathod and colleagues, thoroughly illustrates the recent advancement in the development of natural products as future anti-inflammatory drugs for various chronic inflammatory disorders and diseases.

Chapter 7, *Plant-Derived Antioxidant Nutraceuticals for the Treatment of Neurodegenerative Disorders,* written by Kartik Nakhate and colleague, elaborates on several findings and recent trends in antioxidant nutraceuticals with reference to their potential in the treatment of neurodegenerative disorders.

Chapter 8, *Nutraceutical Antioxidants in the Prevention and Treatment of Diabetes Mellitus,* written by Neha Panchabhai and colleagues, describes few conditions that arise due to diabetes like diabetic retinopathy, diabetic nephropathy, tissue damage, etc. can be controlled by some of the nutraceutical antioxidants. Vitamin E and vitamin D play an important role against diabetic nephropathy and retinopathy.

PART III: FUNCTIONAL FOODS RICH IN ANTIOXIDANTS

Chapter 9, *Antioxidants-Rich Food Sources of Functional and Nutraceutical Values,* written by Preeti Khulbe and colleagues, provides an in-depth discussion on the promotion of older people's health through dietary intake frequency and patterns, as well as the application of a human ecology framework to calculate harmful risk factors for health.

Chapter 10, *Anti-Stress Functional Food,* written by Neelesh Kumar Maurya and colleagues, discusses several antioxidants and neurotransmitters naturally produced in a variety of fruits and vegetables, cereals, nuts and seeds, and beverages that aid in stress reduction and for the benefits of mental health.

Chapter 11, *An Update on the Role of Antioxidants in Health and Disease Prevention,* written by Mrugendra Bhojraj Potdar and colleagues, explains that the “oxidative stress” is a significant element in the pathogenic processes associated with many chronic diseases, and a deficiency in antioxidant-reactive oxygen species balance can lead to this stress. The chapter deals with the potential role of antioxidant for health benefits, as well as it also addresses its potential therapeutic benefits in disease condition.

This book is intended for a wide audience, including health professionals, scientists, and the general public. It provides a valuable resource for anyone interested in learning about the potential health benefits of antioxidants and nutraceuticals and their role in maintaining good health and preventing disease. Whether the reader is a seasoned researcher or just beginning to explore the world of antioxidants and nutraceuticals, this book is an indispensable guide to this fascinating and important field.

PART I

BASICS OF TYPES OF ANTIOXIDANTS AS NUTRACEUTICALS

CHAPTER 1

NATURAL ANTIOXIDANTS AS NUTRACEUTICALS

DATTATRAYA M. SHINKAR[1], AMIT B. PAGE[2], PRASHANT S. MALPURE[3], BHUSHAN RANE[4], and PRASHANT L. PINGALE[1]

[1]*Gokhale Education Society's Sir Dr. M. S. Gosavi College of Pharmaceutical Education and Research, Nashik, India*

[2]*SVKM's NMIMS School of Pharmacy and Technology Management, Shirpur, India*

[3]*KCT's R. G. Sapkal College of Pharmacy, Trimbakeshwar Road, Nashik, India*

[4]*Shri D.D. Vispute College of Pharmacy and Research Center, New Panvel, Maharashtra, India*

ABSTRACT

Natural-source drugs, foods, and dietary supplements have an important role in the global public healthcare system. Nutraceuticals is a broad term that refers to foods, food substances, and dietary supplements that are beneficial to health and disease prevention. These nutraceuticals aid in the fight against the century's key health issues by providing specialized health or pharmaceutical advantages to degenerative and chronic disorders like arthritis, heart diseases, cancer, osteoporosis, diabetes cholesterol, etc. As a result, many researchers have focused their efforts on creating novel treatments, by focusing on the importance of using natural antioxidants such as alkaloids, terpenoids, polyphenols, and carotenoids. The antioxidant activities

Antioxidants as Nutraceuticals. Nayan A. Gujarathi, Raj K. Keservani, Rajesh K. Kesharwani, Bhushan R. Rane, Yogeeta Sameer Goyal (Eds.)

of phytochemicals have been confirmed by a variety of in vitro and in vivo studies. As natural antioxidants, many of these phytochemical substances are important elements of the nutraceutical market, and they aid in the prevention of many degenerative and chronic diseases around the world. Antioxidant shields the body from the harmful effects of reactive oxygen species (ROS), which are produced spontaneously during physiological activities. The chapter summarizes the natural origins of antioxidants, classification, mechanism of action, calculation of the antioxidant potential of nutraceutical substances, safety, toxicity, and their significant involvement in the prevention of many degenerative and chronic diseases.

1.1 INTRODUCTION

Nowadays, a new nutritional health diet model is gaining popularity around the world, with a greater emphasis on the positive components of eating. Consumption of junk food as part of today's new lifestyle has altered basic food habits and multiplied the number of ailments caused by poor nutrition. In most developing countries, the leading cause of death is obesity and heart disease followed by cancer, osteoporosis, arthritis, and a slew of other ailments that are now well-recognized as worldwide problems. All chronic disease patients who are disappointed with the present medical system's pricey and advanced disease-treatment methods are looking for complementary or alternative helpful approaches to health promotion and disease prevention (Carocho and Ferreira, 2013).

As a result of this increased knowledge of the need to live a better lifestyle, organic food products of natural origin and nutritionally rich antioxidants were consumed more frequently than synthetic and processed foods. Furthermore, antioxidants of synthetic nature and preservatives in food have been allied to peroxidation of lipid and a loss of flavor and quality (Brewer, 2011). As a result, the authentication of innovative phytochemicals with appealing biological activity, like antioxidant, anticancer, and antibacterial properties, has become a hot issue in the food sector, with the goal of food researchers developing new functional and therapeutic products (Irshad and Chaudhary, 2002).

In the food, pharmaceutical, and cosmetic industries, researchers are working to produce regular sources of antioxidants that are less expensive and more natural than synthetic supplements (Tiwari, 2001). Although no serious side effects from synthetic supplements have been reported, a prevalent belief that supplementation should be closer to nature is clearly a healthier strategy. As a result, the coming epoch will be called the "Age of

Natural Products," with researchers focusing on natural antioxidants for the use as nutraceuticals (Shebis et al., 2013).

The major objective of this chapter is to deliver an outline of the benefits of natural antioxidants as a nutraceutical and functional food (Keservani et al., 2010a; Keservani et al., 2010b; Keservani et al., 2017; Keservani et al., 2020) in promoting fitness and lowering the possibility of chronic diseases in the modern era of medicine.

1.1.1 NUTRACEUTICALS

People have long used a growing range of natural items that blur the border between food and medication, but recent scientifically backed dietary and medical evidence has allowed them to be beneficial against many chronic diseases. They are produced from plant and animal sources, and they offer the food industry exciting prospects to develop new food products in the future. Rather than focusing on negative elements like microbe amount, adulterants, fatty acids, and inorganic pollutant concentration, nutritional studies are instead looking at foods for their disease-prevention and prevention potential. As a result, researchers from all over the world are working on it. Therefore, scientists across the world are concentrating their efforts on different sources of essential nutrients to promote a healthier and more convenient diet.

Nutraceutical is defined by Health Canada as "a substance extracted or refined from foods that is generally delivered in therapeutic forms not normally associated with food." Many chronic diseases have been biologically benefited or protected from nutraceuticals (Ahad et al., 2017). Stephen DeFelice, creator and head of the Foundation for Innovation in Medicine, an American organization that promotes medical wellness, invented the word "nutraceutical" in 1989 (DeFelice, 1995; Jack, 1995; Brower, 1998; Mannion, 1998). "Neutraceuticals" denotes "any material like nutrients or a component of food that provides therapeutic or health advantages by preventing and treating various degenerative and chronic diseases," according to DeFelice (Pandey et al., 2010; Kalra, 2003; Ferrari, 2004).

Nutraceuticals can originate in a wide range of foodstuffs made by the food, herbal, dietary supplement industry, and pharmaceutical industries. Herbal or natural products, as well as dietary supplements, are two of the fastest-growing areas (Dev et al., 2011). The global nutraceutical market grew up to $74.7 billion dollars in 2007, from $46.7 billion dollars in 2002 (BCC Research). The United States, the United Kingdom, and Japan are the major countries with nutraceutical markets. Herbal preparations (Sharma et al., 2020; Rane et al., 2020a; Rane et al., 2020b; Rane et al., 2020c), isolated nutrients, dietary supplements, and diets are among the nutraceutical items available, as are hereditarily produced "designer" meals and processed foods including cereals, soups, and beverages (Tank et al., 2010; Chaturvedi et al., 2011).

1.1.2 OXIDATION PROCESS

In aerobic organisms' metabolism, oxygen is a critical chemical component. Many foods are made up of a variety of chemical components that are easily oxidized. Fats, oils, and waxes, for example, have the highest inclination for leaking electrons. Lipids present in food are oxidized if exposed to heat, light, ionizable radiation, metal ions, or metalloprotein catalysts, which have been proven to degrade the organoleptic qualities of foods. Triglycerides are found in the fats of functional meals, and their oxidation causes food to become rancid at the unsaturated triglyceride sites.

In biological systems, free radicals are the most common oxidants. Atoms, molecules, and ions have unpaired electrons are known as free radicals and are extremely reactive with other compounds. Free radicals are produced regularly in biological systems from oxygen, nitrogen, and sulfur molecules, and acquire electrons from other elements to stabilize themselves. Even though the first assault pairs the odd electrons, the procedure produces another free radical, culminating in a chain reaction (Angelo et al., 1996; Bandyopadhyay et al., 1999).

However, because oxygen can generate unfavorable reactions, researchers have been looking into the part of its reactive species. Free radicals such as the superoxide anion, singlet oxygen, lipid peroxides, and the hydroxyl radical are examples of reactive oxygen species (ROS). These reactive species are vital in cell signaling, apoptosis, gene expression, and ion transport. They are generated as a by-product of regular cellular energy generation and functional activities. Damage to highly reactive molecules such as proteins, lipids, RNA, and DNA occurs when ROS levels rise. Unsaturated fatty acid double bonds, side chains of amino acids in proteins, and nucleic acid bases are all destroyed by the most powerful oxidant, OH. Oxidative stress is the term for ROS-attacking macromolecules. Cells can generally fight themselves against ROS damage by using internal enzymes to maintain a low level of ROS homeostasis. Free radicals are produced not just by the human body's natural metabolic processes (endogenous sources), but also by external stressors like hassle, pollution, toxic waste, insect killer, and industrial substances (exogenous sources). When the production of ROS exceeds their removal by biological processes, such as antioxidant defence, oxidative stress occurs. Hence, stress due to oxidation plays an important part in a variety of disorders, like cancer, diabetes, arthrosclerosis, neurological diseases, Alzheimer's disease, inflammatory disease, cardiovascular disease, cataracts, autism, and aging. As a result, the body of human and animals have grown a defence system against oxidation that pools metal chelating, enzymatic, and free radical hunting capabilities to neutralize them after they arise, preventing or minimizing ROS-induced oxidative damage. Furthermore, eating natural antioxidants may aid in the maintenance of a sufficient antioxidant state in the body (Giles and Jacob, 2002).

1.1.3 ANTIOXIDANTS

Antioxidants are oxidation inhibitors that eliminate free-radical intermediates by oxidizing themselves (Cornelli, 2009), and protects the organisms from hazardous chain reactions by reducing oxidation reactions through variety of physiological functions in the body. Antioxidants are compounds that slow or prevent oxidation-related degradation, damage, or destruction. According to studies antioxidants are discovered in a number of foods, including beverages. In biological systems, an antioxidant is any chemical that considerably slows or prevents oxidation of an oxidizable substrate or macromolecules if present at low concentrations than oxidizable substrate like DNA, fats, and proteins. Antioxidants are molecules that capture dangerous types of oxygen and prevent them from causing cell damage. Mechanistic descriptions of antioxidants mainly rely on their ability to donate hydrogen or electrons. Many of the most commonly used antioxidant capacity tests can be divided into two categories: based on transfer of hydrogen and distinct electron transfer assays measures the sample radical hunting or reduction capability, but not its preventive activity. The body's natural defence mechanism contrary to free radicals plays an important part, which can be aided by antioxidant supplements in the diet (Beasley et al., 2020).

The nutraceutical sector relies heavily on antioxidants. They make up a large portion of the most well-known nutrients. Many substances have antioxidant activity, either directly or indirectly. These are abundant and diverse in nature, and they protect against oxidation by neutralizing free radicals at low concentrations. Antioxidants are only officially defined in terms of "dietary antioxidants" (De Rijk et al., 1997). Dietary antioxidants and related compounds, as defined by the Panel on Food and Nutrition, are "a molecule in food that considerably reduces the detrimental properties of reactive oxygen and nitrogen species, or both on normal physiology" (Ferrari, 2001).

1.1.3.1 ANTIOXIDANTS PROCESS AND MECHANISM

Antioxidants inhibit the oxidation process by neutralizing free radicals and oxidizing themselves through two different pathways: chain-breaking and preventative action.

i. **Chain-breaking:** A second radical is created when a free radical releases or abstracts one electron and then it repeats the process with a third molecule, resulting in more unstable compounds. The process of antioxidant effect of cycle continues until a chain-breaking antioxidant, such as beta-carotene or vitamins C and E, stabilizes the radical or it decays into a harmless molecule.

ii. **Prevention of oxidation:** Antioxidants inhibit occurrence of oxidation by scavenging free radicals, slowing the onset of chain reactions can prevent an oxidation chain from ever starting. They can also prevent oxidation by stabilizing transition metal radicals like copper and iron (Buttriss et al., 2002).

1.1.3.2 MECHANISM OF ACTION OF ANTIOXIDANTS

Antioxidants reduce the energy of free radicals or limit free radical generation at the cellular level, or they heal damage and reconstitute membranes, as seen in Figure 1.1.

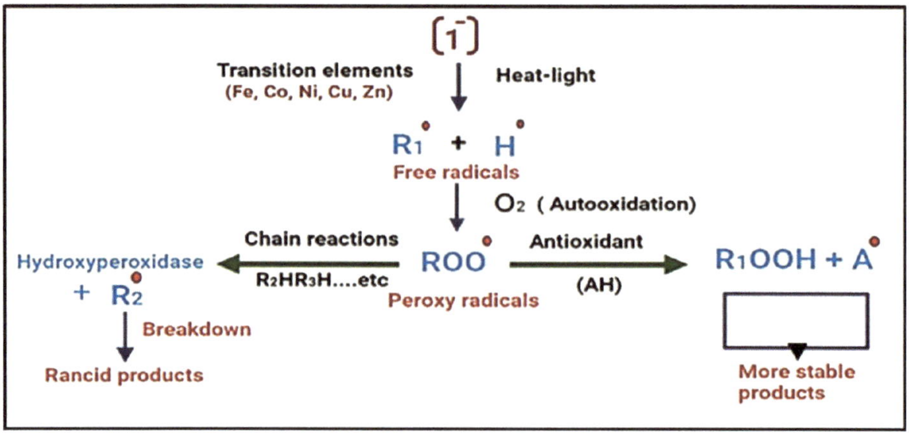

FIGURE 1.1 Antioxidants—mechanism of action.

Antioxidant reduces lipid oxidation by inhibiting the formation of free alkyl radicals at the start of the reaction or stops the free radical chain transmission. The compounds having metal chelating properties, inhibitors of oxygen, and peroxide stabilizers can all help to postpone the onset of free radical production. The transfer of hydrogen from antioxidants and metal chelating agents is the mechanism responsible for the limit the propagation of free radicals.

They are included in fruits and vegetables provide a variety of possible health benefits. The term "nutraceuticals" refer to the recording of health-protectant elements in nutrients and their mode of action, like beta glucan in oat bran, rather than the whole-food notions comprehended in a phrase like functional foods (Brewer, 2011).

1.2 NATURAL ANTIOXIDANTS

Naturally occurring abundant components with endless supply can be utilized as health-promoting agents (Liu et al., 1997; Carocho and Ferreira, 2013). A fruit, vegetables, herbs, spices, and edible mushrooms obtained from natural sources are already part of our daily diet (Ramalakshmi et al., 2008; Duran et al., 2018). A large number of medicinal plants have also been demonstrated to have substantial health-promoting qualities, such as antioxidant capabilities. Antioxidants are classified into two categories: synthetic and natural. Natural antioxidants are phenolic chemicals found in vegetables, fruits, nuts, seeds, leaves, roots, and barks, among other places. Some toxicological investigations studied by many researchers on synthetic antioxidants revealed their unfavorable or negative consequences, recommend that they concentrate their research on natural sources with reasonable antioxidant capacity, such as algae and sea grass from the sea. However, availability and cost are important considerations when employing natural antioxidants (Cao et al., 1998).

Antioxidants derived from natural sources can be divided into several subcategories are from normally consumed or routine natural diet and from plant or herb sources with reasonable antioxidant benefit but are not a common dietary source. As a result, it is critical to identify and publicize these natural sources, which may be evaluated from top to bottom in terms of their antioxidant capacity as a common dietary component that is freely existing and more suitable for nutritional involvements. Many research findings suggested that people who eat vegetables and fruits on a daily basis as part of their meal have been shown to be fewer affected by a variety of chronic diseases due to long-term health benefits of eating a diet rich with natural foods (Slavin and Lloyd, 2012). Dietary supplements containing vitamin E and C from synthetic and natural sources are the most frequent. Citrus fruits are high in vitamin C, as are fruits including oranges, lemons, grapes, strawberry, prunes, blueberry and plums, red beans, spinach, and broccoli flowers (Nahak et al., 2014; Hurrell, 2003). However, because their availability is linked to ecological supply, as well as farming, these are a part of our daily diet. However, because of international trade, they are now available all year round, encouraging the eating of periodic and fresh fruits for a healthy lifestyle (Sonia et al., 2016; August et al., 1996).

1.3 CLASSIFICATION OF NATURAL ANTIOXIDANTS

Natural antioxidants are classified as enzymatic or nonenzymatic depending on the primary site of free radical damage and antioxidant defence mechanism at the cellular level in systemic circulation. Glutathione peroxidase, catalase, superoxide dismutase, and few additional enzymes originated in the body's serum plays a vital as enzymatic antioxidant with greater potential. Nonenzymatic antioxidants include the minerals like zinc and selenium, vitamins, enzyme cofactors (Q10), and peptides. Polyphenolic compounds are the main natural substances that have been shown to have strong antioxidant activity. Figure 1.2 shows a complete classification and sub classification of natural antioxidants (Droge, 2002).

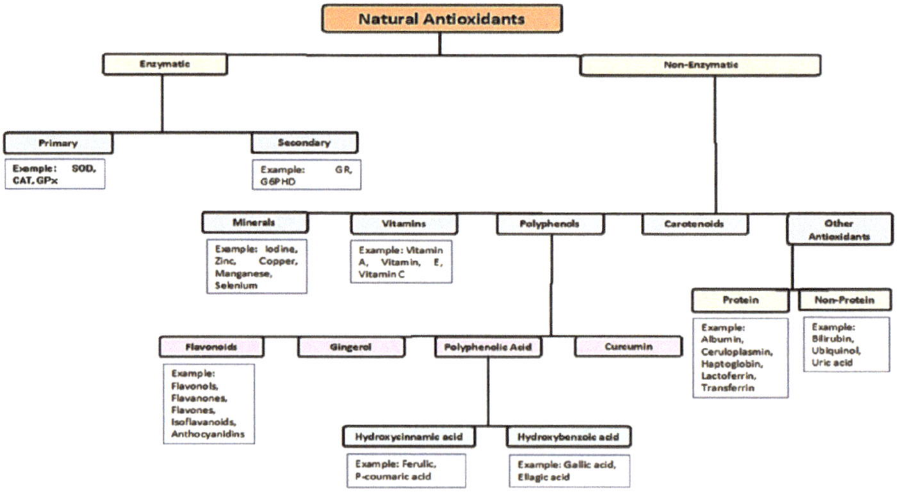

FIGURE 1.2 Classification of natural antioxidants.

1.3.1 *ENZYMATIC ANTIOXIDANTS*

Enzyme-based antioxidants deactivate or stabilize the free radicals before they affect cellular components and minimize cellular network damage by letting free radicals to provide some of their electrons for utilization, allowing them to become stable and disrupting the oxidative chain reaction. Therefore, providing or increasing our consumption of food or supplement with antioxidant enzymes strengthens our bodies ability to resist free radical-related health problems. As a result, antioxidant enzymes are totally life-threatening for a human's proper cellular and systemic health (Droge, 2002).

The principal mechanism of defence against free radicals is antioxidant repair enzymes like superoxide dismutase (SOD), catalase (CAT), glutathione reductase (GR), and glutathione peroxidase (GPx). All the enzymes form jointly a support system of ROS defence mechanisms, as shown in Figure 1.3, with SOD and peroxidase lowers the balanced state level of O_2 and H_2O_2, respectively (Xianquan et al., 2005; Hurrell, 2003).

$$2O_2^- + 2H^+ \xrightarrow{\text{SOD}} H_2O_2 + O_2$$

$$ROOH/H_2O_2 \xrightarrow{\text{GSH Peroxidase}} ROH + H_2O + GSSG + GSH$$

$$H_2O_2 + AH_2 \xrightarrow{\text{Peroxidase}} 2H_2O + A$$

FIGURE 1.3 Mode of action of enzyme antioxidants.

1.3.1.1 COPPER/ZINC AND MANGANESE DEPENDENT

i. **Superoxide dismutase (SOD):** It catalyzes the dismutation of the highly reactive superoxide anion to the less reactive molecule H_2O_2. It is found in our skin and is a necessary enzyme for our bodies to produce enough fibroblasts, which are skin-building cells. The ordinary source of SOD includes broccoli, cabbage, Brussels sprouts, wheat grass, and barley grass. It also protects human body against ageing, heart diseases, peroxidation of lipids, denaturation of protein, and damage due to radiations.

   Humans have three different forms of SOD, each with its own sequence of amino acids, arrangement, and metals factors:

   1. Cu-Zinc SOD is a cytosolic enzyme that has two subunits and is sensitive to H_2O_2 and cyanide.

2. Mitochondrial SOD is a cyanide-insensitive enzyme found in the mitochondrial matrix in prokaryotes.
3. Fluoride Fe SOD is a mineral found in prokaryotes and some medicinal plants' chloroplasts. Hydrogen peroxide inhibits it, but it is unaffected by cyanide (Akinrinmade et al., 2016).

ii. **Catalase (CAT):** It's an enzyme that breaks down and metabolizes hydrogen peroxide, a heme protein with a fast turnover rate. It's a defensive enzyme found in every cell of an animal. The catalase enzyme in human erythrocytes catalyzes the breakdown of H_2O_2 into water and oxygen. Chemical antioxidants protect cells from oxidative damage thanks to an interconnected system of antioxidant enzymes.

iii. **Glutathione peroxidase (GPx):** It is an enzyme that protects cells from harm caused by free radicals such as hydrogen and lipid peroxides. Glutathione lowers H_2O_2 in a GPx-catalyzed enzymatic process present in the vacuole, cystol, and extracellular space. Each of the four identical subunits contains a single selenocysteine residue, which is required for enzyme activity. GPx breaks down lipid hydroperoxides into their alcohols, releasing H_2O_2 and water. Glutathione (GSH), tripeptide a major antioxidant, boosts the immune system and protects cells from the detrimental effects of pollution. It is found in higher concentrations in cells and is essential for keeping them in a reduced state to prevent free radical oxidation damage.

iv. **Glutathione reductase (GR):** It has a secondary vigorous role in the protection of cells damage due to oxidation by maintaining optimal concentration of intracellular glutathione (GSH). It is in conjunction with GPx, works as a reductant, lowering the damaging levels of hydrogen peroxide in the cells. GR uses the hydrogen donor nicotinamide dinucleotide phosphate to catalyze the resuscitation of GSH as well as the reduction of oxidized glutathione (GSSG) to reduced glutathione (NADPH). NADPH has also been proposed to operate as an indirect antioxidant by re-reducing GSSG to GSH and therefore maintaining glutathione's antioxidative effectiveness. Glutathione reductase, a NADPH-dependent enzyme, reduces GSSG.

v. **Glutathione-S-transferases (GST):** It's a group of enzymes that includes cytosolic, mitochondrial, and microsomal proteins that can perform a variety of reactions with a wide range of substrates, both endogenous and xenobiotic. It aids xenobiotic phase II metabolism by conjugating these chemicals with reduced glutathione to make them easier to dissolve in aqueous cellular and extracellular media. It also catalyzes the conjugation of reduced glutathione to electrophilic centers on a number of substrates using the sulfhydryl group. It is a widely distributed enzyme that aids in the detoxification and metabolism of xenobiotics (foreign chemical compounds) as well as endogenous substances like peroxidized lipids.

vi. **Glutathione:** It's a tripeptide that reacts with free radicals exist in more concentrations in maximum eukaryotic cells. Lipid peroxides are reduced directly. Glutathione and vitamin C work together (Cadmak and Horst et al., 1991; Chen and Schopfer, 1999).

1.3.2 NONENZYMATIC ANTIOXIDANTS

Non-enzymatic antioxidants contain directly active antioxidants, like vitamin C, lipoic acid, polyphenols, and carotenoids, all of which are found in foods, are essential in the fight against oxidation stress. A few of these compounds were also produced by the cell. Chelating compounds bind to redox metals and operate as indirect antioxidants, preventing the formation of free radicals. All these biological components quench the free radicals directly or indirectly by assisting in radical scavenging effect (Irshad and Chaudhary, 2002).

i. **Selenium (Se):** Mineral selenium is also found in antioxidant enzymes. It's a crucial trace element found in the human body connected to an elevated risk of ailments including cancer and heart disease (Tinggi, 2008). Large quantities of selenium in supplement form can be hazardous; therefore it's best to acquire it from food. Selenium can be found in fish, shellfish, red meat, grains, eggs, and poultry (Tapiero et al., 2003). If grown in selenium-rich soils, vegetables can also be a good source. The main sources of selenium in the diet are rice and wheat. The amount of selenium in food is determined by the selenium content of the soil, which varies by region. Animals that eat grains or vegetables grown in selenium-rich soil have increased selenium levels in their muscle (Valko et al., 2004; Arner and Holmgren, 2000; Das and Das, 2000). It protects against cancer by assisting in the battle against cell damage caused by oxygen-derived chemicals. Since selenium's discovery as a critical component of antioxidant enzymes there has been a surge in research into selenium-containing proteins or enzymes.

The ROS like hydrogen peroxide, superoxide, hydroxyl radicals, nitric oxide, peroxynitrite, and RNS causes oxidative damage to cells. All the six types of GPx have strong antioxidant activity (Nordberg and Arner, 2001). To preserve the Trx/TrxR system in a reduced state, TrxR is an antioxidant selenoenzyme uses thioredoxin (Trx) as a substrate to allow removal of damaged hydrogen peroxide. TrxR has been detected in three different forms: TrxR1 (cytosolic), TrxR2 (mitochondrial), and SpTrxR (spermatozoa-specific). Selenoprotein may also have a function in the antioxidant defence system, avoiding harmful ROS and RNS attacks, according to new evidence (Gromer et al., 2004; Steinbrenner et al., 2006, Steinbrenner et al., 2006).

ii. **Transferrin:** In the human body, it is a key iron-carrying protein. It's usually loaded to 20–30% capacity.

iii. **Lactoferrin:** It is a protein obtained from milk that aids in iron binding and is comparable to transferrin.

iv. **Ceruloplasmin:** Ceruloplasmin catalyzes the reduction of oxygen to water while oxidizing Fe^{++}–Fe^{+++}.

v. **Vitamin A:** The three most prevalent types of vitamin A are vitamins A1, A2, and A3 and they are abundant in milk, sugary potato, carrot, egg yolks, mozzarella cheese, etc.

vi. **Vitamin C:** It's soluble in water fight against free radicals in the body's aqueous phase. Scurvy is a potentially fatal deficiency situation caused by an absence of vitamin C in the diet. Its antioxidant properties have been shown to stabilize folate in the diet and plasma, as well as to assist the elimination of oxidized folate derivatives in human scurvy. Vitamin C is abundant in citrus fruits, honey melon, cherry, kiwi, mango, papaya, strawberry, tangelo, and watermelon. The vegetables like tomatoes, cabbage, broccoli, Brussels sprouts, beansprouts, cauliflower, kale, mustard greens, red and green peppers, peas, and potatoes are all good sources of iron. Cereals, meat, poultry, and fish all contain vitamin C (Packer et al., 1979).

vii. **Vitamin E:** It is a tocopherol combines with reactive oxygen metabolites to produce lipid hydroperoxide, which the phospholipase-GSPHx system can eliminate. Tocopherol is a potent antioxidant responds far more quickly with the peroxyl radical than other compounds. It prevents future radical reactions by eliminating the radical from the oxidizing fatty acid. During the antioxidant process, tocopherol is transformed to a reasonably stable radical. Wheat germ, sunflower, corn, soyabean oil, almond oil, and cereal seed germ are all polyunsaturated vegetable oils that contain it. Palm oils and aleurone and subaleurone layers of cereal seeds are the good sources of tocotrienols. It is present abundantly in mangoes, almonds, broccoli, and other foods (Herrera and Barbas, 2001).

viii. **Carotenoids (β-Carotene):** It's a wide group of fat soluble colorants found in fruits and vegetables consumed in industrialized countries. It is a carbon-hydrogen orange color carotenoid found in a variety of yellow-orange fruits and also in dark green, leafy vegetables. It is a lipid soluble vitamin A precursor. It prevents lipid peroxidation by working in tandem with tocopherol (Krinsky and Johnson, 2005). β-Carotene inhibits oxidation because the electrons in double bonds are less securely attached to the molecule and thus more easily available for donation. This method is used by antioxidants that are non-polar and have moderately long hydrocarbon chains (Rodriguez-Amaya et al., 2008). Carotene, lycopene, and vitamin A are natural antioxidants that use this approach. Due to their comparable chemical structures and membership in the carotenoid family of compounds, carotene and lycopene have similar antioxidant mechanisms (Voutilainen et al., 2008).

1.3.3 ANTIOXIDANTS FRUITS AND VEGETABLES

Fruits and vegetables are dietary staples with a long history of health benefits and nutritional value. They have a significant historical significance as traditional foods since they contain an abundance of minerals, electrolytes, ascorbic acid, and vitamin E; and some recent research have shown that their phytochemical contents have antioxidant potential (Slavin and Lloyd, 2012). The regular eating of vegetables and fruits drops the oxidation by lowering the threat of mortality associated with a variety of diseases such as diabetes, cancer, and heart diseases (Nahak et al., 2014). The transformation of lipid radicals into more stable compounds by natural antioxidants takes place because of chain breaking mechanism. In fruits and vegetables, the majority of antioxidants have a phenolic structure, which might contain vitamins, minerals, and polyphenols. Minerals including, manganese, copper, iron, and selenium utilized as cofactors for a variety of antioxidant enzymes, and their absence can hinder them from scavenging free radicals (Hurrell, 2003; Sonia et al., 2016).

1.3.3.1 POLYPHENOLS

Polyphenols are a group of antioxidant chemicals with little and high molecular weights that prevent lipid oxidation present abundant in fruits and vegetables (Parr and Bolwell, 2000). Polyphenols, also known as phenolics, are aromatic ring compounds having one or more hydroxyl substituents with esters, methyl ethers, and glycosides are the derivatives (Baxter et al., 1998). Depending on their chemical structure, they are classified as phenolic acids, flavonoids, stilbenes, and lignans. Flavonoids and phenolic acids, which are plentiful in plants, account for around 60% and 30% of total dietary phenols, respectively. The hydroxybenzoic acid generates most common phenolic acids present in plant are gallic acid, vanillic acid, syringic acid, and protocatechuic acid, whereas p-coumaric acid, caffeic acid, and ferulic acid are the derivatives of hydroxycinnamic acid. The most powerful natural chemopreventive agent is ellagic acid, a dimer of gallic acid that protects connective tissue from oxidative damage and restores damaged proteins in blood vessel walls. According to many research findings, polyphenols derived from natural sources such as green tea, red tea, berry, wine, ginkgo, onion, apple, grape, liquorice, rosemary, thyme, fruits, vegetables, and beverages have valuable effects on healthiness. They also prevent the occurrence of many degenerative and chronic diseases. Polyphenols are high in phenols, which help vitamin C work better, cut cancer risk, lower blood pressure, and combat allergies, ulcers, tumors, and platelet aggregation (Urquiaga and Leighton, 2000; Carr et al., 2000; Shahidi, 2000).

1.3.3.2 FLAVONOIDS

Flavonoids (Keservani and Sharma, 2014; Keservani et al., 2016a; Keservani et al., 2016b), also known as bioflavonoids, are a type of polyphenolic secondary metabolite available in a varied range of plants and are thus widely ingested in human diets. It has general structure of fifteen carbons with two phenyl rings (A and B) and heterocyclic moiety in the center, ring C. (2 phenyl-benzo-y-pyrone). Flavonoids are classified as flavonols, flavones, isoflavones, anthocyanidins, and proanthocyanidin. The color of seeds, grains, fruits, vegetables, leaves, flowers, bark, and other parts are determined by flavonoid content of plants (Urquiaga and Leighton, 2000). They are excellent metal chelators and free radical scavengers and also prevent the oxidation of low-density lipoprotein (LDL), assist to reduce plaque formation (Pinho et al., 2000). Binding of flavonoids to transition metals prevents the generation of metal-catalyzed free radicals. Flavonoids are abundant in onions, parsley, blueberry, black, green, bananas, citrus fruits, Ginkgo biloba, red wine, sea buckthorns, buckwheat, and dark chocolate (Quintavalla and Vicini, 2002).

1.3.4 ANTIOXIDANTS DERIVED FROM THE WASTE OF FRUITS AND VEGETABLES

Researchers have been striving to discover strategies to recycle these wastes in order to achieve therapeutic benefits for decades because a huge amount of waste material is generated during the growth, processing, industrial management, preservation, and distribution of fruits and vegetables (Mirabella et al., 2014). Waste materials obtained from vegetables and fruits include peelings, trimmings, grenades, pits, stems, and pulp remnants that persisted after juice removal and processing of starch or sugar (Rudra et al., 2015; Ajila et al., 2010; Goulas and Manganaris, 2012; Fatemeh et al., 2012). According to a study conducted by a group of researchers, these waste scalps have more phenols and ascorbic acids than their pulp, and they include more phenols and ascorbic acids in their unripe form than in their ripened form. The peels of fruits contain more antioxidants than the pulp. The phenolic content of banana peels is higher than that of the pulp. Cucumber peel has been discovered to be an excellent source of antioxidant flavonoids (Guo et al., 2003). Many bioactive chemicals can be retrieved from these wastes and used to produce meals and medicinal preparations (Someya et al., 2002; Agarwal et al., 2012). Many bioactive phytochemicals or molecules with significant antioxidant qualities are obtained from the waste generated during food processing and healing preparations (Baiano, 2014). Mango peel contains a variety of natural antioxidants, including dietary fibers, phenolic compounds, vitamin C, and carotenoids, which have been shown to defend against a variety of diseases like cataracts, cancer, Alzheimer's, and Parkinson's disease (Kalogeropoulos et al., 2012). Various antioxidants derived from wine-making wastes, such as degradable solids including skin, stem, and seeds, have been demonstrated to counteract various progressive processes and have health-promoting properties (Teixeira et al., 2012). Approximately 6% polyphenols and 4% tannins are found in coffee trash (Pujol et al., 2013).

1.3.5 ANTIOXIDANTS FROM MARINE SOURCES

Because of the existence of various fascinating antioxidant molecules as well as other appealing biotechnological compounds such as polysaccharides, pigments, and proteins; food, medicines, nutraceuticals, and cosmetics companies are all paying attention to marine biodiversity. Approximately 25,000 structurally distinct secondary metabolites have been found in various marine sources at this time (Pan et al., 2015).

The richest source of bioactive chemicals with antibacterial and antioxidant properties are seaweeds and sponges (Ngo et al., 2012). Seaweeds and sponges contain organic acids, polysaccharides, and helpful phenolic compounds that promote health and prevent disease. It is the most effective group of food in terms of protecting against pollution and radiation (Wijffels, 2008; Newman and Crag, 2004). Polyphenolic compounds discovered in marine organisms that have antioxidant properties include flavonoid, gallic acid, cinnamic acid, quercy, and phlorotannins (Al-Saif et al., 2014; Anand et al., 2006).

Algae, in particular, are a rich cause of active mixtures with antioxidant potential and biological activities, and are made up of a diverse cluster of photosynthetic organisms with simple reproductive organs, such as macroalgae or seaweeds, and microalgae, which are multicellular and unicellular, respectively. Algae thrive under extremes of temperature, light, and salinity, resulting in the production of a large quantity of ROS. Vitamins (β-carotene and other carotenoids, vitamin C, D), polyphenols (bromophenols, flavonoids, phlorotannins, and phenolic acids), and algae pigments (phycobiliproteins, chlorophylls, and carotenoids) are coping with ROS (Manivannan et al., 2011).

Antioxidant activity has been discovered in fish protein hydrolysate (FPH) generated from a range of marine creatures, including tuna, Alaska Pollock, mackerel, and yellow fin sole (Wu et al., 2003; Jun et al., 2004; Je et al., 2007). Peptides can be found in a variety of forms in fish muscle, bone, skin, and other tissues and are help to remove free radicals, among those that donate hydrogen atoms easily have the most powerful scavenging ability. The antioxidant nature of the FPH is determined by its peptide size and amino acid makeup (Kim and Wijesekara, 2013).

A pigment phycocyanin produced from blue-green algae was tested for antioxidant activity in vitro by luminol-enhanced chemiluminescence (LCL). It produces a light signal when it combines with oxygen (O2), alkoxyl (RO), and hydroxyl (OH) radicals, which can be measured before and after antioxidant addition. The bright signal revealed that phycocyanin may remove OH and RO and prevent oxidation when inflammation was induced in mice paws using glucose oxidase (Romay et al., 1998).

1.3.6 MUSHROOM AS ANTIOXIDANTS

Mushrooms are utilized as substitute vegetables in the nutraceutical industry, but they are not plants and belong to the fungal kingdom (Khatua et al., 2013). Although they have been proven to be an essential supplement, they should be included in one's diet. Many nutritive components found in mushrooms, such as carbohydrates, lipids, vitamins, phenolics, organic acids, and proteins, have been identified as being responsible for antioxidant potential and biological activities such as immunomodulatory, antimicrobial, antitumor, antihypertensive, and hepatoprotective (Rahman and Choudhury, 2013; Ruthes et al., 2016; Valverde et al., 2015). On Earth, there are approximately 1,40,000 mushroom species, of which only 10% are identified, and only 2000 have been confirmed to be safe for human consumption, with only 650 of these having therapeutic characteristics (Rai, 2005). Termitomyces species, Hypsizigus marmoreus, Pleurotus, and Schizophyllum commune all have the potential to prevent oxidation. The presence of phenolic compounds such as gallic acid, cinnamic acid phenolic acid, p-hydroxybenzoic acid, p-coumaric acid, protocatechuic acid, vanillin, rutin, and quercetin gives mushrooms their antioxidant properties. According to recent research, polysaccharide, the mushroom's main component, possesses antioxidant properties (Barros et al., 1998; Wang et al., 2015).

1.3.7 ANTIOXIDANTS FROM MEDICINAL PLANTS AND SPICES

1.3.7.1 ALLIUM SATIVUM

Garlic (Allium sativum) is a perennial herb that grows up to 3 feet tall with a straight blossoming stem belonging to the Alliaceae family (Bhonde and Prakash, 2006). It's a multipurpose herb with a high concentration of minerals, trace elements, and vitamins (Lu et al., 2011). The presence of the entire phenolic content of garlic exhibits antioxidant activity and is the most effective DPPH-scavenger. The antioxidant potential of the plant appears to increase as the plant ages (Rahman and Fazlic, 2012; Park et al., 2009).

1.3.7.2 CAPSICUM ANNUUM

Phytochemical compounds found in Capsicum annuum like organic acids, ascorbic acid, Carotenoids, flavonoids, tocopherols, free sugars, and capsaicinoids have radical-scavenging effects (Hervert-Herandez et al., 2010). High bioactive content of hot dried peppers at the ready stage, such as polyphenols and carotenoids, have significant free radical-scavenging activities (Kim et al., 2011).

1.3.7.3 CURCUMIN

It is a well-known spice from the Zingiberaceae family that is found all over the world in tropical and subtropical climates, but is mostly grown in Asiatic countries such as India, China, and Pakistan (Ferreira et al., 2013). Turmeric, which comes in powder form, has long been utilized as a taste enhancer in both vegetarian and non-vegetarian dishes as part of daily diets. Curcuma longa, the phenolic molecule, is the principal contributor to curcumin's antioxidant activity, and fresh rhizomes containing essential oil have stronger scavenging activities (Singh et al., 2010; Maizura et al., 2011).

1.3.7.4 EUGENIA CARYOPHYLLUS

It is also called as clove, and it’s a medium-sized tree in the Myrtaceae family that’s used as a medicinal and nutritional ingredient. It is primarily grown in Indonesia and Brazil. This plant contains phenolic chemicals such as gallic acid, eugenol, and eugenol acetate, and is one of the greatest sources of these substances (Cortes-Rojas et al., 2014). The major component of plant essential oils, eugenol, has a significant antioxidant capacity (Teixeira et al., 2013). Methanolic extract exhibits stronger scavenging action than acetone and chloroform extracts when compared to other plant extracts (Hemalatha et al., 2016).

1.3.7.5 *GERANIUM SANGUINEUM*

Bloody cranesbill is an herbaceous plant from Asia and Europe that belongs to the Geraniaceae family. The plant is mostly grown in a plot, and methanolic extract demonstrates its free radical-scavenging ability. Pakistan, India, Sri Lanka, Indonesia, Tanzania, the West Indies, and Zanzibar are among the countries that grow it (Bhowmik et al., 2012; Nikolova et al., 2010).

1.3.7.6 *PISTACIA LENTISCUS*

The radical-scavenging activity of extracts of the plant Pistacia lentiscus derived from the leaves displayed is similar to that observed in Algeria, where it is used by rural people. It has a high plummeting power and a strong radical-scavenging effect against DPPH (Atmani et al., 2009; Ghenima et al., 2015).

1.3.7.7 *SALVIA OFFICINALIS*

The presence of polyphenol components in this lawn sage plant from the Lamiaceae family gives it excellent antioxidant properties (Roby et al., 2013). In Iran, it is used to treat seizures, inflammatory diseases, ulcers, dizziness, tremor, paralysis, diarrhea, and hyperglycemia, among other ailments (Hamrouni-Sellami et al., 2013; Walch et al., 2011).

1.3.7.8 *UNCARIA TOMENTOSA*

A timbered plant from the Rubiaceae family found in the tropical forests of South and Central America is utilized to treat rheumatic disorders and cancer and has radical-scavenging effects. Due to its significant antioxidant properties, it reduces free radicals such as H_2O_2, diphenylpicrylhydrazyl, and hypochlorous acid (Goncalves et al., 2005).

1.3.7.9 *LEEA INDICA*

In Malaysia, *L. indica*, a member of the Vitaceae family, is utilized as a natural folk remedy. The phenolic compounds discovered in the leaves of L. indica include ursolic acid, solanesol, farnesol, lupeol, phthalic acid, gallic acid, and 1-eicosanol have antioxidant activity (Srinivasan et al., 2008; Reddy et al., 2012).

1.3.7.10 POLYALTHIA CERASOIDES

It is a traditional Thai medication that contains alkaloid, bidebiline, sesquiterpenes, and other compounds like codamine, laudanosine, laudanidine, and reticuline. Due to its high amount of phenolic compounds, the plant extract showed free radical scavenging action (Kanokmedhakul et al., 2007; Ravikumar et al., 2008; Treeratanapiboon et al., 2011).

1.4 ESTIMATION OF ANTIOXIDANT POTENTIAL

Because of the inherent complexity of oxidative processes in cells, determining the antioxidant capability of molecules is difficult. The following are some methods for determining the antioxidant potential of a given substrate:

1.4.1 CONJUGATED DIENE ASSAY

The oxidation of initial polyunsaturated fatty acid (PUFA) generates conjugated dienes determined by UV method. The conjugated double bonds are formed due to oxidation of linoleic acid are identified at 234 nm and the antioxidant potential was measured as inhibitory concentration (IC50) (David et al., 2004).

1.4.2 1,1 DIPHENYL-2-PICRYLHYDRAZYL (DPPH) METHOD

A free radical scavenger detects the reduction of a methanolic solution of colored free radical DPPH at 516 nm is a regularly used test procedure expressed as EC50; related to the free radical scavenger concentration in the DPPH reagent solution (Sanchez-Moreno et al., 1999).

1.4.3 SUPEROXIDE RADICAL SCAVENGE ACTIVITY

Reduction method using nitro blue tetrazolium (NBT) determines the antioxidant potential of flavonoid, triphala, and Ailanthus. The existence of light can be used to assess riboflavin oxidation as superoxide radical lowers NBT to a blue color at 560 nm by colorimetric determination (Babu et al., 2001; Robak and Gryglewski, 1998).

1.4.4 HYDROXYL RADICAL SCAVENGING ACTIVITY

In the presence of antioxidants, the Fenton reaction is used to assess hydroxyl radical scavenging action, such as iron ion (Fe3+), ascorbate, EDTA, or H_2O_2. The hydroxyl radicals generated by oxidation can also be detected by reacting with dimethyl sulphoxide to give formaldehyde, which displays a strong yellow color when measured spectrophotometrically at 412 nm with Nash reagent (Babu et al., 2001).

1.4.5 NITRIC OXIDE RADICAL INHIBITION ACTIVITY

Griess reagent is used to measure sodium nitroprusside formed in buffer saline solution due to suppression of nitric oxide at 546 nm. Hence, nitric oxide radical inhibition is used to assess antioxidant capacity (Robak and Gryglewski, 1998).

1.4.6 PHOSPHOMOLYBDENUM METHOD

The reduction of phosphomolybdenum Mo (VI)–Mo (V) produces green color Mo (V) complex at acidic pH is used to determine the antioxidant competence of substances by spectroscopic technique (Jayaprakash et al., 2001).

1.4.7 PEROXYNITRITE RADICAL SCAVENGING ACTIVITY

The technique uses a fluorescence spectrophotometer set to 485 nm to observe the dihydrorhodamine oxidation on a microplate to determine antioxidant potential (Kanner, 1994).

1.4.8 2, 2-AZINO-BIS (3-ETHYL BENZOTHIAZOLINE-6-SULFONIC ACID) DIAMMONIUM SALT) ABTS METHOD

Antioxidant $ABTS^+$ radical cation reduced to ABTS is used to assess antioxidant capability resulted in a decline in color reported at 645, 734, and 815 nm by colorimetric reaction (Kanner, 1994; Choi, 2002; Simonetti et al., 1997).

1.4.9 DMPD (N, N-DIMETHYL-P-PHENYLENEDIAMINE DIHYDROCHLORIDE) METHOD

The colored buffered solution of DMPD in acetate buffer and ferric chloride in presence of scavengers was used to measure the antioxidant potential at 505 nm (Vinson and Hontz, 1995).

1.4.10 OXYGEN RADICAL ABSORBANCE CAPACITY (ORAC)

It's a novel way to look into the antioxidant capacity of foods and other chemical compounds. The Trolox equivalent (TE) equivalent is calculated using vitamin E water soluble analog as a reference and given as oxygen radical absorbance capacity unit or value. Hence, the greater the value, the more the antioxidant potential of chemical (Ronald, 1998).

1.4.11 CAROTENOID LINOLEATE MODEL

The assay is based on the premise that oxygenated water produces ROS, which oxidizes linoleic acid, an unsaturated fatty acid. As a result, the substance generated will initiate β-carotene oxidation, resulting in discoloration. Antioxidant activity is measured using a colorimetric technique at 434 nm, which reduces discoloration (Kanner, 1994).

1.4.12 TOTAL RADICAL TRAPPING ANTIOXIDANT POTENTIAL (TRAP) TECHNIQUE

The technique determines the quenching of fluorescence degradation of R-phytocoerythrin during an oxidation reaction by 2,2′-azobis (2-amidinopropane) hydrochloride. The antioxidant potential is assessed by the time it takes for discoloration to occur (Ghiselli, 1995).

1.5 HEALTH BENEFITS AND POTENTIAL ROLE OF ANTIOXIDANTS IN DIFFERENT DISEASES

Today, the study and application of the disease-fighting properties of a variety of photochemical substances found in both food and non-food plants as antioxidants has resulted in a resurgence in human health and nutritional research, including disease prevention and therapy. Nutraceuticals have been shown to have a positive control on health, mostly in the hindrance of cardiovascular, metabolic, neurodegenerative, and cancer disorders, according to numerous research findings.

1.5.1 NEURODEGENERATIVE DISEASES

Neurodegenerative disorders are excruciatingly painful conditions caused by oxidative stress and the inflammatory process. Antioxidants have been studied and proven to aid in the treatment of Alzheimer's, Parkinson's, Huntington's, brain ageing, and multiple sclerosis, to name a few.

Flavonoids have been found to play a special attention in the CNS to maintain homeostasis by acting as an anti-anxiety and anti-convulsant agent via altering metabolism due to oxidation and neurotransmitters (Kavitha et al., 2019; Velmurugan et al., 2018). Tea leaves contain a polyphenol called epigallocatechin-3-galate, which appears to prevent the degeneration of neurons. In Alzheimer's disease, a medication combination with epigallocatechin-3-galate was found to reduce amyloid plaques (Walker et al., 2015; Wobst et al., 2015). In a Parkinson's disease study, Koh SH et al discovered that polyphenol and tea prevents the loss of cells in the significant nigra (Koh et al., 2003). Quercetin dramatically reduces apoptosis, increases viability of cells and inhibits ROS and MDA formation in PC-12 cells toxicity influenced by peroxide and hippocampal neurons (Kavitha et al., 2019).

Curcumin is helpful in Alzheimer's disease due to its ability to bind to amyloid plaques by inhibiting nuclear factor (Zhang et al., 2010). An ethanolic extract of curcuma longa L. has shown decrease in stress due to oxidation by lowering MDA concentration in blood and brain. It also increases GSH intensity and activity of enzymes like SOD, CAT, and GPx in brain (Yuliani et al., 2019).

By avoiding the death of neuronal cell and increasing the utility of brain capillary endothelial monolayers, Yang et al. (2018) found evidence of Ginkgo biloba extract's neuroprotective effects. According to Wu et al. (2014), astaxanthin can alleviate brain aging by reducing oxidative stress, enriching hippocampal damage, and raising brain-derived neurotrophic factor levels, which can help to prevent age-related neurodegenerative disorders.

Goodwin discovered that higher levels of β-carotene and ascorbic acid in the plasma of healthy human volunteers improved memory function and performance (Goodwin et al., 1983).

1.5.2 DIABETES MELLITUS

It's a long-term metabolic condition marked by high blood glucose levels and an inability to create and use insulin. It has become a leading cause of death worldwide. Diabetes in humans increases the peroxidation of lipids and decreases the antioxidant potential of a few enzyme systems like SOD, CAT, and GSH-PX. Tannins, cinnamic acid, polyphenols, coumarins, diterpenes, flavonoids, lignans, prophenylphenols, monoterpenes, and triterpenes are natural antioxidants that have been demonstrated to protect against diabetes and its consequences (Bacanli et al., 2019).

1.5.3 CARDIOVASCULAR DISEASES

Stress, smoking, diabetes, hypercholesterolemia, hypertension, poor diet, and physical inactivity are the leading causes of cardiovascular disease. Daily use of green vegetables, whole grain, honey, walnuts, black tea and green tea boosted hepatic antioxidant enzymes, lowering the risk of numerous cardiovascular illnesses. Cardiovascular disease caused by oxidative stress is prevented by the presence of particular dietary antioxidant components in some fruits, vegetables, and legumes.

The results of a seven-year study on flavonoid consumption in the United States indicated that flavonoid consumption reduced the threat of death from cardiovascular disease (McCullough et al., 2012). Eating plant-based diets lowers the threat of heart diseases studied by Patel et al. (2017). A cohort study on 75,000 individuals conducted by Zhang and discovered that soy diet consumption reduced the risk of coronary heart disease (Zhang et al., 2003).

High blood pressure causes a variety of cardiac and vascular issues. In hypertensive rats, seed powder Moringa oleifera did not lower blood pressure but lowers the heart rate at night-time and improves cardiac diastolic function (Randriamboavonjy et al., 2016). A diet high in lycopene lowers blood pressure, enhances vascular function, increases metabolic syndrome, reduces oxidative stress, and maintains a normal blood glucose level by preventing insulin resistance (McCullough et al., 2012).

1.5.4 CANCER

Several studies, similar to those on cardiovascular illnesses, have shown that natural antioxidants can help prevent and treat cancer. Curcumin, a polyphenol molecule, has anticancer characteristics via controlling cell cycle, death, oncogene expression, and metastasis. Green tea use has been shown to aid in the management of low-grade B-cell tumors (Shanafelt et al., 2006; Hosseini et al., 2015). Panax ginseng also reduces the risk of pharyngeal, laryngeal, and esophageal cancers, as well as their inflammation. Flavonoids such as catechin, apigenin, kaempferol, and quercetin have demonstrated to be good for health and have been employed as a chemoprotective therapeutic agents for cancer treatment (Yun et al., 2001; Patil and Masand, 2018). Few dietary flavonoids have anticancer activity and have been found to be strong aromatase inhibitors in breast cancer. In the therapy of prostate cancer, quercetin inhibited cell growth, and death by down regulating heat-shock protein 90 (Aalinkeel et al., 2008).

1.6 CONCLUSION

Many researchers have now investigated and employed many phytochemical substances with antioxidant potential derived from plants, fruits, vegetables, and marine sources, resulting in a resurgence in human health and nutritional study. Nutraceuticals, which come in the form of isolated nutrients, dietary supplements, and particular diets, have been scientifically proven to be useful in treating and preventing a variety of diseases. Hippocrates, who lived over 2000 years ago, thought, "Let food be your medicine, and medicine be your nourishment." Indians, Egyptians, and Chinese are just a few of the people who have supplied evidence that food may be utilized as medicine to treat and prevent disease, and this fact is confirmed by Ayurveda, a 5000-year-old ancient health system. Scientists from all over the world are working to develop a non-synthetic alternative source that will be safer and more convenient as a natural dietary component.

Nutraceuticals are therapeutic foods that aid in the maintenance of good health, well-being, and immunity. As a result, ailments like cancer, cardiovascular, metabolic, and neurogenetic diseases can be prevented as well as treated. Natural herbs, vegetables, fruits, spices, and plant substances have been employed as preservatives, aromas, and flavors in medicines since ancient times. This chapter examines the potential for several phytochemicals produced from natural sources to have a significant antioxidant effect. Approximately 75–80% of the world's residents cannot afford current supplements and treatments for many disorders and diseases due to high cost; hence people can easily arrange and consume their daily nutritional diet with antioxidants. Nutraceuticals have been proven to provide health benefits, and their use will help humans avoid diseases and preserve overall good health.

CONFLICT OF INTEREST

Authors have no conflict of interest.

KEYWORDS

- **natural antioxidants**
- **nutraceutical**
- **phytochemical**
- **chronic disease**
- **dietary supplement**
- **food**

REFERENCES

Aalinkeel, R.; Bindukumar, B.; Reynolds, J. L.; Sykes, D. E.; Mahajan, S. D.; Chadha, K. C. Thedietary Bioflavonoid, Quercetin, Selectively Induces Apoptosis of Prostate Cancer Cells by Down-Regulating the Expression of Heat Shock Protein 90. *Prostate* **2008,** *68* (16), 1773–1789.

Agarwal, M.; Kumar, A.; Gupta, R.; Upadhyaya, S. Extraction of Polyphenol, Flavonoid from Emblica officinalis, Citrus limon, Cucumis sativus and Evaluation of their Antioxidant Activity. *Orient. J. Chem.* **2012,** *28* (2), 993.

Ahad, T.; Nissar, J.; Rather, A. H. Nutraceuticals-Health Benefits: A Review. *Int. J. Eng. Technol. Sci. Res.* **2017,** *4* (12), 262–267.

Ajila, C. M.; Aalami, M.; Leelavathi, K.; Rao, U. P. Mango Peel Powder: A Potential Source of Antioxidant and Dietary Fiber in Macaroni Preparations. *Innov. Food Sci. Emerg. Technol.* **2010,** *11* (1), 219–224.

Akinrinmade, F. J.; Akinrinde, A. S.; Soyemi, O. O.; Oyagbemi, A. A. Antioxidant Potential of the Methanol Extract of Parquetina nigrescens Mediates Protection Against Intestinal Ischemia-Reperfusion Injury in Rats. *J. Diet. Suppl.* **2016,** *13* (4), 420–432.

Al-Saif, S. S. A. L.; Abdel-Raouf, N.; El-Wazanani, H. A.; Aref, I. A. Antibacterial Substances from Marine Algae Isolated from Jeddah Coast of Red Sea, Saudi Arabia. *Saudi J. Biol. Sci.* **2014,** *21* (1), 57–64.

Anand, T. P.; Bhat, A. W.; Shouche, Y. S.; Roy, U.; Siddharth, J.; Sarma, S. P. Antimicrobial Activity of Marine Bacteria Associated with Sponges from the Waters off the Coast of South East India. *Microbiol. Res.* **2006,** *161* (3), 252–262.

Angelo, A. J.; Vercellotti. J.; Jacks, T.; Legendre, M. Lipid Oxidation in Foods. *Crit. Rev. Food Sci. Nutr.* **1996,** *36* (3), 175–224.

Arner, E. S.; Holmgren, A. Physiological Functions of Thioredoxin and Thioredoxin Reductase. *Euro. J. Biochem.* **2000,** *267* (20), 6102–6109.

Atmani, D.; Chaher, N.; Berboucha, M.; Ayouni, K.; Lounis, H.; Boudaoud, H.; Atmani, D. Antioxidant Capacity and Phenol Content of Selected Algerian Medicinal Plants. *Food Chem.* **2009,** *112* (2), 303–309.

August, J. T.; Murad, F.; Anders, M. W.; Coyle, J. T.; Packer, L. In *Antioxidants in Disease Mechanisms and Therapy*; Academic Press, Dec 10, 1996.

Babu, B. H.; Shylesh, B. S.; Padikkala, J. Antioxidant and Hepatoprotective Effect of *Alanthus icicifocus*. *Fitoterapia* **2001,** *72*, 272–277.

Bacanli, M.; Dilsiz, S. A.; Basaran, N.; Başaran, A. A. Effects of Phytochemicals against Diabetes. In *Advances in Food and Nutrition Research*; Academic Press Inc., 2019; vol *89*, pp 209–238.

Baiano, A. Recovery of Biomolecules from Food Wastes-A Review. *Molecules* **2014,** *19* (9), 14821–14842.

Bandyopadhyay, U.; Das, D.; Banerjee, R. K. Reactive Oxygen Species: Oxidative Damage and Pathogenesis. *Curr. Sci.* **1999,** *10*, 658–666.

Barros, L.; Dueñas, M.; Ferreira, I. C.; Baptista, P.; Santos-Buelga, C. Phenolic Acids Determination by HPLC–DAD–ESI/MS in Sixteen Different Portuguese Wild Mushrooms Species. *Food Chem. Toxicol.* **2009,** *47* (6), 1076–1079.

Baxter, H.; Harborne, J. B.; Moss, G. P. In *Phytochemical Dictionary: A Handbook of Bioactive Compounds from Plants*; CRC Press: Philadelphia (PA), USA, 1998

Beasley, J. M.; Rillamas, S. E.; Tinker, L. F.; Wylie, R. J.; Mossavar, R. Y.; Datta, M.; Caan, B. J; LaCroix, A. Z. Dietary Intakes of Women's Health Initiative Long Life Study Participants Falls Short of the Dietary Reference Intakes. *J. Acad. Nutr. Diet.* **2020,** *120* (9), 1530–1537.

Bhonde, S.; Prakash, H. In *Garlic Cultivation in India*; National Horticultural Research and Development Foundation; Nashik, India, 2006.

Bhowmik, D.; Kumar, K. S.; Yadav, A.; Srivastava, S.; Paswan, S.; Dutta, A. S. Recent Trends in Indian Traditional Herbs Syzygium Aromaticum and its Health Benefits. *J. Pharmacogn. Phytochem.* **2012,** *1* (1), 13–22.

Brewer, M.S. Natural Antioxidants: Sources, Compounds, Mechanisms of Action, and Potential Applications. *Compr. Rev. Food Sci. Food Saf.* **2011,** *10* (4), 221–247.

Brower, V. Nutraceuticals: Poised for a Healthy Slice of the Healthcare Market. *Nat. Biotechnol.* **1998,** *16* (8), 728–731.

Buttriss, J. L.; Hughes, J.; Kelly, C. N.; Stanner, S. Antioxidants in Food: A Summary of the Review Conducted for the Fod Standards Agency. *Nutr. Bull.* **2002,** *27* (4), 227–236.

Cadmak, L.; Horst, W. J. Effect of Aluminium on Lipid Peroxidation, Superoxide Dismutase, Catalase and Peroxidase Activities in Root Tips of Soybean. *Plant Physiol.* **1991,** *83*, 463–468.

Cao, G.; Russell, R. M.; Lischner, N.; Prior, R. L. Serum Antioxidant Capacity is Increased by Consumption of Strawberries, Spinach, Red Wine or Vitamin C in Elderly Women. *J. Nutr.* **1998,** *128* (12), 2383–2390.

Carocho, M.; Ferreira, I. C. A Review on Antioxidants, Prooxidants and Related Controversy: Natural and Synthetic Compounds, Screening and Analysis Methodologies and Future Perspectives. *Food Chem. Toxicol.* **2013,** *51*, 15–25.

Carr, A.C.; Zhu, B.Z.; Frei, B. Potential Antiatherogenic Mechanisms of Ascorbate (Vitamin C) and α-tocopherol (Vitamin E). *Circ. Res.* **2000,** *87* (5), 349–354.

Chaturvedi, S.; Sharma, P. K.; Garg, V. K.; Bansal, M. Role of Nutraceuticals in Health Promotion. *Int. J. Pharm. Tech. Res.* **2011,** *3* (1), 442À8.

Chen, S.; Schopfer, P. Hydroxyl Radical Production in Physiological Reactions: A Novel Functions of Peroxidase. *Euro. J. Biochem.* **1999,** *260*, 726–735

Choi, H. R. Peroxynitrite Scavenging Activity of Herb Extracts. *Phytother. Res.* **2002,** *16*, 364–367.

Cornelli, U. Antioxidant use in Nutraceuticals. *Clin. Dermatol.* **2009,** *27* (2), 175–194.

Cortes-Rojas, D. F.; de Souza, C. R. F.; Oliveira, W. P. Clove (Syzygium aromaticum): A Precious Spice. *Asian Pac. J. Trop. Biomed.* **2014,** *4* (2), 90–96.

Das, K. C.; Das, C. K. Thioredoxin, A Singlet Oxygen Quencher and Hydroxyl Radical Scavenger: Redox Independent Functions. *Biochem. Biophys. Res. Commun.* **2000,** 277 (2), 443–447.

David, G. B.; Erik, E.A.; Rohini, S. A. Antioxidant Enzyme Expression and ROS Damage in Prostatic Intraepithelial Neoplasia and Cancer. *Cancer* **2000,** *89*, 124–134.

de Rijk, M. C.; Breteler, M. M.; den Breeijen, J. H.; Launer, L. J.; Grobbee, D. E.; van der Meché, F. G.; Hofman, A. Dietary Antioxidants and Parkinson Disease: The Rotterdam Study. *Arch. Neurol.* **1997,** *54* (6), 762–765.

DeFelice, S. L. The Nutraceutical Revolution: Its Impact on Food Industry R&D. *Trends Food Sci. Technol.* **1995,** *6* (2), 59–61.

Dev, R.; Kumar, S.; Singh, J.; Chauhan, B. Potential Role of Nutraceuticals in Present Scenario: A Review. *J. Appl. Pharm. Sci.* **2011,** *1*, 26–28.

Droge, W. Free Radicals in the Physiological Control of Cell Function. *Physiol. Rev.* **2002,** *82*, 47–95.

Duran, C.; Arce-Johnson, P.; Aquea, F. Methylboronic Acid Fertilization Alleviates Boron Deficiency Symptoms in Arabidopsis thaliana. *Planta* **2018,** *248* (1), 221–229.

Fatemeh, S. R.; Saifullah, R.; Abbas, F. M. A.; Azhar, M. E. Total Phenolics, Flavonoids and Antioxidant Activity of Banana Pulp and Peel Flours: Influence of Variety and Stage of Ripeness. *Int. Food Res. J.* **2012,** *19* (3), 1041.

Ferrari, C. K. Oxidative Stress Pathophysiology: Searching for an Effective Antioxidant Protection. *Int. Med. J. Tokyo* **2001,** *8* (3), 175–184.

Ferrari, C. K. Functional Foods, Herbs and Nutraceuticals: Towards Biochemical Mechanisms of Healthy Aging. *Biogerontology* **2004,** *5* (5), 275–289.

Ferreira, F. D.; Kemmelmeier, C.; Arrotéia, C. C.; da Costa, C. L.; Mallmann, C. A.; Janeiro, V.; Machinski, Jr. M. Inhibitory Effect of the Essential Oil of Curcuma longa L. and Curcumin on Aflatoxin Production by Aspergillus flavus Link. *Food Chem.* **2013,** *136* (2), 789–793.

Ghenima, A. I.; Idir, M.; Nadjet, M. G.; Samia, M. A.; Mihoub, Z. M.; Karim, H. In Vitro Evaluation of Biological Activities of Pistacia lentiscus aqueous Extract. *Int. J. Pharm. Pharm. Sci.* **2015,** *7* (11), 133–139.

Ghiselli, A. Fluorescence Based Method for Measuring Total Plasma Antioxidant Capability. *Free Radic. Biol. Med.* **1995,** *18*, 29–36.

Giles, G. I.; Jacob, C. Reactive Sulfur Species: An Emerging Concept in Oxidative Stress. *Biol. Chem.* **2002,** *383*, 375–388.

Goncalves, C.; Dinis, T.; Batista, M. T. Antioxidant Properties of Proanthocyanidins of Uncaria tomentosa Bark Decoction: A Mechanism for Anti-inflammatory Activity. *Phytochemistry* **2005,** *66* (1), 89–98

Goodwin, J. S; Goodwin, J. M.; Garry, P. J. Association between Nutritional Status and Cognitive Functioning in a Healthy Elderly Population. *J. Am. Med. Assoc.* **1983,** *249*, 2917–2921.

Goulas, V.; Manganaris, G. A. Exploring the Phytochemical Content and the Antioxidant Potential of Citrus Fruits Grown in Cyprus. *Food Chem.* **2012,** *131* (1), 39–47.

Gromer, S.; Urig, S.; Becker, K. The Thioredoxin System-From Science to Clinic. *Med. Res. Rev.* **2004,** *24*, 40–89.

Guo, C.; Yang, J.; Wei, J.; Li, Y.; Xu, J.; Jiang, Y. Antioxidant Activities of Peel, Pulp and Seed Fractions of Common Fruits as Determined by FRAP Assay. *Nutr. Res.* **2003,** *23* (12), 1719–1726.

Hamrouni-Sellami, I.; Rahali, F. Z.; Rebey, I. B.; Bourgou, S.; Limam, F.; Marzouk, B. Total Phenolics, Flavonoids, and Antioxidant Activity of Sage (Salvia officinalis L.) Plants as Affected by Different Drying Methods. *Food Bioproc. Technol.* **2013,** *6* (3), 806–817.

Hemalatha, R.; Nivetha, P.; Mohanapriya, C.; Sharmila, G.; Muthukumaran, C.; Gopinath, M. Phytochemical Composition, GC-MS Analysis, in vitro Antioxidant and Antibacterial Potential of Clove Flower Bud (Eugenia caryophyllus) Methanolic Extract. *J. Food Sci. Technol.* **2016,** *53* (2), 1189–1198.

Herrera, E.; Barbas, C. Vitamin E: Action, Metabolism and Perspectives. *J. Physiol. Biochem.* **2001,** *57* (2), 43–56.

Hervert-Herandez, D.; Sáyago-Ayerdi, S. G.; Goni, I. Bioactive Compounds of Four Hot Pepper Varieties (Capsicum annuum L.), Antioxidant Capacity, and Intestinal Bioaccessibility. *J. Agric. Food Chem.* **2010,** *58* (6), 3399–3406.

Hosseini, A.; Ghorbani, A. Cancer Therapy with Phytochemicals: Evidence from Clinical Studies. *Avicenna J. Phytomed.* **2015,** *5* (2), 84–97.

Hurrell, R. F. Influence of Vegetable Protein Sources on Trace Element and Mineral Bioavailability. *J. Nutr.* **2003,** *133* (9), 2973S–2977S.

Irshad, M.; Chaudhary, P. S. Oxidant- Antioxidant System: Role and Significant in Human Body. *Indian J. Exp. Biol.* **2002,** *40*, 1233–1239.

Jack, D. B. Keep Taking the Tomatoes-the Exciting World of Nutraceuticals. *Mol. Med. Today* **1995,** *1* (3), 118–121.

Jayaprakash, G. K.; Singh, R. P.; Sakariah, K. K. Antioxidant Activity of Grape Seed Extracts on Peroxidation Models in-vitro. *J. Agric. Food Chem.* **2001,** *55*, 1018–1022.

Je, J. Y.; Qian, Z. J.; Byun, H. G.; Kim, S. K. Purification and Characterization of an Antioxidant Peptide Obtained from Tuna Backbone Protein by Enzymatic Hydrolysis. *Process Biochem.* **2007,** *42* (5), 840–846.

Jun, S. Y.; Park, P. J.; Jung, W. K.; Kim, S. K. Purification and Characterization of an Antioxidative Peptide from Enzymatic Hydrolysate of Yellowfin Sole (Limanda aspera) Frame Protein. *Euro. Food Res. Technol.* **2004,** *219* (1), 20–26.

Kalogeropoulos, N.; Chiou, A.; Pyriochou, V.; Peristeraki, A.; Karathanos, V. T. Bioactive Phytochemicals in Industrial Tomatoes and their Processing Byproducts. *LWT Food Sci. Technol.* **2012,** *49* (2), 213–216.

Kalra, E. K. Nutraceutical-Definition and Introduction. *Aaps Pharmsci.* **2003,** *5* (3), 27–28.

Kanner, J. Natural Antioxidants in Grapes and Wines. *J. Agric. Food Chem.* **1994,** *42*, 64–69.
Kanokmedhakul, S.; Kanokmedhakul. K.; Lekphrom, R. Bioactive Constituents of the Roots of Polyalthia cerasoides. *J. Natl. Prod.* **2007,** *70* (9), 1536–1538.
Kavitha, R. V.; Kumar, J. R; Egbuna, C.; Ifemeje, J. C. Phytochemicals as Therapeutic Interventions in Neurodegenerative Diseases. In *Phytochemicals as Lead Compounds for New Drug Discovery*; Elsevier, 2019; pp 161–178.
Keservani, R. K.; Kesharwani, R. K.; Sharma, A. K.; Vyas, N.; Chadoker, A. Nutritional Supplements: An Overview. *Int. J. Curr. Pharm. Rev. Res.* **2010b,** *1* (1), 59–75.
Keservani, R. K.; Kesharwani, R. K.; Vyas, N.; Jain, S.; Raghuvanshi, R.; Sharma, A. K. Nutraceutical and Functional Food as Future Food: A Review. *Der Pharmacia Lettre* **2010a,** *2* (1), 106–116.
Keservani, R. K.; Sharma, A. K. Flavonoids: Emerging Trends and Potential Health Benefits. *J. Chinese Pharm. Sci.* **2014,** *23* (12), 815.
Keservani, R. K.; Sharma, A. K.; Kesharwani, R. K. Nutraceutical and Functional Foods for Cardiovascular Health. In *Food Process Engineering*; Apple Academic Press, CRC Press, 2016a; pp 291–312, pp 257–278. ISBN: 9781771884020.
Keservani, R. K.; Sharma, A. K.; Kesharwani, R. K. Medicinal Effect of Nutraceutical Fruits for the Cognition and Brain Health. *Scientifica* 2016b, *2016*, 3109254. doi:10.1155/2016/3109254.
Keservani, R. K.; Sharma, A. K.; Kesharwani, R. K. An Overview and Therapeutic Applications of Nutraceutical and Functional Foods. *Rec. Adv. Drug Deliv. Technol.* **2017,** 160–201. ISBN: 9781522507543.
Keservani, R. K.; Sharma, A. K.; Kesharwani, R. K. Eds.; In *Nutraceuticals and Dietary Supplements: Applications in Health Improvement and Disease Management*; CRC Press, 2020; pp 1–342. ISBN: 9781771888738.
Khatua, S.; Paul, S.; Acharya, K. Mushroom as the Potential Source of New Generation of Antioxidant: A Review. *Res. J. Pharm. Technol.* **2013,** *6* (5), 496–505.
Kim, J. S.; Ahn, J.; Lee, S. J.; Moon, B.; Ha, T. Y.; Kim, S. Phytochemicals and Antioxidant Activity of Fruits and Leaves of Paprika (Capsicum annuum L., var. Special) Cultivated in Korea. *J. Food Sci.* **2011,** *76* (2), C193–C198.
Kim, S. K.; Wijesekara, I. Marine-Derived Nutraceuticals. Marine Nutraceuticals: Prospects and Perspectives. *Marine Drugs* **2013,** *11*, 1300–1303.
Koh, S. H.; Kim, S. H.; Kwon, H.; Park, Y.; Kim, K. S.; Song, C. W.; Jung, H. K. Epigallocatechin Gallate Protects Nerve Growth Factor Differentiated PC12 Cells from Oxidative-Radical-Stress-Induced Apoptosis through its Effect on Phosphoinositide 3-kinase/Akt and Glycogen Synthase Kinase-3. *Mol. Brain Res.* **2003,** *118* (1-2), 72–81.
Krinsky, N. I.; Johnson, E. J. Carotenoid Actions and their Relation to Health and Disease. *Mol. Aspects Med.* **2005,** *26*, 459–516.
Liu, F.; Ooi, V. E.; Chang, S. T. Free Radical Scavenging Activities of Mushroom Polysaccharide Extracts. *Life Sci.* **1997,** *60* (10), 763–771.
Lu, X.; Ross, C. F.; Powers, J. R.; Aston, D. E.; Rasco, B. A. Determination of Total Phenolic Content and Antioxidant Activity of Garlic (Allium sativum) and Elephant Garlic (Allium ampeloprasum) by Attenuated Total Reflectance Fourier Transformed Infrared Spectroscopy. *J. Agric. Food Chem.* **2011,** *59* (10), 5215–5221.
Maizura, M.; Aminah, A.; Wan Aida, W. Total Phenolic Content and Antioxidant Activity of Kesum (Polygonum minus), Ginger (Zingiber officinale) and Turmeric (Curcuma longa) Extract. *Int. Food Res. J.* **2011,** *18* (2), 529–534.

Manivannan, K.; Anantharaman, P.; Balasubramanian, T. Antimicrobial Potential of Selected Brown Seaweeds from Vedalai Coastal Waters, Gulf of Mannar. *Asian Pac. J. Trop. Biomed.* **2011,** *1* (2), 114–120.

Mannion, M. Nutraceutical Revolution Continues at Foundation for Innovation in Medicine Conference. *Am. J. Nat. Med.* **1998,** *5*, 30–33.

McCullough, M. L.; Peterson, J. J.; Patel, R.; Jacques, P. F.; Shah, R.; Dwyer, J. T. Flavonoid Intake and Cardiovascular Disease Mortality in a Prospective Cohort of US Adults. *Am. J. Clin. Nutr.* **2012,** *95* (2), 454–464.

Mirabella, N.; Castellani, V.; Sala, S. Current Options for the Valorization of Food Manufacturing Waste: A Review. *J. Clean. Prod.* **2014,** *65*, 28–41.

Nahak, G.; Suar, M.; Sahu, R. K. Antioxidant Potential and Nutritional Values of Vegetables: A Review. *Res. J. Med. Plant* **2014,** *8* (2), 50–81.

Newman, D. J, Cragg, G. M. Marine Natural Products and Related Compounds in Clinical and Advanced Preclinical Trials. *J. Natl. Prod.* **2004,** *67* (8), 1216–1238.

Ngo, D. H.; Vo, T. S.; Ngo, D. N.; Wijesekara, I.; Kim, S. K. Biological Activities and Potential Health Benefits of Bioactive Peptides Derived from Marine Organisms. *Int. J. Biol. Macromol.* **2012,** *51* (4), 378–383.

Nikolova, M.; Tsvetkova, R.; Ivancheva, S. Evaluation of Antioxidant Activity in some Geraniacean species. *Bot. Serb.* **2010,** *34* (2), 123–125.

Nordberg, J.; Arner, E. S. Reactive Oxygen Species, Antioxidants, and the Mammalian thioredoxin System. *Free Radic. Biol. Med.* **2001,** *31*, 1287–1312.

Packer, J. E.; Slater, T. F.; Wilson, R. S. Direct Observation of Free Radical Interaction between Vitamin E and Vitamin C. *Nature* **1979,** *278*, 737–738.

Pan, H.; Han, Y.; Huang, J.; Yu, X.; Jiao, C.; Yang, X.; Yang, B. B. Purification and Identification of a Polysaccharide from Medicinal Mushroom Amauroderma Rude with Immunomodulatory Activity and Inhibitory Effect on Tumor Growth. *Oncotarget* **2015,** *6* (19), 17777.

Pandey, M.; Verma, R. K.; Saraf, S. A. Nutraceuticals: New Era of Medicine and Health. *Asian J. Pharm. Clin. Res.* **2010,** *3* (1), 11–15.

Park, J. H.; Park, Y. K.; Park, E. Antioxidative and Antigenotoxic Effects of Garlic (Allium sati- vum L.) Prepared by Different Processing Methods. *Plant Foods Human Nutr.* **2009,** *64* (4), 244–278.

Parr, A. J.; Bolwell, G. P. Phenols in the Plant and in Man. The Potential for Possible Nutritional Enhancement of the Diet by Modifying the Phenols Content or Profile. *J. Sci. Food Agric.* **2000,** *80* (7), 985–1012.

Patel, H.; Chandra, S.; Alexander, S.; Soble, J.; Williams, K. A. Plant-Based Nutrition: An Essential Component of Cardiovascular Disease Prevention and Management. *Curr. Cardiol. Rep.* **2017,** *19* (10), 104–116.

Patil, V. M.; Masand, N. Anticancer Potential of Flavonoids: Chemistry, Biological Activities, and Future Perspectives. In *Studies in Natural Products Chemistry*; Elsevier, 2018; vol 59, pp 401–430.

Pinho, O.; Ferreira, I. M. P. L. V. O.; Oliveira, M. B. P. P.; Ferreira, M. A. Quantification of Synthetic Phenolic Antioxidants in Liver Pates. *Food Chem.* **2000,** *68* (3), 353–357.

Pujol, D.; Liu, C.; Gominho, J.; Olivella, M.; Fiol, N.; Villaescusa, I.; Pereira, H. The Chemical Composition of Exhausted Coffee Waste. *Ind. Crops Prod.* **2013,** *50*, 423–429.

Quintavalla, S.; Vicini, L. Antimicrobial Food Packaging in Meat Industry. *Meat Sci.* **2002,** *62* (3), 373–380.

Rahman, T.; Choudhury, M. Shiitake Mushroom: A Tool of Medicine. *Bangladesh J. Med. Biochem.* **2013,** *5* (1), 24–32.
Rahman, M.; Fazlic, V. S. Antioxidant Properties of Raw Garlic (Allium sativum) Extract. *Int. Food Res. J.* **2012,** *19* (2), 589–591.
Rai, M.; Tidke, G.; Wasser, S. P. Therapeutic Potential of Mushrooms, 2005.
Ramalakshmi, K.; Kubra, I. R.; Rao, L. J. Antioxidant Potential of Low-Grade Coffee Beans. *Food Res. Int.* **2008,** *41* (1), 96–103.
Randriamboavonjy, J. I.; Loirand, G.; Vaillant, N.; Lauzier, B.; Derbrr, S.; Michalet, S.; Tesse, A. Cardiac Protective Effects of Moringa oleifera Seeds in Spontaneous Hypertensive Rats. *Am. J. Hypertens.* **2016,** *29* (7), 873–881.
Rane, B. R.; Bharath, M. S.; Patil, R. R.; Keservani, R. K.; Jain, A. S. Novel Approaches in Nutraceuticals, Chapter 11. In *Enhancing the Therapeutic Efficacy of Herbal Formulations through Novel Drug Delivery Systems*; Kesharwani, R. K., Keservani, R. K., Sharma, A. K., IGI Global International Publisher: Pennsylvania, USA, 2020b; pp 241–266. ISBN13: 9781799844532.
Rane, B. R.; Patil, A. S.; Keservani, R. K.; Jain, A. S. Novel Approaches in Herbal Formulation, Chapter 2. In *Enhancing the Therapeutic Efficacy of Herbal Formulations through Novel Drug Delivery Systems*; Kesharwani, R. K., Keservani, R. K., Sharma, A. K., IGI Global International Publisher: Pennsylvania, USA, 2020a; pp 43–68. ISBN13: 9781799844532.
Rane, B. R.; Tadavi, S. A.; Keservani, R. K. Naturopathy, Chapter 12. In *Herbal Product Development*; Sharma, A. K., Keservani, R. K., Gautam, S. P., Apple Academic Press, CRC Press, Taylor & Francis Group, 2020c; pp 321–347. ISBN: 9781771888776.
Ravikumar, Y. S.; Mahadevan, K. M.; Kumaraswamy, M. N.; Vaidya, V. P.; Manjunatha, H.; Kumar, V.; Satyanarayana, N. D. Antioxidant, Cytotoxic and Genotoxic Evaluation of Alcoholic Extract of Polyalthia cerasoides (Roxb.) Bedd. *Environ. Toxicol. Pharmacol.* **2008,** *26* (2), 142–146.
Reddy, N. S.; Navanesan, S.; Sinniah, S. K.; Wahab, N. A.; Sim, K. S. Phenolic Content, Antioxidant Effect and Cytotoxic Activity of Leea indica Leaves. *BMC Complement. Altern. Med.* **2012,** *12* (1), 1–7.
Robak, J.; Gryglewski, R. J. Flavonoids are Scavengers of Superoxide Anions. *Biochem. Pharmacol.* **1998,** *37*, 837–841.
Roby, M. H. H.; Sarhan, M. A.; Selim, K. A. H.; Khalel, K. I. Evaluation of Antioxidant Activity, Total Phenols and Phenolic Compounds in Thyme (Thymus vulgaris L.), Sage (Salvia officinalis L.), and Marjoram (Origanum majorana L.) Extracts. *Ind. Crops Prod.* **2013,** *43*, 827–831.
Rodriguez-Amaya, D. B.; Kimura, M.; Godoy, H. T.; Amaya-Farfan, J. Updated Brazilian Database on Food Carotenoids: Factors Affecting Carotenoid Composition. *J. Food Compos. Anal.* **2008,** *21*, 445–463.
Romay, C. H.; Armesto, J.; Remirez, D.; González, R.; Ledon, N.; Garcia, I. Antioxidant and Anti-inflammatory Properties of C-phycocyanin from Blue-Green Algae. *Inflamm. Res.* **1998,** *47* (1), 36–41.
Ronald, L. P. Antioxidant Capacity as Influenced by Total Phenolic & Anthocyanin Content Maturity and Variety of *Vaccinium* Species. *J. Agric. Food Chem.* **1998,** *46*, 2686–2693.
Rudra, S. G.; Nishad, J.; Jakhar, N.; Kaur, C. Food Industry Waste: Mine of Nutraceuticals. *Int. J. Sci. Environ. Technol.* **2015,** *4* (1), 205–229.
Ruthes, A. C.; Smiderle, F. R.; Iacomini, M. Mushroom Heteropolysaccharides: A Review on their Sources, Structure and Biological Effects. *Carbohydr. Polym.* **2016,** *136*, 358–375.

Sanchez-Moreno, C.; Larrauri, J.; Saura-Calixto, F. Free Radical Scavenging Capacity of Selected Red and White Wine. *J. Sci. Food Agric.* **1999,** *79*, 1301–1304.
Shahidi, F. Antioxidants in Food and Food Antioxidants. *Mol. Nutr. Food Res.* **2000,** *44* (3), 158–163
Shanafelt, T. D.; Lee, Y. K.; Call, T. G.; Nowakowski, G. S.; Dingli, D.; Zent, C. S.; Kay, N. E. Clinical Effects of Oral Green Tea Extracts in Four Patients with Low Grade B-Cell Malignancies. *Leukemia Res.* **2006,** *30* (6), 707–712.
Sharma, A. K.; Keservani, R. K.; Gautam, S. P. In *Herbal Product Development*; Apple Academic Press, CRC Press, Taylor & Francis Group, 2020; pp 1–376. ISBN: 9781771888776.
Shebis, Y.; Iluz, D.; Kinel-Tahan, Y.; Dubinsky, Z.; Yehoshua, Y. Natural Antioxidants: Function and Sources. *Food Nutr. Sci.* **2013,** *4* (06), 643.
Simonetti, P.; Pietta, P.; Testolin, G. Polyphenol Content and Total Antioxidant Potential Selected Italian Wines. *J. Agric. Food Chem.* **1997,** *45*, 1152–1155.
Singh, G.; Kapoor, I. P. S.; Singh, P.; de Heluani, C. S.; de Lampasona, M. P.; Catalan, C. A. Comparative Study of Chemical Composition and Antioxidant Activity of Fresh and Dry Rhizomes of Turmeric (Curcuma longa Linn.). *Food Chem. Toxicol.* **2010,** *48* (4), 1026–1031.
Slavin J. L.; Lloyd, B. Health Benefits of Fruits and Vegetables. *Adv. Nutr.* **2012,** *3* (4), 506–516.
Someya, S.; Yoshiki, Y.; Okubo, K. Antioxidant Compounds from Bananas (Musa Cavendish). *Food Chem.* **2002,** *79* (3), 351–354.
Sonia, N.; Mini, C.; Geethalekshmi, P. Vegetable Peels as Natural Antioxidants for Processed Foods–A Review. *Agric. Rev.* **2016,** *37* (1), 35–41.
Srinivasan, G.; Ranjith, C.; Vijayan, K. Identification of Chemical Compounds from the Leaves of Leea indica. *Acta Pharm.* **2008,** *58* (2), 207–214.
Steinbrenner, H.; Alili, L.; Bilgic, E.; Sies, H.; Brenneisen, P. Involvement of Selenoprotein P in Protection of Human Astrocytes from Oxidative Damage. *Free Radic. Biol. Med.* **2006,** *40*, 1513–1523.
Steinbrenner, H.; Bilgic, E.; Alili, L.; Sies, H.; Brenneisen, P. Selenoprotein P Protects Endothelial Cells from Oxidative Damage by Stimulation of Glutathione Peroxidase Expression and Activity. *Free Radic. Res.* **2006,** *40*, 936–943.
Tank, D. S.; Gandhi, S.; Shah, M. Nutraceuticals-Portmanteau of Science and Nature. *Int. J. Pharm. Sci. Rev. Res.* **2010,** *5* (3), 33–38.
Tapiero, H.; Townsend, D. M.; Tew, K. D. The Antioxidant Role of Selenium and Selenocompounds. *Biomed. Pharm.* **2003,** *57*, 134–144.
Teixeira, A.; Baenas, N.; Dominguez-Perles, R.; Barros, A.; Rosa, E.; Moreno, D. A.; Garcia-Viguera, C. Natural Bioactive Compounds from Winery By-products as Health Promoters: A Review. *Int. J. Mol. Sci.* **2014,** *15* (9), 15638–15678.
Teixeira, B.; Marques, A.; Ramos, C.; Serrano, C.; Matos, O.; Neng, N. R.; Nunes, M. L. Chemical Composition and Bioactivity of Different Oregano (Origanum vulgare) Extracts and Essential Oil. *J. Sci. Food Agric.* **2013,** *93* (11), 2707–2714.
Tinggi, U. Selenium: Its Role as Antioxidant in Human Health. *Environ. Health Prevent. Med.* **2008,** *13* (2), 102–108.
Tiwari, A.K. Imbalance in Antioxidant Defence and Human Diseases: Multiple Approach of Natural Antioxidants Therapy. *Curr. Sci.* **2001,** *10*, 1179–1187.

Treeratanapiboon, L.; Worachartcheewan, A.; Suksrichavalit, T.; Kiatfuengfoo, R.; Prachayasittikul, S.; Ruchirawat, S.; Prachayasittikul, V. Bioactive 4-hydroxycinnamide and Bioactivities of Polyalthia cerasoides. *EXCLI J.* **2011,** *10*, 16.

Urquiaga, I.; Leighton, F. Plant Polyphenol Antioxidants and Oxidative Stress. *Biol. Res.* **2000,** *33* (2), 55–64.

Valko, M.; Rhodes, C. J.; Moncol, J.; Izakovic, M.; Mazur, M. Free Radicals, Metals and Antioxidants in Oxidative Stress-Induced Cancer. *Chem. Biol. Interact.* **2006,** *160*, 1–40.

Valverde, M. E.; Hernández-Pérez, T.; Paredes-López, O. Edible Mushrooms: Improving Human Health and Promoting Quality Life. *Int. J. Microbiol.* **2015,** *3* (7), 392–442.

Velmurugan, B. K.; Rathinasamy, B.; Lohanathan, B. P.; Thiyagarajan, V.; Weng, C. F. Neuroprotective Role of Phytochemicals. *Molecules* **2018,** *23* (10), 2485–2524.

Vinson, J. A.; Hontz, B. A. Phenol Antioxidant Index: Comparative Antioxidant Effectiveness of Red and White Wines. *J. Agric. Food Chem.* **1995,** *43*, 401–403.

Voutilainen, S.; Nurmi, T.; Mursu, J.; Rissanen, T. H. Carotenoids and Cardiovascular Health. *Am. J. Clin. Nutr.* **2006,** *83*, 1265–1271.

Walch, S. G.; Ngaba Tinzoh, L.; Zimmermann, B. F.; Stühlinger, W.; Lachenmeier, D. W. Antioxidant Capacity and Polyphenolic Composition as Quality Indicators for Aqueous Infusions of Salvia officinalis L. (sage tea). *Front. Pharmacol.* **2011,** *2*, 79.

Walker, J. M.; Klakotskaia, D.; Ajit, D.; Weisman, G. A.; Wood, W. G.; Sun, G. Y.; Schachtman, T. R. Beneficial Effects of Dietary EGCG and Voluntary Exercise on Behavior in an Alzheimer's Disease Mouse Model. *J. Alzheimer's Dis.* **2015,** *44* (2), 561–572.

Wang, J. H.; Zhang, B. W.; Sun, Y. H.; Zhang, J. C. Structure of Polysaccharide Dips-2 from Dictyophora Indusiata and its Effect on Anti-fatigue Activities. *Curr. Top. Nutraceut. Res.* **2015,** *13* (4).

Wijffels, R. H. Potential of Sponges and Microalgae for Marine Biotechnology. *Trends Biotechnol.* **2008,** *26* (1), 26–31.

Wobst, H. J.; Sharma, A.; Diamond, M. I; Wanker, E. E.; Bieschke, J. The Green Tea Polyphenol (−)-epigallocatechin Gallate Prevents the Aggregation of Tau Protein into Toxic Oligomers at Substoichiometric Ratios. *FEBS Lett.* **2015,** *589* (1), 77–83.

Wu, H. C.; Chen, H. M.; Shiau, C. Y. Free Amino Acids and Peptides as Related to Antioxidant Properties in Protein Hydrolysates of Mackerel (Scomber austriasicus). *Food Res. Int.* **2003,** *36* (9-10), 949–957.

Wu, W.; Wang, X.; Xiang, Q.; Meng, X.; Peng, Y; Du, N. Astaxanthin Alleviates Brain Aging in Rats by Attenuating Oxidative Stress and Increasing BDNF Levels. *Food Funct.* **2014,** *5* (1), 158–166.

Xianquan, S.; Shi, J.; Kakuda, Y.; Yueming, J. Stability of Lycopene during Food Processing and Storage. *J. Med. Food* **2005,** *8* (4), 413–422.

Yang, X.; Zheng, T.; Hong, H.; Cai. N.; Zhou, X, Sun, C.; Jin, F. Neuroprotective Effects of Ginkgo Biloba Extract and Ginkgolide B Against Oxygen–Glucose Deprivation/Reoxygenation and Glucose Injury in a New in vitro Multicellular Network Model. *Front Med.* **2018,** *12* (3), 307–318.

Yuliani, S.; Mustofa, P. G. The Neuroprotective Effects of an Ethanolic Turmeric (Curcuma longa L.) Extract against Trimethyltin-Induced Oxidative Stress in Rats. *Nutr. Neurosci.* **2019,** *22* (11), 797–804.

Yun T. K.; Choi, S. Y.; Yun, H. Y. Epidemiological Study on Cancer Prevention by Ginseng: Are All Kinds of Cancers Preventable by Ginseng? *J. Korean Med. Sci.* **2001,** 19–27.

Zhang, C.; Browne, A.; Child, D.; Tanzi, R. E. Curcumin Decreases Amyloid-β Peptide Levels by Attenuating the Maturation of Amyloid-β Precursor Protein. *J. Biol. Chem.* **2010,** *285* (37), 28472–28480.

Zhang, X.; Shu, X. O.; Gao, Y. T.; Yang, G.; Li, Q.; Li, H.; Zheng, W. Soy Food Consumption is Associated with Lower Risk of Coronary Heart Disease in Chinese Women. *J. Nutr.* **2003,** *133* (9), 2874–2878.

CHAPTER 2

IMPORTANCE OF PHYTOCHEMICAL ANTIOXIDANTS

YOGEETA GOYAL[1], MRUNALI PATIL[2], KAMINI MORE[1], and KIRAN PATIL[1]

[1]*Department of Pharmaceutics, Shri Vile Parle Kelavani Mandal's Institute of Pharmacy, Dhule, Maharashtra, India*

[2]*Department of Pharmaceutical Chemistry, Shri Vile Parle Kelavani Mandal's Institute of Pharmacy, Dhule, Maharashtra, India*

ABSTRACT

The etiology of several illnesses is triggered by a superfluous of oxidants (reactive oxygen and nitrogen species) in the human body. The process of neutralizing these oxidants can be considered a useful strategy for reducing organisms' oxidative stress levels. The substances that balance these oxidants are called antioxidants. They can be obtained both naturally and synthetically. Natural antioxidants the secondary plant metabolite are recommended over synthetic antioxidants, which have been discovered to have adverse effects. Numerous foods and botanicals contain antioxidant phytochemicals, which are crucial in the management and cure of chronic illnesses driven by oxidative stress. This chapter's goal is to provide an overview of the significance, necessity, and enumeration of the medical advantages of various phytochemical antioxidants.

2.1 INTRODUCTION

Phytochemicals are chemical substances obtained from plants. As the name implies, it has been originated from the Greek word phyto, which means

Antioxidants as Nutraceuticals. Nayan A. Gujarathi, Raj K. Keservani, Rajesh K. Kesharwani, Bhushan R. Rane, Yogeeta Sameer Goyal (Eds.)

"plant." They are usually the primary or secondary metabolic products of plants. They exhibit biological action in the host plant and are crucial for plant development or defense (Altemimi et al., 2017; Zhang et al., 2015).

Antioxidants are compounds that prevent oxidation. Although oxygen is essential for the respiration process some amount of inhaled oxygen is converted to reactive oxygen species (ROS) on account of the rigorous oxidative process, which is responsible for the degradation of nucleic acids, proteins, lipids, and carbohydrates that ultimately affects immune functions causing degenerative diseases. Antioxidants being inhibitors, oxidize themselves to remove these free radicals. When the level of free radicals exceeds our bodies' antioxidant defense system, it results in oxidative stress (OS). Antioxidants guard the body against harmful chain reactions (Margaritelis et al., 2018; Mason et al., 2020).

It is quite interesting to study the beneficial effects of the number of phytochemicals with an antioxidant capacity which will serve as protection to human health from oxidative stress. Primary antioxidants are the body's own natural defense against free radicals. The probable mechanism by which these antioxidants may provide safety is limiting the amount of free radicals produced, capturing free radicals, assisting in the repair, and harnessing a conducive environment. They protect against cellular damage by scavenging them before they have a chance to harm cells (Baby et al., 2018; Ghosia et al., 2019; Saleem et al., 2020).

These natural antioxidants can be classified based on many points like forms, method of action, environment, solubility, structural dependency, and source (Liguori et al., 2018; Neha et al., 2019). Here, we try to explain the importance of phytochemical antioxidants by classifying them broadly as enzymatic and non-enzymatic antioxidants. Primary antioxidants are engaged in the avoidance of oxidant production; secondary antioxidants are recognized to be ROS scavengers whereas tertiary antioxidants are known to restore the oxidized molecules through sources such as dietary or subsequent antioxidants. Some of the examples of primary enzymatic antioxidants include Superoxide dismutase (SOD) and common antioxidant enzyme (CAT) (Anto Suganya and Jeya Jothi, 2020). Examples of secondary enzymatic antioxidants are glutathione reductase (GR), glucose-6-phosphate dehydrogenase (G6PHD). Non-enzymatic antioxidant includes minerals, vitamins, polyphenols, carotenoids, and other antioxidants. This chapter will focus on the importance of all these phytochemicals (Moon and Shibamoto, 2009).

2.2 NEED FOR ANTIOXIDANTS

Biological antioxidants were developed to combat the risk of harm caused by oxidants. Small antioxidant molecules and antioxidant enzymes, which are mostly consumed from fruits and vegetables, are present in abundance in cells (Grover, 2013). The following are some examples of antioxidant defenses:

1. Catalase, glutathione peroxidase (GPx), and SOD, speed up the disproportionation of O_2 to H_2O_2, to produce water from H2O2.
2. Urate, ascorbate, and glutathione are used as hydrophilic radical scavengers.
3. Carotenoids, tocopherols, ubiquinol, and flavonoids are used as lipophilic radical scavenger.
4. Enzymes that reduce small-molecule antioxidants in their oxidised state (such as GSH reductase and ascorbate reductase) or maintain protein thiols (thioredoxin reductase).

Diverse antioxidant systems work together to reduce ROS burden. Additionally, it is beneficial to redirect ROS to different reaction pathways that result in less reactive products, to preferentially inactivate ions from transition metals (in redox terms), and, if all else fails, to provide sacrificial molecules that serve as a reproducible or recycled content "buffer" to soak up oxidative hits and energy generated (Li et al., 2015; Veurink et al., 2020).

2.3 IMPORTANCE OF PHYTOCHEMICAL ANTIOXIDANTS

2.3.1 VITAMINS

2.3.1.1 VITAMINS A

Retinoic acid is another name for vitamin A and it belongs to the family of unsaturated lipo-soluble organic compounds including retinol, retinal, retinyl palmitate, carotenoids like beta-carotene. Carotenoids are a collection of about 600 chemicals (Benzie and Choi, 2014). Of them, only 50 or so exhibit provitamin A activity. Green and yellow vegetables, dairy products, fruits, and organ meats all are the richest sources of vitamin A. Carotenoids are said to be protective and effective for heart diseases (Baranowska and Bartoszek, 2016). They have further reported to possess the capacity to restrain viral hepatitis. Its activity is discussed to be due to the hydrophobic chain of polyene units that may neutralize thiyl radicals, quench singlet oxygen, and interact with and stabilize peroxyl radicals (Koekkoek and van Zanten, 2016). Due to its structure, vitamin A and carotenoids can autoxidize when O2 tension increases, hence they can be said effective antioxidants (Dao et al., 2017).

2.3.1.2 VITAMIN C

L-ascorbic acid, a form of vitamin C, is an optically active hydro soluble powerful antioxidant with free radical scavenging ability (Chakraborthy et al., 2014). This vitamin's proton loss from the 3-hydroxyl group is quick, resulting in a resonance-stabilized ascorbate anion. By directly interacting with peroxyl radicals or by reacting indirectly by increasing the antioxidant property of vitamin E, ascorbate promotes free radicals both inside and beyond the cell (Padayatty et al., 2003). This aids in regulating the lipid peroxidation of cellular membranes and nuclear components. The co-factor vitamin C also has a role in several metabolic processes that perform essential functions in humans, plants, and animals. Vitamin C safeguards proteins necessary for DNA repair due to its potent antioxidant activity. It also stops nitrosamine from forming which is responsible for producing ROS. It is also said to have a pro-oxidant impact that kills cancer cells. It is also claimed to be crucial in protein thiol group protection by elevating glutathione levels in the cell (Caritá et al., 2020).

2.3.1.3 VITAMIN E

Vitamin E is an optically active methylated phenolic. Tocopherols and tocotrienols are fat-soluble substances that come in alpha, beta, gamma, and delta forms, respectively. They are lipid soluble and possess unique antioxidant qualities. Vitamin E is exogenous, it is only biosynthesized by plants, photosynthetic algae, and certain cyanobacteria. In exercise-induced oxidative stress, protective effect was seen by rise in the amount of alpha-tocopherol in the liver (Jiang, 2014; Lee and Han, 2018). Alpha-tocopherol is said to prevent lipid peroxidation by cellular membranes by scavenging superoxide radical anion and lipid peroxyl free radicals. The adverse effects that is oxidative stress induced due to exposure to lead by the workers were also reduced by the use of alpha-tocopherol. In diabetic wounds, gamma-tocopherol can reduce oxidative stress, inflammatory response, and apoptosis via nuclear factor kappa B, nuclear factor (erythroid-derived 2)-like 2, and sirtuin-1 (Miyazawa et al., 2019).

2.3.2 VITAMIN COFACTORS AND MINERALS

2.3.2.1 COENZYME Q 10

CoQ-10, sometimes referred to as coenzyme Q-10 or ubiquinone, is a naturally occurring Quinone, in which 10 denotes the quantity of repeated isoprene. It was first found in mitochondria and its level is highest in organs such as the heart, kidney, and liver with a high metabolic rate for transferring energy. CoQ10's main biochemical function is as an electron-transport chain cofactor in the series of redox processes necessary to produce adenosine triphosphate. Since nearly all cellular processes require an appropriate amount of adenosine triphosphate (ATP), CoQ10 is crucial for the well-being of all human tissues and organs (Raizner, 2019). One of the most important lipid antioxidants, coenzyme Q10 guards against the formation of free radicals and their alterations to proteins, lipids, and DNA. The concentration of coenzyme Q10 in the human body declines in many diseases associated with increased production and action of ROS, and a lack of coenzyme Q10 results in the dysfunction of the respiratory chain, which is caused by the insufficient production of highly energetic compounds, which lowers the efficiency of cells (Pastor-Maldonado et al., 2020). CoQ10 boosts immunity, increases energy, and functions as an antioxidant. Heart disease, high blood pressure, cancer, periodontal disease, mitochondrial disorders, radiation injury, obesity, diabetes, Parkinson's disease, acquired immune deficiency syndrome (AIDS), gastric ulcers, allergy, migraine headaches, kidney failure, muscular dystrophy, and aging are among the conditions that coenzyme Q10 has been shown to be helpful in treating. Given that the tissues and cells involved in immune function are highly energy-dependent and need an appropriate supply of CoQ10 to function at their best, CoQ10 has a substantial impact on enhancing the immune system and enhancing physical performance (Hargreaves and Mantle, 2019).

2.3.2.2 MINERALS

Minerals are little trace components in diet that are necessary for growth and help in various functions of life. The fundamental minerals included in our food are manganese, copper, zinc, selenium, iron, potassium, magnesium, calcium, phosphorus, iron, and sodium (Ugboaja et al., 2012). Numerous microelements, including zinc, copper, manganese, iron, selenium, and selenium, function as cofactors for a variety of antioxidant enzymes and contribute to redox metabolism, which helps to slow down the aging process by reducing ROS in cells (Sarker et al., 2020). Since they give muscles strength and are needed for the formation of bones, minerals are scientifically acknowledged as essential nutrients for end-user health. These essential minerals are engaged in a variety of physiological processes in people (Catania et al., 2009).

2.3.2.3 MANGANESE

Numerous biological processes, such as the metabolism of amino acids, cholesterol, glucose, and carbohydrates, are aided by manganese. Additionally, it aids in blood coagulation, bone development, and inflammation reduction. Manganese is primarily used in the production and activation of enzymes, protein, and vitamins C and B. Examples of these enzymes are oxidoreductases, transferases, hydrolases, lyases, and isomerases. It also has a significant impact in the metabolism of carbohydrate and lipids, keeping the production and secretion of insulin at normal levels. MnSOD together with Cu/Zn SOD is involved in mitochondrial oxidative stress to clear ROS. Manganese is also reported to catalyze hematopoiesis and improve immune function. The liver, pancreas, bones, kidneys, and brain may all store manganese, which the human body cannot make. Typically, a person gets manganese via their food (Avila et al., 2013; Fukai and Ushio-Fukai, 2011; Lingappa et al., 2019).

2.3.2.4 SELENIUM

Selenium, a sulphur analogue is an essential trace element with high chemical activity. It is also an important constituent of some selenoproteins and enzymes like GPx , blood, and tissue proteins. Selenium is found to have antioxidant property; it is an active immunomodulator too. It is reported to have greater power antioxidant than vitamin E, C, and A (Burk, 2002). It actively participates in the transformation of thyroxine into triiodethyonine during the manufacture of thyroid hormone. Additionally, selenium promotes sperm motility and fertility. Selenium is also said to protect DNA and chromosomes, vascular endothelium, and low-density lipoproteins. Selenium, is also reported to contribute remarkably as a food component (Steinbrenner and Klotz, 2020). It helps in protection from diseases like cancer, atherosclerosis, and coronary ischemic diseases. Selenium deficiency can cause serious health effects such as Keshan disease, cardio muscular malfunctions, osteoarthritis and viral infections. The selenoproteins acts as antioxidants and helps to maintain the intracellular redox status which in turn aids for normal physiological processes in the cell (Wang et al., 2017).

2.3.2.5 COPPER

Humans require the trace mineral copper, which is an important nutrient. It helps the body use iron. It must be available in adequate through diet or supplements. An essential component of several significant enzymes and a mineral that balances zinc, copper is engaged in a variety of crucial biological processes. It has been reported that a deficiency in copper raises the risk of oxidative damage to cells. Numerous known copper proteins catalyze processes that need contact with oxygen or ROS. Since they are thought to be crucial in defending tissues against some of the pathological responses that are known to occur when ROS become excessively high, these processes are known as antioxidant functions. It also plays an important role in the production of hemoglobin for oxygen transportation. It is said to display key role in action of prostate gland and the activity of oil glands which helps to prevent acne. Also copper is needed for the healthy performance of joints and nerves and it may lower cholesterol level. But if copper intake is above limit it can cause neurological and mental symptoms as it can involve in electron transfer and production of ROS and act as pro-oxidants. Deficiency of copper can also lead to various symptoms like iron deficient anemia, fatigue, and skin rashes (Allen and Klevay, 1994; Medhat Hegazy et al., 2020; Sharif et al., 2021).

2.3.2.6 ZINC

Zinc is a redox-inert metal, known as a vital trace element necessary for human health. It controls a crucial aspect of cell-mediated immunity and is reported as a powerful anti-inflammatory and antioxidant agent. The stability of membrane structure, protection of the protein sulfhydryl groups, protection of the protein sulfhydryl groups, and induction of metallothionein production are all factors contributing to its antioxidant effect. It also acts as a co-factor for a few enzymes that add to the appropriate working of the antioxidant defense system. It has been widely observed experimentally that zinc supplements decrease the level of oxidative stress biomarkers and inflammatory cytokines (Powell, 2000; Prasad, 2009). Additionally, it has been suggested that zinc functions as a chemical signal for immune cells and other transcription factors involved in the gene development of adhesion molecules and inflammatory cytokines. Many chronic diseases like aging, atherosclerosis, cardiac disorders, cancer, neurodegeneration, and immunologic disorders are affected by this oxidative stress and chronic inflammation. ROS are greatly reduced by zinc. Growth retardation, impaired immunological function, immune dysfunctions, increased oxidative stress, and increased production of inflammatory cytokines are all symptoms of zinc deficiency (Skrajnowska and Bobrowska-Korczak, 2019).

2.3.2.7 IODINE

Iodine is a beneficial micronutrient. Iodine is well recognized for its action in the thyroid, but its many non-thyroidal uses—mostly those based on its antioxidant properties—are less well known. It is evaluated to protect against free radicals and peroxides. It is demonstrated by in vivo experiments that malondialdehyde and peroxide levels are decreased and antioxidant enzyme activity is boosted when iodine is administered. It has a well-established role in thyroid hormone production by converting iodide to iodine (organification). According to reports, iodine shortage may generate an oxidative stress state with high TSH levels that produce a level of H2O2 that is not used to create thyroid hormones because of the deficiency in iodide. The generation of free radicals may be a prerequisite for the excess iodide's cytotoxic effects in thyroid cells, which may be linked to both necrotic and apoptotic pathways. One Japanese study also showed a protective benefit toward breast cancer for a diet high in iodine seaweed. Balneotherapeutic application of iodine/iodide is also well evidenced to have positive effect on oxidative stress induced diseases like cardiac diseases, respiratory disorders, eye diseases, and other degenerative diseases (Aceves et al., 2013; Smyth, 2003).

2.3.3 POLYPHENOLS

Flavonoids: These are the secondary metabolite bioactives synthesized by plants. These are believed to be responsible for the flavor, color, and pharmacological activities. These have potential antioxidant properties and are therefore they been studied extensively, in various oxidative stress related diseases. Cocoa products, black and green tea, fruits, vegetables, and red wine are believed to be the main sources of flavonoids. Several studies have exhibited the free radical scavenging capability of flavonoids and prevent oxidative stress-related diseases in the long term. Along with this, flavonoids are also believed in regulating cellular metabolism, anticancer effect, etc. In the case of cancer, flavonoids are believed to bring changes in the ROS-scavenging activities of cell cycle enzymes responsible for arresting the cell cycle, apoptosis induction, autophagy, and suppression of cancer cell proliferation and invasion (Keservani and Sharma, 2014; Keservani et al., 2016a; Keservani et al., 2016b). The impairment of cellular homeostasis between pro-oxidant happenings and antioxidant defense leads to amplified ROS production leading to the accumulation of free radicals (Rodríguez-García et al., 2019). Mostly ROS, the by-products of oxidative phosphorylation, are engendered in the electron transport chain in the cell. Oxidative stress is produced by the virtue of elevated amounts of ROS (Murphy, 2009). This oxidative stress results in an upsurge in inflammation which results in conditions like cancer and degenerative diseases. Flavonoids act dually, as antioxidants in normal conditions and as potent pro-oxidants triggering apoptotic pathways in cancer cells. The phenolic hydroxyl groups in flavonoids possess the ability to stabilize the free radicals. This enables the flavonoids to directly scavenge chelate metals ions and ROS (Chirumbolo et al., 2018). Activation of antioxidant enzymes, stimulant production of antioxidant enzymes and phase II detoxification enzymes and suppression of pro-oxidant enzymes are the other effects related to flavonoids (Fig. 2.1).

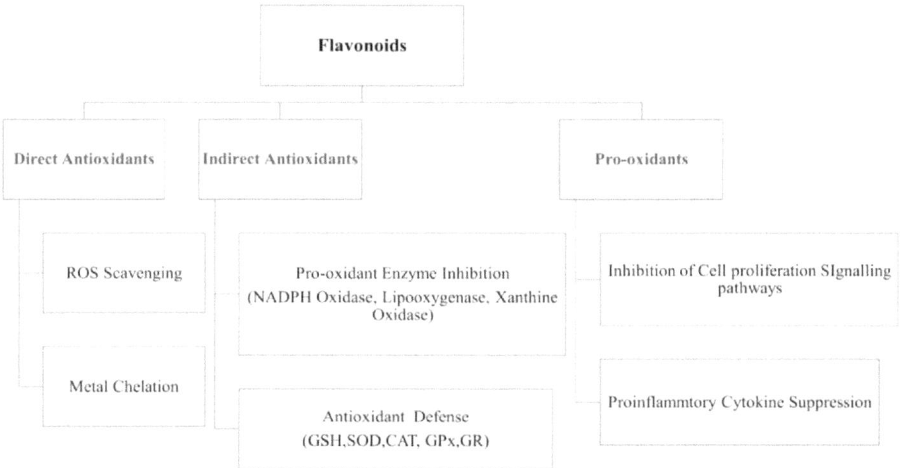

FIGURE 2.1 Antioxidant and pro-oxidant activities of flavonoids in oxidative stress.

2.3.3.1 GINGEROL

Ginger is well known for its use as customary medicine and as a spice in South Asian countries. Its use has been practiced in muscle discomfort, nausea, vomiting, and abdominal pain. It is believed that the afore listed chemical constituents of ginger possess various therapeutic properties like anti-cancer, as antioxidant, anti-inflammatory, and analgesic (Oboh et al., 2012). One of the key active constituents of fresh ginger, 6- Gingerol was found to show a decrement in IL-1β-induced inflammation along with the oxidative stress in ROS/NF-κB/COX-2 signaling pathway as studied in human HuH7 hepatocyte cells (Li et al., 2013). Shogaols are one of the major constituents of ginger which are the dehydration products of gingerols. It has been established through various studies that shogaols have antiproliferative, anti-inflammatory, and anti-cancer properties (Tuorkey, 2015). Another study showed the inhibition of LPS-induced TNF-α, IL-1β, IL-6, and PGE2 production and NF-κB activation by the virtue of 6-Shogaol in BV2 microglia cells. Another molecule 1-Dehydro-10-gingerdione, also derived from ginger, was found to have more potency than 6-Shogaol in context of constraining the NO production along with activation of NF-κB macrophages previously activated by LPS (Han et al., 2017).

2.3.4 POLYPHENOLIC ACID

2.3.4.1 HYDROXYCINNAMIC ACID

Studies have shown the potential antioxidant property in hydroxycinnamic acids (HCA). These include caffeic, ferulic, sinapic acid, and flavonoids. Moreover, studies have shown that the antioxidant property of HCAs is strongly structural feature dependent, essentially on the presence of hydroxyl functional group (Silva et al., 2000).

2.3.4.2 FERULIC ACID

Phytochemically classified as HCA, Ferulic acid is a phenolic nearly ubiquitous constituent abundantly found abundantly in fruits, vegetables, and grains. In plants, these are found covalently bound to biopolymers of cell wall including polysaccharides, lignin, and glycoproteins (Zhuang et al., 2017).

Ferulic acid is believed to exhibit antibacterial, antiallergic, hepato-protective anti-cancer, and antiviral properties (Angiolella et al., 2018). It is also well known for metal chelation, enzymatic activities modulation, free radicals scavenging properties along with signal transduction and gene expression (Sudheer et al., 2005). It is also believed to have radical's chain response management property. Another important role of ferulic acid is to construct other crucial secondary metabolites like vanillin, sinapic acid, curcumin, coniferyl liquor, and di-ferulic acid. Along with this ferulic acid is also involved in maintaining the rigidity of cell wall. The mechanism of antioxidant property exhibited by ferulic acid is dependent on hindering ROS or Nitrogen formation along with neutralization of free radicals. Ferulic acid also possesses metal chelation property in context of Cu (II) or Fe (II) protonated metal ions. It not only scavenges free radical by enhancing the scavenging enzyme activity but also inhibit free radical generation catalysing enzyme.

2.3.5 CAROTENOIDS

Structure of carotenoids consists of 40 carbons united in eight isoprene units covalently linked together. Furthermore, carotenoids are categorized into two categories the ones that have provitamin-A activity (-carotene and -cryptoxanthin) and others that do not (lycopene and lutein). Carotenoids can decrease the health menace of macular degeneration, some forms of cancer, and cardiovascular diseases. This is estimated to be the result of antioxidant properties. Thus carotenoid consumption is vital and fruitful to human health. The main targets of carotenoids involve ROS, inactivation of free radicals and modulation of expression of gene by intonation of intracellular signaling pathway further affecting gene expression and protein translation. Studies have confirmed that carotenoid intake may considerably decrease the menace of nonalcoholic fatty liver disease (NAFLD) and nonalcoholic steatohepatitis (NASH) and used in their treatment and prevention (Dewanjee et al., 2021). NAFLD is characterized by oxidative stress and inflammation as a result of lipid peroxidation. Lipid peroxidation is the result of disparity in lipid metabolism which further causes fat accumulation in Hepatocyte (Stahl and Sies, 2003). Accumulation of carotenoids and their metabolites may improve hepatocyte metabolism. This helps in controlling and modulating cellular oxidative state in some hepatic conditions. Studies have demonstrated that dietary carotenoids exhibit a free radical scavenging effect in cardiovascular disease. These also improve LDL cholesterol resistance to oxidation (Ciccone et al., 2013). Oxidative stress has a vital role in the progression of ischaemic brain damage. Studies have confirmed that carotenoids have essential role as antioxidant in lowering stroke risk. It is well known that the higher blood concentrations of carotenes are associated with lowering the risk of many chronic conditions (Bahonar et al., 2017). Carotenoids are believed to be very efficient physical quenchers of singlet oxygen and ROS. They can also act as an antioxidant by chemically quenching through irreversible oxygenation. To sum up, carotenoid intake provides beneficial effects in oxidative stress as a part of conditions like cancer, cardiovascular, and photosensitivity disorders (Fiedor and Burda, 2014).

2.3.5.1 β-CAROTENE

β-Carotene acts as an antioxidant by scavenging singlet oxygen. β-Carotene is also known to produce positive photoprotective influence in photooxidative damage and sunburn. A decrement in serum β-carotene levels is known to be associated with an increased risk of congestive cardiac failure. It is also known to reduce erythema when treated with β-carotene applied transdermally (Padmanabhan et al., 2016). The effect of β-carotene on the progression and metastatis of melanoma is still to be studied further (Madhunapantula and Robertson, 2012). β–Carotene shows a direct effect against ROS and prevents oxidative stress. Studies have observed a significant reduction in the risk of hepatic steatosis and oxidative damage. Oxidative stress so generated altered malondialdehyde (MDA), Glutathione (GSH), catalyze, SOD, and GSH peroxidase levels. Through its Provitamin A activity, β–Carotene is established to inhibit ROS. β–carotene is also well known to improve the diseased conditions in hepatice steatosis, fibrosis, oxidative stress, inflammation, and apoptosis as a result of its protective and preventive actions. Another study confirmed that β–carotene defends physiological antioxidants against aflatoxin-induced carcinogenesis. Other effects of β–Carotene include increase in the levels of vitamin C, glutathione, and enzymes related to glutathione thus aiding in reducing the toxicity of aflatoxin-B1. Studies have also established additional pharmacological effects produced by β-carotene are reduction in plasma cholesterol and atherogenesis index; reduction in fat accumulation and inflammation due to transcriptional regulation of inflammatory cytokines; prevention of development of carcinoma hepatocellular; improved diet-induced obesity and dyslipidemia. Moreover β-carotene may also improve liver fibrosis and inflammatory response in Non -alcoholic Steatohepatitis and cellular steatosis (Mueller and Boehm, 2011).

2.3.5.2 LYCOPENE

Lycopene is established to inactivate ROS and extinct free radicals leading to antioxidant effect. Lycopene is recognized to defend against chronic ailments by gene expression regulation, anti-proliferative capacity, gap junctions, immune, and modulation of hormone, etc. A study stated that lycopene intake in rats helped in recuperating the enzymes like SOD, glutathione reductase, and catalase and demonstrating the preventive role contrary to NDEA persuaded oxidative stress. As a natural neuroprotective, lycopene is believed to contribute to cognitive longetivity. Thus lycopene is found useful in the management of conditions like cerebral ischemia, Parkinson's disease (PD), Alzheimer's disease (AD), subarachnoid haemorrhage, epilepsy, Huntington's disease, and depression (Imran et al., 2020a). Another study investigated the protective effect of lycopene in hepatocarcinogenesis promoted by NASH in an in vivo study where single dose Diethylnitrosamine was administered to rats. It was found to inhibit hepatocarcinogenesis by reducing oxidative stress. A group study on two groups of rat, one fed with high fats and tomato juice and another fed with only high-fat diet suggested significant increase in the levels of high density lipoproteins and also decreased oxidative stress by the reduction in isoprostances (Park et al., 2020). Chronic obstructive pulmonary disease co-morbidities are worsened more by systemic inflammation. Lycopene's antioxidant properties help alleviate this condition (Naveen Kumar et al., 2017). It was also indicated that lycopene as an antioxidant, improved hepatotoxicity. By reducing protein carbonylation. Lycopene is also known to ease aflatoxin B1 induced liver injuries resulting in improved hepatic oxidation. It can also improve detoxification potential by activating Nrf2 (Du et al., 2015). Tomato juice intake in rats with fat induced steatosis increased the levels of metabolites related to its antioxidant effect (Elvira-Torales et al., 2019).

2.3.5.3 CURCUMIN

Curcumin is a yellow colorant, is an important constituent of turmeric. It has been traditionally used as a spice and in cosmetics. Its use as an antioxidant and anti-inflammatory is well-established. Studies have allied curcumin in numerous chronic pathological conditions like atherosclerosis, cancer, and neurodegenerative diseases by the virtue of its effects against peroxidation mediated by free radicals of membranous lipids and oxidative damage of proteins and DNA. It has been established through studies that curcumin exhibits anti-inflammatory property by the inhibition of lipoxygenase (LOX), cyclooxygenase-2 (COX-2), and inducible nitric oxide synthase (iNOS) which facilitate the inflammatory process. It also exhibits protective influence against peroxidative damages on biomembranes. This protective action of curcumin is a result of the reactive free radical scavenging. (Abrahams et al., 2019; Menon and Sudheer, 2007).

2.3.5.4 LUTEIN

Lutein has antioxidant properties due to its ability to uptake free radicals thereby being effective against oxidative damage. It is also found to inhibit viral transcription producing an anti-viral effect in hepatitis B (Imran et al., 2020a). A study on guinea pigs (fed on a hypercholesterolemic diet) concluded that 0.1% lutein for 12 weeks resulted in the decrement of oxidative stress & inflammation in the liver and eyes and also had lower DNA-binding activity of NF-κB (Park et al., 2020). Lutein may prevent liver degenerative conditions as a result of decrement in the levels of attenuate lipid peroxidation, free cholesterol, and production of proinflammatory cytokines and showed protective effects against NAFLD. Its nanoemulsion showed protective effects in hepatic steatosis (Naveen Kumar et al., 2017). Studies have shown that Lutein can contribute to defend against LPS-induced uveitis. The partial mechanism for this outcome is through interference with inflammation progression (Du et al., 2015). Natural significance of lutein as an antioxidant is demonstrated by its crucial role in anticipation in cases like age-related macular degeneration and cancer (Elvira-Torales et al., 2019).

2.3.5.5 β-CRYPTOXANTHIN

As per the established scientific evidence, in concern with its antioxidant activity, it was found that its plasma concentration is inversely proportional to oxidative DNA damage & lipid peroxidation rate. Additionally, its anti-inflammatory properties were witnessed affecting the immune response of macrophages. Thus to conclude, β-cryptoxanthin has antioxidant and anti-inflammatory activities in patients with NAFLD (Elvira-Torales et al.,

2019). Studies also suggest that dietary intake of β-cryptoxanthin leads to a decline in oxidative stress. Obesity, diabetes mellitus, and atherosclerotic vascular diseases together form metabolic syndrome. This metabolic syndrome is the key cause of oxidative stress generation. Thus we can conclude that β-cryptoxanthin supplementation can prevent and improve metabolic syndrome through its antioxidant activity. Serum concentrations of β-cryptoxanthin are indirectly correlated with lipid peroxidation, DNA damage, and oxidative stress (Roche et al., 2008).

2.3.5.6 OTHER CAROTENOIDS

Other carotenoids, such as β-carotene and zeaxanthin, also showed positive effects in chronic liver injury. Studies show that β-carotene has a restraining result on spontaneous hepatic carcinogenesis in male mice, with a significant reduction in the average number of hepatomas. Zeaxanthin showed protective effects against NAFLD, decrement in liver fibrosis, and oxidative stress (Elvira-Torales et al., 2019).

2.3.6 PROTEINS

2.3.6.1 ALBUMIN

Albumin exerts antioxidant properties through its multiple-binding sites and free radical trapping properties. Albumin exhibits alterations in the redox state in various physiological and pathological conditions. Albumin administration in conditions like acute respiratory distress syndrome shows positive influence on the redox state. This results in reduced oxidative stress. Thus albumin is responsible for conferring robust protection against oxidative stress regulating inflammation (Roche et al., 2008). Studies have shown the correlation of the protein antioxidant capacity of albumin with the progression of various conditions like obstructive sleep apnoea (Faure et al., 2008) and diabetic neuropathy (Medina-Navarro et al., 2014). Studies have shown correlation of oxidized human serum albumin can be directly correlated with Acute Ischemic Stroke. In such cases, albumin exhibits better protection from ROS (Rael et al., 2019). Evidence has demonstrated that human serum albumin interferes with functions like microcirculation and endothelium role. This is the result of specific antioxidant properties and interaction with glycocalyx (Taverna et al., 2013). The redox state of albumin may be used as a biomarker for various pathological conditions since albumin is believed to be one of the first few proteins to be affected by oxidative stress (Belinskaia et al., 2020). Studies have shown that albumin exhibits an antioxidant effect after intracerebral hemorrhage. Additionally, it is also believed to show anti-apoptotic effects. Other effects include neuroprotective action on neuronal cells. Albumin is believed to inhibit oxidative stress injury. The mechanism behind this effect is neutralization of free $Cu^{2+}$and iron (Imran et al., 2020b).

2.3.6.2 CERULOPLASMIN

Ceruloplasmin, one of the important chain-breaking peroxyl radical scavengers, is effective against a variety of radicals (Atanasiu et al., 1998). Ceruloplasmin, α-globulin, facilitates cellular energy production and prevents oxygen radical formation. It is well-established that ceruloplasmin has its role as an antioxidant and prooxidant and is hence called "the moonlighting protein." It is an acute-phase protein as an antioxidant in inflammation, pregnancy, diabetes, myocardial infarction, and trauma. Studies have also confirmed that ceruloplasmin acts as a prooxidant by enhancing the oxidation of density lipoproteins in the vasculature. It is believed to produce an antioxidant effect in the CNS protecting it from iron-mediated free radical injury by oxidative modifications in ceruloplasmin. It is also believed to protect against excessive generation of free radicals in inflammatory states and CHF. Its antioxidant property is mainly related to ferroxidase I activity, Myeloperoxidase activity and GPx activity. Liver diseases may lead to decrement in ceruloplasmin further leading to copper deficiency accompanied by a hypochromic and microcytic anemia (Harris, 2019). Studies suggest that ceruloplasmin as a scavenger of peroxyl radical is more effective than SOD, deferoxamine and BSA. It was found to less effective against peroxyl radical than catalase. Heat denaturation of protein was found to increase the radical absorbing capacity of ceruloplasmin in concern with peroxyl radical (Harris, 2019). It is well-established that ceruloplasmin is associated with conditions like burn and trauma. It is observed that in burn and trauma cases, ceruloplasmin oxidase activity is decreased. This results in hypoferremia and inflammation (Dubick et al., 2015).

2.3.6.3 HAPTOGLOBIN

Studies have shown that haptoglobin is a potent antioxidant. It is also believed to be associated with the risk of cardiovascular diseases and diabetes mellitus in patients. Haptoglobin is said to protect the low-density lipoproteins against the $Cu2^{+}$-induced oxidation. It is well established that Haptoglobin has greater antioxidant activity than probucol and vitamin E. Haptoglobin plays a provocative antioxidant (Tseng et al., 2004). It's antioxidant effect is the outcome of prevention of hemoglobin-driven oxidative tissue damage. It was found that an allelic polymorphism in the Haptoglobin gene can predict the possibility of various micro and macrovascular diabetic complications. This can be due to the increase in oxidative stress (Melamed-Frank et al., 2001). Studies have shown that there is a strong link between the proinflammatory cytokines on muscle mass and ROS production. Evidence has been provided that the reduction of the deteriorating effect of systemic inflammation and oxidative stress may be a result of inflammatory cytokines which are responsible for activating the Haptoglobin response pathway (Bertaggia et al., 2014).

2.3.6.4 LACTOFERRIN

Lactoferrin is believed to possess antioxidant property against oxidative stress. Lactoferrin is a food-derived multifunctional glycoprotein and has shown antioxidant capacity on erythrocytes through the prevention of inhibition of lipid peroxidation and hemolysis. Studies have shown a decline in intracellular levels of ROS followed by lactorferrin treatment indicating its ability to reduce oxidative stress-induced apoptosis. Lactoferrin produced a protective effect against iron-catalyzed hydroxyl radicals by iron scavenging and inhibition of iron-catalyzed formation of ROS (Safaeian et al., 2015). It is also well-established through studies that the antioxidant effect of lactoferrin could be used to normalize systolic blood pressure. Thus studies confirm the antihypertensive effect of lactoferrin against the prevention or treatment of oxidative stress in hypertension (Safaeian and Zabolian, 2014). Studies suggest that levels of lactoferrin in plasma may predict endothelial dysfunction in some diseases. It is also known to increase HDL level (Safaeian et al., 2015). Studies have shown that human lactoferrin more effectively inhibits free radical processes than histidine and mannitol, the usual free radical scavengers. It is well-established that lactoferrin affects the proliferation, maturation, and activity of immune cells at the cellular level by scavenging free iron in fluids and inflamed areas. Complete saturation of lactoferrin with iron decreases its antioxidation property (Belizi et al., 1999). LF plays a significant protective role in inflammation, oxidative stress, fibrosis, endoplasmic reticulum (ER) stress, autophagy dysfunction, and mitochondrial dysfunction (Ahmed et al., 2021).

2.3.6.5 TRANSFERRIN

Transferrin reduces oxidative stress and lipid peroxidation produced in diabetes mellitus. This effect is achieved as a result of the sequestration of iron in a redox inactive form (van Campenhout et al., 2003). It can also decrease the oxidative damage. This oxidative damage may be induced by Cumulus Oocyte Complexes. This results in imperative damage to endometrial fluid (101) An increased serum transferrin level may significantly reduce oxidative damage. This is believed to occur due to the decrement in ROS as in patients suffering from thalassemia and immunocompromised infants. Transferrin can be used to determine the extent of superoxide-based lipid peroxidation and cellular damage (Siotto et al., 2019). Transferrin is found in lung epithelial fluid (ELF) which is a locally secreted substance. Transferrin in the ELF acts as an antioxidant. This provides the front-line defense for the lower respiratory tract epithelium. It is observed to act as a potent inhibitor of lipid peroxidation. The antioxidant activity of transferrin may be eradicated due to preincubation with Fe^{3+} (Pacht and Davis, 1988).

2.3.7 NON-PROTEIN

2.3.7.1 BILIRUBIN

Bilirubin is highly lipophilic. Bilirubin is the end product of heme metabolism. It is a potent antioxidant that may provide cytoprotection (Sedlak et al., 2009). It is believed to be a physiologic antioxidant. It is well-established that bilirubin is also a neuroprotectant. Studies have established that bilirubin prevents neurotoxic damage. It is also believed to protect against seizures, stroke damage, and traumatic brain injury. The antioxidant actions of bilirubin are dramatically amplified by BVR in a biliverdin–bilirubin cycle. Bilirubin also protects against lipid peroxidation of cell membranes since it is highly lipophilic (Jansen and Daiber, 2012; Sedlak et al., 2009). Bilirubin has been established to have antioxidant and anti-inflammatory activity. This effect is inversely related to the risk of various conditions like hypertension, metabolic syndrome, ischaemic heart disease, diabetes type II, and obesity (DiNicolantonio et al., 2018; Kim and Park, 2012; Nag et al., 2009). Bilirubin effect on vascular endothelium may depict a clearer picture of its role in the above conditions. In case of neonatal jaundice, bilirubin acts as an antioxidant and a strong prooxidant. This prevents against oxidative stress as a result of phototherapy. Phototherapy is the most accepted treatment for neonatal jaundice. Bilirubin also attributes cardioprotective as a result of its antioxidant and vasodilator properties. This can prove beneficial in endothelial dysfunction. Besides, it is also believed that bilirubin has a protective effect against ischemic-reperfusion injury. Studies have shown that bilirubin has anti-proliferative effect which aids in protecting against ischaemic-reperfusion injury. Bilirubin is a source antioxidant. It prevents oxidant production by suppressing superoxide generation at its source. Hydrogen peroxide has proinflammatory effect on cellular signaling. Source antioxidants like bilirubin play a vital role in opposing the proinflammatory effect of hydrogen peroxide. Nitric oxide converts to peroxynitrite, a potent oxidant, to generate oxidative stress. Bilirubin is believed to prevent this conversion of nitric oxide to peroxynitrite (Ziberna et al., 2016). Oxidative stress can develop many untoward responses in the body. One such response is insulin sensitivity in adipocytes. This sensitivity is a result majorly of NADPH oxidase enzyme activity. Bilirubin and heme oxygenase aid in adipocyte insulin sensitivity induced due to oxidative stress in adipocytes. This effect is found to be inversely related to conditions like metabolic syndrome and Diabetes. Bilirubin may function both to prevent adipocyte hypertrophy—via its hypothalamic effects—and to improve the function of adipocytes that have already hypertrophied. In biological systems, bilirubin shows potent antioxidant properties, especially against peroxyl radicals. When bilirubin acts as an antioxidant, it is itself oxidized to biliverdin which is rapidly reduced by BVR to bilirubin, which increases its bioavailability (Ernster and Forsmark-Andre, 1993).

2.3.7.2 UBIQUINOL

Ubiquinone (ubiquinone, 2-methyl-5,6-dimethoxy-1,4-benzoquinone) is vital for the finest biological function (Tasaki et al., 2017). Ubiquinone acts in its reduced form (ubiquinol) as an antioxidant, preventing the initiation and propagation of lipid peroxidation in biological membranes and in serum low-density lipoprotein. In addition, ubiquinol can efficiently sustain the antioxidant effect of vitamin E by regenerating the vitamin from the tocopheroxyl radical. Ubiquinol, the reduced form of Ubiquinone-10, is the only known lipid-soluble antioxidant that animal cells can synthesize. This indicates an important role of ubiquinol in cellular defense against oxidative damage. Degenerative diseases and aging may be manifestations of a decreased capacity to maintain adequate ubiquinol levels (Frei et al., 1990). Ubiquinol-10 efficiently scavenges free radicals generated chemically within liposomal membranes (Tasaki et al., 2017). Studies have suggested the important role of ubiquinol and ubiquinone in cellular defense against oxidative damage as antioxidants. Altered levels of ubiquinol clearly indicate their role in the pathogenesis and cellular mechanism of Cancer, Alzheimer's disease, diabetes mellitus, and neurodegenerative disorders. Studies have shown the impact of ubiquinol in the instigation, evolution, management & anticipation of neurodegenerative, cardiovascular, and carcinogenenic diseases. It is an amphipathic molecule as a result of presence of a hydrophilic benzoquinone ring and the lipophilic poly isoprenoid side-chain. As an antioxidant (as ubiquinol), it regulates membrane fluidity. Studies have shown that it protects membrane phospholipids against lipid peroxidation. It is also believed to recycle radical forms of Vit C and E. In serum, it is demonstrated to prevent lipid peroxidation of low-density lipoproteins (Tasaki et al., 2017). Ubiquinol's antioxidant characteristic is not dependent on the presence of Vit E, where the latter inhibits lipid peroxidation by acting as a chain-breaking antioxidant. Additionally, it can extend the antioxidation produced by vitamin E by regenerating its antioxidant radical form. Due to lipid solubility, ubiquinol has widespread occurrence in biological membranes and serum. Aging and degenerative diseases can be an outcome of a decrement in competence to keep up enough ubiquinol levels. Studies have also shown that ubiquinol-10 is as effective as the antioxidant radical form of Vit E (Frei et al., 1990).

2.3.7.3 URIC ACID

Studies have shown that uric acid scavenges the free radical activity in plasma and also prevents lipid peroxidation. Out of the overall antioxidation by free radical scavenging uric acid is believed to cover 2/3rd portion. It is specifically efficient against quenching hydroxyl, superoxide, and peroxynitrite radicals (Kurajoh et al., 2021). It is observed that in conditions like oxidative stress and ischaemia, the local uric acid concentration increase in vascular and organ beds. The increase in the concentration clearly indicates the activation of a complementary mechanism focused on protecting against the increment in free radical activity. Similar significantly increased local concentration was observed in cases of acute brain injury, middle cerebral artery occlusion, and acute ischaemic stroke in animal model studies. Studies have shown that increased system concentration of uric acid protects hippocampal neurons against excitotoxic and metabolic injury. Uric acid showed a protective effect in cerebral diseases mediated by free radicals, protecting against neurological deficit and ischemia infarct. Uric acid is also believed to correlate inversely the ischemic symptoms with neurological impairment and final infarction size (Settle, 2014). Uric acid has a protective role in acute ischaemic stroke. Acute elevation in levels of uric acid is also known to be associated with antioxidant effects in central nervous system-related conditions like Parkinson's, multiple sclerosis, Alzheimer's disease, and acute stroke (Settle, 2014). Studies have confirmed that there is a close connection between the levels of serum uric acid and the progression of conditions like lupus nephritis and systemic lupus erythematosus (Hafez et al., 2021).

2.4 CONCLUSION

The information included in this chapter illustrates the intense interest in phytochemicals and their applicability in treating human disorders linked to oxidative stress. They have a wide range of biological functions and health advantages, including antioxidant and free radical scavenging properties, anti-inflammatory properties, anti-cancer properties, anti-aging properties, and protective properties for cardiovascular diseases, diabetes mellitus, obesity, and neurodegenerative diseases. Future research should focus on separating and identifying more antioxidant phytochemicals, as well as on their bioactivities and mechanisms of action. Further investigation should also include the possible negative effects of antioxidant phytochemicals on humans.

KEYWORDS

- **ubiquinone**
- **ceruloplasmin**
- **coenzyme Q 10**
- **β-cryptoxanthin**
- **haptoglobin**

REFERENCES

Abrahams, S.; Haylett, W. L.; Johnson, G.; Carr, J. A.; Bardien, S. Antioxidant Effects of Curcumin in Models of Neurodegeneration, Aging, Oxidative and Nitrosative Stress: A Review. *Neuroscience* **2019,** *406*, 1–21.

Aceves, C.; Anguiano, B.; Delgado, G. The Extrathyronine Actions of Iodine as Antioxidant, Apoptotic, and Differentiation Factor in Various Tissues. *Thyroid* **2013,** *23*, 938–946.

Ahmed, K.; Saikat, A.; Moni, A.; Kakon, S.; Islam, M.; Uddin, M. Lactoferrin: Potential Functions, Pharmacological Insights, and Therapeutic Promises. *J. Adv. Biotechnol. Exp. Ther.* **2021,** *4*, 223.

Allen, K. G. D.; Klevay, L. M. Copper: An Antioxidant Nutrient for Cardiovascular Health. *Curr. Opin. Lipidol.* **1994,** *5*, 22–28.

Altemimi, A.; Lakhssassi, N.; Baharlouei, A.; Watson, D.; Lightfoot, D. Phytochemicals: Extraction, Isolation, and Identification of Bioactive Compounds from Plant Extracts. *Plants* **2017,** *6*, 42.

Angiolella, L.; Sacchetti, G.; Efferth, T. Antimicrobial and Antioxidant Activities of Natural Compounds. *Evid. Based Complement. Altern. Med.* **2018,** *2018*, 1–3.

Anto Suganya, R.; Jeya Jothi, G. Enzymatic and Non-enzymatic Antioxidant, Anti-inflammatory and Anticancer Activities of Floscopa Scandens Lour. *J. Tradit. Chin. Med.* **2020,** *40*, 473–483.

Atanasiu, R. L.; Stea, D.; Mateescu, M. A.; Vergely, C.; Dalloz, F.; Briot, F.; Maupoil, V.; Nadeau, R.; Rochette, L. Direct Evidence of Caeruloplasmin Antioxidant Properties. *Mol. Cell. Biochem.* **1998,** *189*, 127–135.

Avila, D. S.; Puntel, R. L.; Aschner, M. In *Manganese in Health and Disease*, 2013; pp 199–227.

Baby, B.; Antony, P.; Vijayan, R. Antioxidant and Anticancer Properties of Berries. *Crit. Rev. Food Sci. Nutr.* **2018,** *58*, 2491–2507.

Bahonar, A.; Saadatnia, M.; Khorvash, F.; Maracy, M.; Khosravi, A. Carotenoids as Potential Antioxidant Agents in Stroke Prevention: A Systematic Review. *Int. J. Prev. Med.* **2017,** *8*, 70.

Baranowska, M.; Bartoszek, A. Antioxidant and Antimicrobial Properties of Bioactive Phytochemicals from Cranberry. *Postępy Higieny i Medycyny Doświadczalnej* **2016,** *70*, 1460–1468.

Belinskaia, D. A.; Voronina, P. A.; Shmurak, V. I.; Vovk, M. A.; Batalova, A. A.; Jenkins, R. O.; Goncharov, N. V. The Universal Soldier: Enzymatic and Non-Enzymatic Antioxidant Functions of Serum Albumin. *Antioxidants* **2020,** *9*, 966.

Belizi, S.; Nazarova, I. A.; Klimova, I. A.; Prokof'ev, V. N.; Pushkina, N. V. Antioxidant Properties of Lactoferrin from Human Milk. *Bull. Exp. Biol. Med.* **1999,** *127*, 471–473.

Benzie, I. F. F.; Choi, S. W. Antioxidants in Food: Content, Measurement, Significance, Action, Cautions, Caveats, and Research Needs. *Adv. Food Nutr. Res.* **2014,** *71*, 1–53.

Bertaggia, E.; Scabia, G.; Dalise, S.; Lo Verso, F.; Santini, F.; Vitti, P.; Chisari, C.; Sandri, M.; Maffei, M. Haptoglobin Is Required to Prevent Oxidative Stress and Muscle Atrophy. *PLoS One*. **2014,** *9*, e100745.

Burk, R. F. Selenium, an Antioxidant Nutrient. *Nutr. Clin. Care* **2002,** *5*, 75–79.

Caritá, A. C.; Fonseca-Santos, B.; Shultz, J. D.; Michniak-Kohn, B.; Chorilli, M.; Leonardi, G. R. Vitamin C: One Compound, Several Uses. Advances for Delivery, Efficiency and Stability. *Nanomed. Nanotechnol. Biol. Med.* **2020** *24*, 102117.

Catania, A. S.; Barros, C. R. de; Ferreira, S. R. G. Vitaminas e Minerais Com Propriedades Antioxidantes e risco Cardiometabólico: Controvérsias e Perspectivas. *Arquivos Brasileiros de Endocrinologia & Metabologia* **2009,** *53*, 550–559.

Chakraborthy, A.; Ramani, P.; Sherlin, H.; Premkumar, P.; Natesan, A. Antioxidant and Pro-Oxidant Activity of Vitamin C in Oral Environment. *Indian J. Dent. Res.* **2014,** *25*, 499.

Chirumbolo, S.; Bjørklund, G.; Lysiuk, R.; Vella, A.; Lenchyk, L.; Upyr, T. Targeting Cancer with Phytochemicals via Their Fine Tuning of the Cell Survival Signaling Pathways. *Int. J. Mol. Sci.* **2018,** *19*, 3568.

Ciccone, M. M.; Cortese, F.; Gesualdo, M.; Carbonara, S.; Zito, A.; Ricci, G.; De Pascalis, F.; Scicchitano, P.; Riccioni, G. Dietary Intake of Carotenoids and Their Antioxidant and Anti-Inflammatory Effects in Cardiovascular Care. *Mediators Inflamm.* **2013,** *2013*, 1–11.

Dao, D. Q.; Ngo, T. C.; Thong, N. M.; Nam, P. C. Is Vitamin A an Antioxidant or a Pro-oxidant? *J. Phys. Chem. B* **2017,** *121*, 9348–9357.

Dewanjee, S.; Bhattacharjee, N.; Chakraborty, P.; Bhattacharjee, S. Carotenoids as Antioxidants. In *Carotenoids: Structure and Function in the Human Body*; Springer International Publishing: Cham, 2021; pp 447–473.

DiNicolantonio, J. J.; McCarty, M. F.; O'Keefe, J. H. Antioxidant Bilirubin Works in Multiple Ways to Reduce Risk for Obesity and its Health Complications. *Open Heart* **2018,** *5*, e000914.

Du, S. Y.; Zhang, Y. L.; Bai, R. X.; Ai, Z. L.; Xie, B. S.; Yang, H. Y. Lutein Prevents Alcohol-Induced Liver Disease in Rats by Modulating Oxidative Stress and Inflammation. *Int. J. Clin. Exp. Med.* **2015,** *8*, 8785–8793.

Dubick, M.; Barr, J.; Keen, C.; Atkins, J. Ceruloplasmin and Hypoferremia: Studies in Burn and Non-Burn Trauma Patients. *Antioxidants* **2015,** *4*, 153–169.

Elvira-Torales, L. I.; García-Alonso, J.; Periago-Castón, M. J. Nutritional Importance of Carotenoids and Their Effect on Liver Health: A Review. *Antioxidants* **2019,** *8*, 229.

Ernster, L.; Forsmark-Andre, P. Ubiquinol: An Endogenous Antioxidant in Aerobic Organisms. *Clin. Investig.* **1993,** *71* (8 Suppl), S60–S65.

Faure, P.; Tamisier, R.; Baguet, J. P.; Favier, A.; Halimi, S.; Levy, P.; Pepin, J. L. Impairment of Serum Albumin Antioxidant Properties in Obstructive Sleep Apnoea Syndrome. *Eur. Respir. J.* **2008,** *31*, 1046–1053.

Fiedor, J.; Burda, K. Potential Role of Carotenoids as Antioxidants in Human Health and Disease. *Nutrients* **2014,** *6*, 466–488.

Frei, B.; Kim, M. C.; Ames, B. N. Ubiquinol-10 is an Effective Lipid-Soluble Antioxidant at Physiological Concentrations. *Proc. Natl. Acad. Sci. U. S. A.* **1990,** *87*, 4879–4883.

Fukai, T.; Ushio-Fukai, M. Superoxide Dismutases: Role in Redox Signaling, Vascular Function, and Diseases. *Antioxid. Redox Signal.* **2011,** *15*, 1583–1606.

Ghosia, L.; Asma, S.; Kafeel, A.; Jamila, H. Phytochemical Screening, Antioxidant and Antibacterial Properties of Daphne Mucronata. *J. Tradit. Chin. Med* **2019,** *39*, 764–771.

Grover, A. K. Why Fruits are Rich in Antioxidants? An Opinion Review. *Can. J. Physiol. Pharmacol.* **2013,** *91*, 191–197.

Hafez, E. A.; Hassan, S. A. E.; Teama, M. A. M.; Badr, F. M. Serum Uric Acid as a Predictor for Nephritis in Egyptian Patients with Systemic Lupus Erythematosus. *Lupus* **2021,** *30*, 378–384.

Han, Q.; Yuan, Q.; Xie, G. 6-Shogaol Attenuates LPS-Induced Inflammation in BV2 Microglia Cells by Activating PPAR-γ. *Oncotarget* **2017,** *8*, 42001–42006.

Hargreaves, I. P.; Mantle, D. Coenzyme Q10 Supplementation in Fibrosis and Aging, 2019; pp 103–112.
Harris, Z. L. Ceruloplasmin. In *Clinical and Translational Perspectives on WILSON DISEASE*; Elsevier, 2019; pp 77–84.
Imran, M.; Ghorat, F.; Ul-Haq, I.; Ur-Rehman, H.; Aslam, F.; Heydari, M.; Shariati, M. A.; Okuskhanova, E.; Yessimbekov, Z.; Thiruvengadam, M.; et al. Lycopene as a Natural Antioxidant Used to Prevent Human Health Disorders. *Antioxidants* **2020a,** *9*, 706.
Imran, M.; Ghorat, F.; Ul-Haq, I.; Ur-Rehman, H.; Aslam, F.; Heydari, M.; Shariati, M. A.; Okuskhanova, E.; Yessimbekov, Z.; Thiruvengadam, M.; et al. Lycopene as a Natural Antioxidant Used to Prevent Human Health Disorders. *Antioxidants* **2020b,** *9*, 706.
Jansen, T.; Daiber, A. Direct Antioxidant Properties of Bilirubin and Biliverdin. Is there a Role for Biliverdin Reductase? *Front. Pharmacol.* **2012,** *3*, 30.
Jiang, Q. Natural Forms of Vitamin E: Metabolism, Antioxidant, and Anti-inflammatory Activities and their Role in Disease Prevention and Therapy. *Free Radic. Biol. Med.* **2014,** *72*, 76–90.
Keservani, R. K.; Sharma, A. K. Flavonoids: Emerging Trends and Potential Health Benefits. *J. Chinese Pharm. Sci.* **2014,** *23* (12), 815.
Keservani, R. K.; Sharma, A. K.; Kesharwani, R. K. Nutraceutical and Functional Foods for Cardiovascular Health. In *Food Process Engineering*; Apple Academic Press, CRC Press, 2016a; pp 291–312, pp 257–278. ISBN: 9781771884020.
Keservani, R. K.; Sharma, A. K.; Kesharwani, R. K. Medicinal Effect of Nutraceutical Fruits for the Cognition and Brain Health. *Scientifica* **2016b,** *2016*, 3109254. DOI: 10.1155/2016/3109254.
Kim, S. Y.; Park, S. C. Physiological Antioxidative Network of the Bilirubin System in Aging and Age-Related Diseases. *Front. Pharmacol.* **2012**, *3*, 45.
Koekkoek, W. A. C. (Kristine); van Zanten, A. R. H. Antioxidant Vitamins and Trace Elements in Critical Illness. *Nutr. Clin. Pract.* **2016,** *31*, 457–474.
Kurajoh, M.; Fukumoto, S.; Yoshida, S.; Akari, S.; Murase, T.; Nakamura, T.; Ishii, H.; Yoshida, H.; Nagata, Y.; Morioka, T.; et al. Uric Acid Shown to Contribute to Increased Oxidative Stress Level Independent of Xanthine Oxidoreductase Activity in MedCity21 Health Examination Registry. *Sci. Rep.* **2021,** *11*, 7378.
Lee, G.; Han, S. The Role of Vitamin E in Immunity. *Nutrients* **2018,** *10*, 1614.
Li, X. H.; McGrath, K. C. Y.; Tran, V. H.; Li, Y. M.; Duke, C. C.; Roufogalis, B. D.; Heather, A. K. Attenuation of Proinflammatory Responses by S -[6]-Gingerol via Inhibition of ROS/NF-Kappa B/COX2 Activation in HuH7 Cells. *Evid. Based Complement. Alternat. Med.* **2013,** *2013*, 1–8.
Li, S.; Tan, H. Y.; Wang, N.; Zhang, Z. J.; Lao, L.; Wong, C. W.; Feng, Y. The Role of Oxidative Stress and Antioxidants in Liver Diseases. *Int. J. Mol. Sci.* **2015,** *16*, 26087–26124.
Liguori, I.; Russo, G.; Curcio, F.; Bulli, G.; Aran, L.; Della-Morte, D.; Gargiulo, G.; Testa, G.; Cacciatore, F.; Bonaduce, D.; et al. Oxidative Stress, Aging, and Diseases. *Clin. Interv. Aging* **2018,** *13*, 757–772.
Lingappa, U. F.; Monteverde, D. R.; Magyar, J. S.; Valentine, J. S.; Fischer, W. W. How Manganese Empowered Life with Dioxygen (and Vice Versa). *Free Radic. Biol. Med.* **2019,** *140*, 113–125.
Madhunapantula, S. V.; Robertson, G. P. Chemoprevention of Melanoma. *Adv. Pharmacol.* **2012,** *65*, 361–398.

Margaritelis, N. V.; Paschalis, V.; Theodorou, A. A.; Kyparos, A.; Nikolaidis, M. G. Antioxidants in Personalized Nutrition and Exercise. *Adv. Nutr.* **2018,** *9*, 813–823.
Mason, S. A.; Trewin, A. J.; Parker, L.; Wadley, G. D. Antioxidant Supplements and Endurance Exercise: Current Evidence and Mechanistic Insights. *Redox Biol.* **2020,** *35*, 101471.
Medhat Hegazy, A.; Hafez, A. S.; Eid, R. M. Protective and Antioxidant Effects of Copper-Nicotinate Complex against Glycerol-Induced Nephrotoxicity in Rats. *Drug Chem. Toxicol.* **2020,** *43*, 234–239.
Medina-Navarro, R.; Corona-Candelas, I.; Barajas-González, S.; Díaz-Flores, M.; Durán-Reyes, G. Albumin Antioxidant Response to Stress in Diabetic Nephropathy Progression. *PLoS One* **2014,** *9*, e106490.
Melamed-Frank, M.; Lache, O.; Enav, B. I.; Szafranek, T.; Levy, N. S.; Ricklis, R. M.; Levy, A. P. Structure-Function Analysis of the Antioxidant Properties of Haptoglobin. *Blood* **2001,** *98*, 3693–3698.
Menon, V. P.; Sudheer, A. R. Antioxidant and Anti-Inflammatory Properties of Curcumin. In *The Molecular Targets and Therapeutic Uses of Curcumin in Health and Disease*; Springer: Boston, MA, US; 2007, pp 105–125.
Miyazawa, T.; Burdeos, G. C.; Itaya, M.; Nakagawa, K.; Miyazawa, T. Vitamin E: Regulatory Redox Interactions. *IUBMB Life* **2019,** *71*, 430–441.
Moon, J. K.; Shibamoto, T. Antioxidant Assays for Plant and Food Components. *J. Agric. Food Chem.* **2009,** *57*, 1655–1666.
Mueller, L.; Boehm, V. Antioxidant Activity of β-Carotene Compounds in Different in Vitro Assays. *Molecules* **2011,** *16*, 1055–1069.
Murphy, M. P. How Mitochondria Produce Reactive Oxygen Species. *Biochem. J.* **2009,** *417*, 1–13.
Nag, N.; Halder, S.; Chaudhuri, R.; Adhikary, S.; Mazumder, S. Role of Bilirubin as Antioxidant in Neonatal Jaundice and Effect of Ethanolic Extract of Sweet Lime Peel on Experimentally Induced Jaundice in Rat. *Indian J. Biochem. Biophys.* **2009,** *46*, 73–78.
Naveen Kumar P. V.; Elango, P.; Kavimani, S. A Systematic Review on Lycopene and its Beneficial Effects. *Biomed. Pharmacol. J.* **2017,** *10*, 2113–2120.
Neha, K.; Haider, M. R.; Pathak, A.; Yar, M. S. Medicinal Prospects of Antioxidants: A Review. *Eur. J. Med. Chem.* **2019,** *178*, 687–704.
Oboh, G.; Akinyemi, A. J.; Ademiluyi, A. O. Antioxidant and Inhibitory Effect of Red Ginger (Zingiber Officinale var. Rubra) and White Ginger (Zingiber officinale Roscoe) on Fe2+ Induced Lipid Peroxidation in Rat Brain in vitro. *Exp. Toxicol. Pathol.* **2012,** *64*, 31–36.
Pacht, E. R.; Davis, W. B. Role of Transferrin and Ceruloplasmin in Antioxidant Activity of Lung Epithelial Lining Fluid. *J. Appl. Physiol.* **1988,** *64*, 2092–2099.
Padayatty, S. J.; Katz, A.; Wang, Y.; Eck, P.; Kwon, O.; Lee, J. H.; Chen, S.; Corpe, C.; Dutta, A.; Dutta, S. K.; et al. Vitamin C as an Antioxidant: Evaluation of Its Role in Disease Prevention. *J. Am. Coll. Nutr.* **2003,** *22*, 18–35.
Padmanabhan, P.; Cheema, A.; Paliyath, G. Solanaceous Fruits Including Tomato, Eggplant, and Peppers. In *Encyclopedia of Food and Health*; Elsevier, 2016; pp 24–32.
Park, H.; Kim, Y. J.; Shin, Y. Estimation of Daily Intake of Lycopene, Antioxidant Contents and Activities from Tomatoes, Watermelons, and their Processed Products in Korea. *Appl. Biol. Chem.* **2020,** *63*, 50.
Pastor-Maldonado, C. J.; Suárez-Rivero, J. M.; Povea-Cabello, S.; Álvarez-Córdoba, M.; Villalón-García, I.; Munuera-Cabeza, M.; Suárez-Carrillo, A.; Talaverón-Rey, M.;

Sánchez-Alcázar, J. A. Coenzyme Q10: Novel Formulations and Medical Trends. *Int. J. Mol. Sci.* **2020,** *21*, 8432.
Powell, S. R. The Antioxidant Properties of Zinc. *J. Nutr.* **2000,** *130*, 1447S–1454S.
Prasad, A. S. Zinc: Role in Immunity, Oxidative Sstress and Chronic Inflammation. *Curr. Opin. Clin. Nutr. Metab. Care* **2009,** *12*, 646–652.
Rael, L. T.; Leonard, J.; Salottolo, K.; Bar-Or, R.; Bartt, R. E.; Wagner, J. C.; Bar-Or, D. Plasma Oxidized Albumin in Acute Ischemic Stroke Is Associated With Better Outcomes. *Front. Neurol.* **2019,** *10*, 709.
Raizner, A. E. Coenzyme Q10. *Methodist DeBakey Cardiovasc. J.* **2019,** *15*, 185.
Roche, M.; Rondeau, P.; Singh, N. R.; Tarnus, E.; Bourdon, E. The Antioxidant Properties of Serum Albumin. *FEBS Lett.* **2008,** *582*, 1783–1787.
Rodríguez-García, C.; Sánchez-Quesada, C.; Gaforio, J. J. Dietary Flavonoids as Cancer Chemopreventive Agents: An Updated Review of Human Studies. *Antioxidants* **2019,** *8*, 137.
Safaeian, L.; Javanmard, S. H.; Mollanoori, Y.; Dana, N. Cytoprotective and Antioxidant Effects of Human Lactoferrin Against H2O2-Induced Oxidative Stress in Human Umbilical Vein Endothelial Cells. *Adv. Biomed. Res.* **2015,** *4*, 188.
Safaeian, L.; Zabolian, H. Antioxidant Effects of Bovine Lactoferrin on Dexamethasone-Induced Hypertension in Rat. *ISRN Pharmacol.* **2014,** *2014*, 943523.
Saleem, H.; Htar, T. T.; Naidu, R.; Zengin, G.; Ahmad, I.; Ahemad, N. Phytochemical Profiling, Antioxidant, Enzyme Inhibition and Cytotoxic Potential of Bougainvillea glabra Flowers. *Natl. Prod. Res.* **2020,** *34*, 2602–2606.
Sarker, U.; Oba, S.; Daramy, M. A. Nutrients, Minerals, Antioxidant Pigments and Phytochemicals, and Antioxidant Capacity of the Leaves of Stem Amaranth. *Sci. Rep.* **2020,** *10*, 3892.
Sedlak, T. W.; Saleh, M.; Higginson, D. S.; Paul, B. D.; Juluri, K. R.; Snyder, S. H. Bilirubin and Glutathione have Complementary Antioxidant and Cytoprotective Roles. *Proc. Natl. Acad. Sci.* **2009,** *106*, 5171–5176.
Settle, T. The Role of Uric Acid as an Antioxidant in Selected Neurodegenerative Disease Pathogenesis: A Short Review. *Brain Disord. Ther.* **2014,** *03*, 3.
Sharif, M.; Rahman, M. A.; Ahmed, B.; Abbas, R. Z.; Hassan, F. Copper Nanoparticles as Growth Promoter, Antioxidant and Anti-Bacterial Agents in Poultry Nutrition: Prospects and Future Implications. *Biol. Trace Elem. Res.* **2021,** *199*, 3825–3836.
Silva, F. A. M.; Borges, F.; Guimarães, C.; Lima, J. L. F. C.; Matos, C.; Reis, S. Phenolic Acids and Derivatives: Studies on the Relationship Among Structure, Radical Scavenging Activity, and Physicochemical Parameters. *J. Agric. Food Chem.* **2000,** *48*, 2122–2126.
Siotto, M.; Filippi, M. M.; Simonelli, I.; Landi, D.; Ghazaryan, A.; Vollaro, S.; Ventriglia, M.; Pasqualetti, P.; Rongioletti, M. C. A.; Squitti, R.; et al. Oxidative Stress Related to Iron Metabolism in Relapsing Remitting Multiple Sclerosis Patients With Low Disability. *Front. Neurosci.* **2019,** *13*, 86.
Skrajnowska, D.; Bobrowska-Korczak, B. Role of Zinc in Immune System and Anti-Cancer Defense Mechanisms. *Nutrients* **2019,** *11*, 2273.
Smyth, P. P. A. Role of Iodine in Antioxidant Defence in Thyroid and Breast Disease. *BioFactors* **2003,** *19*, 121–130.
Stahl, W.; Sies, H. Antioxidant Activity of Carotenoids. *Mol. Aspects Med.* **2003,** *24*, 345–351.
Steinbrenner, H.; Klotz, L. O. Selen und Zink: „Antioxidanzien" für ein gesundes Altern? *Zeitschrift Für Gerontologie Und Geriatrie.* **2020,** *53*, 295–302.

Sudheer, A. R.; Chandran, K.; Marimuthu, S.; Menon, V. P. Ferulic Acid Modulates Altered Lipid Profiles and Prooxidant/Antioxidant Status in Circulation During Nicotine-Induced Toxicity: A Dose-Dependent Study. *Toxicol. Mech. Methods* **2005,** *15*, 375–381.

Tasaki, E.; Sakurai, H.; Nitao, M.; Matsuura, K.; Iuchi, Y. Uric Acid, An Important Antioxidant Contributing to Survival in Termites. *PLoS One* **2017,** *12*, e0179426.

Taverna, M.; Marie, A. L.; Mira, J. P.; Guidet, B. Specific Antioxidant Properties of Human Serum Albumin. *Ann. Intensive Care* **2013,** *3*, 4.

Tseng, C. F.; Lin, C. C.; Huang, H. Y.; Liu, H. C.; Mao, S. J. T. Antioxidant Role of Human Haptoglobin. *Proteomics* **2004,** *4*, 2221–2228.

Tuorkey, M.J. Cancer Therapy with Phytochemicals: Present and Future Perspectives. *Biomed. Environ. Sci.* **2015,** *28*, 808–819.

Ugboaja, O. C.; Bielory, L.; Bielory, B. P.; Ehiorobo, E. S. Antioxidant Vitamins, Minerals and Cataract. *Curr. Opin. Allergy Clin. Immunol.* **2012,** *12*, 517–523.

van Campenhout, A.; van Campenhout, C. M.; Lagrou, A. R.; Manuel-y-Keenoy, B. Transferrin Modifications and Lipid Peroxidation: Implications in Diabetes Mellitus. *Free Radic. Res.* **2003,** *37*, 1069–1077.

Veurink, G.; Perry, G.; Singh, S. K. Role of Antioxidants and a Nutrient Rich Diet in Alzheimer's Disease. *Open Biol.* **2020,** *10*, 200084.

Wang, N.; Tan, H. Y.; Li, S.; Xu, Y.; Guo, W.; Feng, Y. Supplementation of Micronutrient Selenium in Metabolic Diseases: Its Role as an Antioxidant. *Oxid. Med. Cell. Longev.* **2017,** *2017*, 1–13.

Zhang, Y. J.; Gan, R. Y.; Li, S.; Zhou, Y.; Li, A. N.; Xu, D. P.; Li, H. B. Antioxidant Phytochemicals for the Prevention and Treatment of Chronic Diseases. *Molecules* **2015,** *20*, 21138–21156.

Zhuang, X. M.; Chen, L.; Tan, Y.; Yang, H. Y.; Lu, C.; Gao, Y.; Li, H. Identification of Human Cytochrome P450 and UGT Enzymes Involved in the Metabolism of Ferulic Acid, A Major Bioactive Component in Traditional Chinese Medicines. *Chinese J. Natl. Med.* **2017,** *15*, 695–702.

Ziberna, L.; Martelanc, M.; Franko, M.; Passamonti, S. Bilirubin is an Endogenous Antioxidant in Human Vascular Endothelial Cells. *Sci. Rep.* **2016,** *6*, 29240.

CHAPTER 3

EPIGALLOCATECHIN GALLATE: NUTRITIONAL AND PHARMACOLOGICAL INTERVENTION IN THE TREATMENT OF DISEASE

MYRENE ROSELYN D'SOUZA[1] and KHALID MOHAMMED NAJI[2,3]

[1]*Department of Biochemistry, Mount Carmel College Autonomous, Karnataka, India*

[2]*Department of Chemistry, Faculty of Science, Sana'a University, Sana'a, Yemen*

[3]*Department of Chemical Ecology/Biological Chemistry, Konstanz University, Konstanz, Germany*

ABSTRACT

The rise of new ailments, such as heart disease, cancer, diabetes, obesity, and neurodegenerative disease, is putting the health of the society in jeopardy. As a result, it is critical to make investments that benefit the general public's health. Many plants, including tea, contain the flavonoid epigallocatechin gallate (EGCG). EGCG has been shown in multiple trials to help combat these diseases. However, the low intestinal absorption and volatility of EGCG are the key drawbacks to using this chemical for both prevention and treatment. Increased therapeutic efficacy can be achieved by encapsulating EGCG in nanocarriers, which enhances its long-term stability. This chapter will have an in-depth investigation of nanocarrier-based encapsulation of EGCG.

Antioxidants as Nutraceuticals. Nayan A. Gujarathi, Raj K. Keservani, Rajesh K. Kesharwani, Bhushan R. Rane, Yogeeta Sameer Goyal (Eds.)

3.1 INTRODUCTION

Throughout the course of human history, the beverage that has been consumed the most frequently is brewed tea. This can be ascribed to its pleasant flavor as well as its aromatic odor and the beneficial effects it has on the human body. Based on the fermentation process of the leaves of *Camellia sinensis*, we obtain green, oolong, or black tea. Green tea is prepared from fresh tea shoots by heating them to a high temperature, deactivating the enzyme polyphenol oxidase (PPO) that causes oxidation while preserving polyphenols in their natural state. This process does not require fermentation. Chlorogenic acid, flavanols, theogallin, coumarylquinic acid, caffeine, alkaloids, theobromine, vitamin P, theophylline, theanine, fluoride, minerals, volatile compounds, trace elements, and other uncharacterized compounds are among the many ingredients that remain in green tea products. The fermentation process causes these polyphenolic compounds to go through an oxidative polymerization process that is accelerated by PPO. This process results in the creation of thearubigins and theaflavins, which are the primary antioxidants (Singh et al., 2017) found in black tea (Bokuchava and Skobeleva, 1980). Some of the many health benefits of green tea include free-radical scavenging, antioxidative, anti-inflammatory, iron-chelating, weight-lowering, antihyperglycemic, antiaging, thrombosis-inhibitory, neuroprotective, hepatoprotective, and exercise-endurance increasing. To a greater extent than other types of tea, green tea demonstrates extraordinary biological and pharmacological properties, which are dependent on a number of specific active phytochemical constituents, in particular catechins. Tea products in general offer benefits such as reviving the body, diuresis, and feeling of alertness. In today's world, crude extracts of green tea, refined catechin fractions, and synthesized catechin derivatives can all be used in complementary medicine for the treatment, prevention, and cotherapy of several disorders.

Catechins found in green tea are stable in water at about 25°C; nevertheless, they are degraded by 20% while brewing at 98°C for 7 h. In addition, some compounds are epimerized to their respective derivatives when subjected to autoclaving at 120°C for 20 min (Chen et al., 2001). The fresh leaves of tea have an extraordinarily high concentration of the polyphenolic catechins, making up as much as 30% of the leaf's dry weight (Rababah et al., 2004). Since the PPO enzyme is immediately rendered inactive during the production of green tea, the catechin profiles of green tea are comparable with those of fresh tea leaves in terms of their composition. Condensation reactions lead to the production of theaflavins, bisflavanols, thearubigens, epitheaflavic acids, and several quinines that are subsequently created via enzymatic oxidative reactions. These chemicals are responsible for giving black and oolong tea their distinctive flavor and color (Graham, 1992).

3.2 DISPOSITION OF GREEN TEA BIOACTIVES

After ingestion, it is absolutely necessary to have a thorough understanding of the effective concentrations as well as the forms of catechins that are present in plasma and tissues. Following administration of a substance, pharmacokinetics is the study of how that substance is absorbed, distributed, metabolized, eliminated, and how bioavailable it is. In a nutshell, when green tea or its extract is taken orally, the catechins in the tea are absorbed in the small intestine, and any excess catechins move on to the colon. Conjugation of catechins can take place in the small intestine through the action of glucuronic acid, sulfate, or O-methylation. During the process of enterohepatic recirculation, some catechins and secreted bile make their way into the colon, where the resident microorganisms break down the catechins into various flavonoid rings. The phenolic acids that were broken down can be reabsorbed into the circulation and then eliminated through the urine. Catechins, their conjugated metabolites, and a significant amount of small phenolic acids that have been catabolized are all capable of being distributed to a wide variety of organs and tissues, absorbed by tissue cells, further metabolized, and performing a wide variety of biological actions (Fig. 3.1).

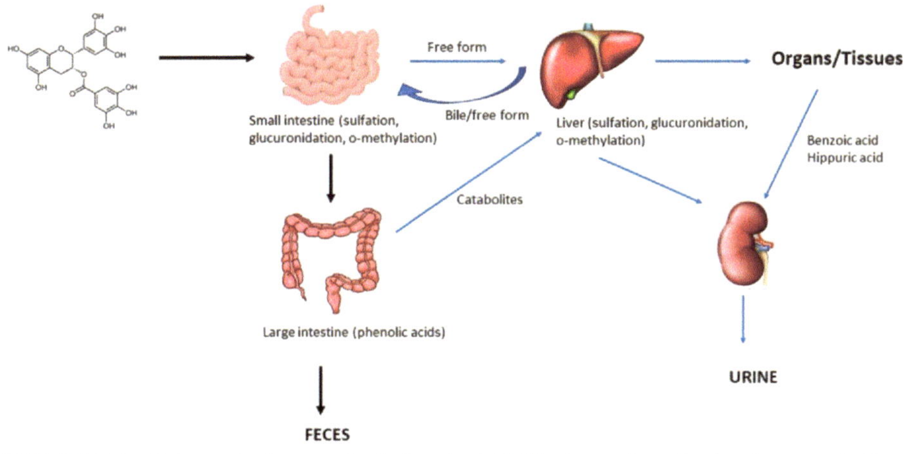

FIGURE 3.1 Schematic diagram depicting the ADME (absorption, distribution, metabolism, and elimination) of catechins in the body. Thick black arrows imply the flow of a large amount of metabolites. Thin blue arrows depict a low amount of catechins.

3.2.1 ABSORPTION AND DISTRIBUTION

There is a hierarchy of antioxidant activity among these polyphenolic chemicals, and it goes as follows: epicatechin 3-gallate (ECG) > epigallocatechin 3-gallate (EGCG) > epigallocatechin (EGC) > gallic acid (GA) > epicatechin (EC) (Salah et al., 1995). Green tea has the ability to reduce the amount of nonheme iron that is absorbed from the diet due to the chelating activity of pro-oxidant metals like Fe^{2+} (Samman et al., 2001). The ratio of EGC to iron was 3:1, EGCG to iron was 2:1, ECG to iron was 2:1, and EC to iron was 3:1 (Guo et al., 1996). In contrast to the majority of flavonoids, tea catechins are absorbed into the bloodstream after oral consumption and are subsequently metabolized in the liver by sulfation, methylation, and glucuronidation processes (Valcic et al., 2000). Structure-based activity investigations prove the existence of a galloyl ring at position 3 and the trihydroxyphenyl B ring, which are crucial with respect to the antioxidant activities of catechins (Guo et al., 1996).

Intravenous administration of pure EGCG fractions and green tea to rats was done to investigate their pharmacokinetic properties. Clearances were found to be 2.0 and 13.9 mL•min kg^{-1}, and apparent distribution volumes (Vds) were found to be 1.5 and 3.6 dL/kg for EGCG and EC, respectively. EGCG demonstrated a shorter half-life ($T_{1/2}$) of 135 min. When administered intragastrically, there was a detection of approximately 0.1% and 31.2% of EGCG and EC in the plasma, respectively. It was discovered that the gut samples contained the highest levels of EGCG, which thereafter began to drop off at a rate of 173 min/h. The levels of EGCG and EC measured in the gut and kidney are much higher than those observed in the liver and the lungs (Chen et al., 1997). Hence, it indicates that EGCG is mostly eliminated through the bile, but EC is excreted through the urine as well as the bile. Variations in the normal flora of the colon and genetic polymorphisms in polyphenol metabolic enzymes contribute to substantial differences among individuals with respect to the bioavailability of catechins from green tea (Scalbert and Williamson, 2000). Different genotypes may have different responses to drinking green tea (Loktionov et al., 1998). High levels of EGCG have been reported in the prostate gland, kidneys, and lungs, while lower levels were reported in the spleen, liver, thyroid gland, and heart (Kim et al., 2000). The largest amount of EGC was seen in the bladder, while the highest levels of EGCG were reported in the colon.

3.2.2 METABOLISM

Glucuronidation of EC does not occur due to the absence of uridine diphosphate-glucuronosyltransferases (UGTs) in the human liver and microsomes of the enterocyte. It, however, undergoes glucuronidation effectively in the microsomes of rat liver, which results in two different glucuronides. It also undergoes sulfation in the human liver cytosol by the SULT1A1 isoform and in the intestine via the SULT1A1 and SULT1A3 isoforms. EGCG and ECG of green tea competitively inhibit SULT1A1 and SULT1A3 activities needed for presystemic inactivation in the liver and intestine, respectively (Nishimuta et al., 2007). This can be accomplished through competitive inhibition. Since the glucuronidation of ECG and EGCG in liver microsomes is fairly low, glucuronidation is not a significant metabolic pathway. Because of the galloyl ring, it is known that the two powerful catechins circulate as unconjugated forms in the plasma (Crespy et al., 2004). According to the findings of one study, catechins were toxic to rat hepatocytes due to the collapse of the mitochondrial membrane potential.

3.2.3 EXCRETION

There is a possibility that the small intestine is unable to absorb the majority of the polyphenolic catechins found in green tea. The nonabsorbed catechins will be converted into simpler phenolic compounds, like hippuric acid, by the bacterial flora in the large intestine. These compounds will then be taken to the blood circulation and excreted in the urine (Mulder et al., 2005). According to pharmacokinetics investigations, the main route for EGCG excretion is through bile, while EGC and EC are excreted via bile and urine. Catechins are eliminated from the body primarily via the urinary and biliary systems. The parent and conjugated forms of nongalloylated catechins are the primary forms in which they are eliminated from the body via the urinary tract. The majority of galloylate catechins are eliminated from the body via biliary drainage into the colon. After drinking green tea, a small amount of epi- or gallocatechin-O-sulfates was found in the urine of the participants (Nakagawa and Miyazawa, 1997), but aglycones, including ECG and EGCG, were not present. It was found that urine contained no conjugates of ECG or EGCG, which suggests that the derivatives of gallate did not go through phase II of biotransformation. The flavan-3-ol metabolites that are eliminated from the body are equivalent to 8.1% of those consumed in green tea (Nakagawa and Miyazawa, 1997). Since EGCG cannot be found in urine, we know that its elimination does not involve the kidneys. On the other hand, after being absorbed through the small intestine, it is degalloylated in the liver to produce other catechins, which are then metabolized and eliminated through the urine, leaving no EGCG behind. Furthermore, nongallated catechins, such as EGC and EC, possess significantly shorter half-lives than those of gallated catechins, such as EGCG and ECG (Hung et al., 2003). There is a possibility that this is due to the fact that the more hydrophobic gallated catechins bind to serum proteins with greater affinity and exist in nonconjugated free forms, neither of which are ideal for renal excretion (Ishii et al., 2010).

3.3 ADVANTAGES TO HEALTH

3.3.1 HEALTH AND WELLNESS

The catechins found in green tea may have positive effects on one's health, but those effects are contingent not only on the quantity that is ingested but also on the catechins' bioavailability. In rats, oral administration of tea catechins resulted in the identification of all four primary catechins in the portal vein (Okushio et al., 1996). This finding suggests that tea catechins are intestinally absorbed. When compared to other tea catechins, the bioavailability of EGCG appears to vary depending on the specific species. The isomers of epicatechin isolated from green tea were effective agents in preventing oxidative alteration of human LDL and erythrocyte membranes (Zhang et al., 1997). The ability of these compounds to scavenge free radicals and the iron-chelating capabilities they possess make these effects possible. The compounds bind to any accessible iron, which significantly lowers the bioavailability of the iron. In addition, they have a wide variety of pharmacological actions, such as those that are hypocholesterolemic (Imai and Nakachi, 1995), anticarcinogenic (Wang et al., 1994), and antihypertensive (Henry and Stephens-Larson, 1984).

Surprisingly, catechins were found to inhibit the activity of xanthine oxidase in vitro (Lam et al., 2006). Furthermore, the inhibition constant of EGCG for xanthine oxidase was found to be equivalent to allopurinol (Aucamp et al., 1997). Consumption of green tea extract for 7 days significantly lowers the levels of serum uric acid in humans (Kimura et al., 2002). It was also reported that consumption of 2 g/day of green tea extract decreased serum uric acid by 3.5% and at the same time augmented serum trolox-equivalent antioxidant capacity (TEAC) values, indicating either a hypouricemic effect due to inhibition of xanthine oxidase or an increase in the urinary urate excretion (Kimura et al., 2002).

3.3.2 HEMATOLOGIC DISEASES

Its potential for iron chelation, low toxicity, significant antioxidant capacity, and the fact that it can be administered orally make it an excellent agent in the therapy of disorders connected to an overload of iron. The elimination of iron might, in theory, lessen the oxidative damage to the cellular macromolecules; as a consequence, this could both inhibit and enhance essential organ dysfunction (Fraga and Oteiza, 2002). Orally effective compounds like EGCG products quickly penetrate and mobilize nonheme iron from the erythrocytes of beta-thalassemic patients.

Even though the harmful role of redox iron in hemosiderosis has been well-recognized, excessive buildup of iron results in severe organ dysfunction. Recent research on the discovery of gene mutations associated with iron metabolism in the brain has offered valuable insights into the processes of iron homeostasis as well as the pathology of neurodegenerative diseases. The accumulation of iron in the brain, which is already abundant in fatty acids and oxygen, creates an environment that is optimal for the development of oxidative stress and potentially permanent tissue injury. It is a widely held belief that neuronal death in brain illnesses is connected with oxidative stress, which is caused by elevated levels of iron in the brain and possibly also by abnormalities in the processes that protect against free radicals (Fraga and Oteiza, 2002).

It has been established that an excessive amount of iron in the body can have a negative impact on the antioxidant capacity of the body, particularly with regard to vitamins C and E. The ability of vitamin E to afford protection against the consequences of iron toxicity has been the subject of a significant amount of research (Fraga and Oteiza, 2002). Patients showed an enhancement in plasma antioxidant–oxidant balance and diminished lipid peroxidation in RBCs in reaction to vitamin E oral therapy, while the high amounts of reactive oxygen species (ROS) normalized as a result of this treatment (Tesoriere et al., 2001). Patients diagnosed with beta-thalassemia intermedia who were given vitamin E over an extended period of time did not experience any substantial alterations in their Hb levels (Rachmilewitz et al., 2005). Hence, vitamin E alone is not enough to induce large modifications to the rate of hemolysis of RBC and to prolong their survival, which would result in increased Hb levels. This conclusion is supported by the evidence (Tesoriere et al., 2001).

The relationship between iron and vitamin C is not as well understood. Vitamin C can convert free ferric into the ferrous form, which facilitates the induction and progression of free-radical reactions. For those who are at risk of iron overload, which is characterized by higher levels of iron that have the potential to result in higher concentrations of "free iron," an excessive amount of vitamin C may have adverse effects. Another class of antioxidants that may have application in the treatment of thalassemia is known as flavonoids, which are found in plants and include rutin and curcumin (Vyas et al., 2010; Kesharwani et al., 2015; Kesharwani et al., 2018; Mishra et al., 2019; Singh et al., 2013a; Singh et al., 2013b; Singh et al., 2015; Upadhyaya et al., 2009; Singh et al., 2016; Kesharwani and Misra, 2011). However, despite what appear to be beneficial effects that antioxidants have on RBCs, it has not been demonstrated that antioxidants can improve anemia (Rund and Rachmilewitz, 2006). It is possible that using antioxidants in conjunction with an iron chelator will make them more effective. If it is successful, this strategy has the potential to be of particular help to nations that have restricted access to financial resources.

The possibility that drinking green tea can help prevent or alleviate the symptoms of chronic diseases is the topic of a significant amount of research at the moment. The free-radical scavenging capability of catechins from green tea is commonly recognized as a key factor, even though a number of different pathways have been hypothesized for the positive effects of green tea. Emerging data have demonstrated that catechins possess varied mechanisms of action (Otsuka et al., 1998). These additional mechanisms of action include influencing various locations, potentiating endogenous antioxidants, and evoking dual activities in response to oxidative stress. A significant amount of evidence that catechins in green tea have an antioxidant role has been gained from studies of their antioxidant activity that have been performed in vitro. On the other hand, there is less evidence to suggest that catechins in green tea work as antioxidants in vivo, either directly or indirectly. It has been demonstrated that the catechins protect culture cells from the damage caused by iron (Raza and John, 2007). In animal models, the accumulation of iron has been observed to block iron-induced lipid oxidation in the liver (Higuchi et al., 2003), causing a reduction in the amount of labile iron in the plasma, which in turn reduces the amount of oxidative stress (Ounjaijean et al., 2008). However, none of the treatments that were administered over the course of 2 months had any effect on the blood hemoglobin levels in wild-type (WT), knockout (BKO), or deficient (DH) mice that were given an iron-rich diet. The survival rate of erythrocytes of both the wild-type and the BKO mice was dramatically boosted after consuming either of these two green teas. Therapy with green tea extract and EGCG immediately improves the rate of erythropoiesis in both normal and thalassemic mice; nonetheless, it most likely safeguards red cells against ROS-induced hemolysis.

NSF60 leukemic cell lines had a dose- and time-dependent reduction in their ability to survive when treated with EGCG (Otsuka et al., 1998). There is also evidence of the chemopreventive effects that EGCG can have in multistep carcinogenesis (Surh, 1999). EGCG was found to inhibit vascular endothelial growth factor (VEGF) receptor phosphorylation, which is a powerful angiogenic cytokine necessary for tumor cell survival (Béliveau and Gingras, 2004). This resulted in the death of the chronic lymphocytic leukemia B cells. EGCG increases the binding of E2F-1, an hTERT repressor, at the promoter of MCF-7 breast cancers (Berletch et al., 2008). Patients with early-stage chronic lymphocytic leukemia who took green tea extract for a period of 6 months exhibited reductions in absolute lymphocyte counts and lymphadenopathy according to the findings of the Phase 2 clinical investigation (Shanafelt et al., 2013).

3.3.3 CARDIOVASCULAR DISEASES

The several risk factors for atherosclerosis include hypercholesterolemia, hypertension, diabetes, epigenetics, physical inactivity, stress, heavy smoking, and obesity. The antiobesity effects of catechins include reducing the differentiation and proliferation of adipocytes; a reduction in lipogenesis; a reduction in fat mass; a reduction in body weight; a decrease in fat absorption; a decrease in plasma triglycerides, free fatty acids, cholesterol, glucose, and insulin; and an increase in β-oxidation and thermogenesis. ECG and EGCG from Chinese green tea significantly reduced serum cholesterol and the atherogenic index in rats. Additionally, ECG and EGCG reduced the weight caused by lipid deposition (Yang and Koo, 1997). When compared to rats that were fed a control diet, rats that were given a diet that was enhanced with green tea powder at a concentration of 20 g/kg body weight demonstrated a 33% rise in the lag-phase oxidation of plasma containing VLDL and LDL (Anderson et al., 1998). It was hypothesized that EGCG competitively inhibits β-ketoacyl reductase (Wang and Tian, 2001). EGCG and ECG reduce the activity of FAS and malate enzymes in the rat liver cytosol, leading to a considerable reduction in the amount of deposition of hepatic triglyceride and visceral fat (Ikeda et al., 2005). Chinese green tea was found to lower cholesterol levels by raising fecal bile acids and cholesterol excretion (Yang and Koo, 2000). However, this study did not find a reduction in plasma cholesterol levels by inhibiting the activities of cholesterol 7-hydroxylase, HMG-CoA reductase, and FAS.

Catechins from green tea in micelles were found to be effective in preventing peroxidation of membrane phospholipid, have potent synergistic antioxidant activity with alpha-tocopherol (Zhou et al., 2005), and protect HDL from endothelial cell-dependent vasodilatation (Liu et al., 2000). They exhibit a wide variety of pharmacological properties, some of which include the ability to lower blood pressure and prevent atherosclerosis. It is abundantly clear that catechins, in particular EGCG, have the potential to have a hypolipidemic effect. This effect may take place, at least in part, as a result of catechins' interference with digestion (Koo and Noh, 2007), emulsification, and micellar solubilization of lipids, all of which are needed for intestinal absorption of dietary lipids. Green tea extract with 2% catechins reduces total cholesterol by 60%, IDL and VLDL by 70%, LDL by 80% in plasma, total cholesterol by 10%, and unesterified cholesterol by 15%, but biomarkers for cardiovascular disease were not affected (Frank et al., 2009).

3.3.4 NEUROLOGICAL DISEASES

It has been discovered that the disruptions in iron metabolism in the brain that are associated with neurological illnesses are due to a combination of factors; however, the conditions of treatment appear to be particularly significant. Epilepsy, a disorder of the brain that is oxidatively connected, has been used as a model for the inquiry into the function of iron in neurological disorders. Iron has recently become the focus of research into neurodegenerative illnesses due to the latest genetic and pharmacological modifications of iron overload. This is reinforced by the identification of genetic and nongenetic dysregulation of the iron metabolism in various illnesses. It has been found that unusually elevated levels of iron can be seen in certain parts of the brain in patients who suffer from a variety of neurodegenerative diseases (Snyder and Connor, 2009). Evidence that iron contributes to pathological conditions by amplifying the effects of oxidative stress has prompted researchers to investigate whether or not iron also has a role in the pathogenesis of other conditions, such as epilepsy, in which oxidative stress may play a role. Identification of whether accumulated iron from the labile iron pool (LIP) is responsible for participation in the Fenton reaction to form the reactive hydroxyl radical is still not clear. It is possible that the existence of free iron can be inferred from the fact that there is a decrease in GSH both during the progression of the disease and reaction to neurotoxins, as well as an increase in the accumulation of iron and the production of ROS (Zecca et al., 2004).

It is widely believed that oxidative stress, which is caused by the elevation of iron in the brain and also due to defects in antioxidant defensive mechanisms, is associated with the death of neurons in these disorders (Halliwell, 2001). In addition, decreased levels of GSH and other antioxidants in the brain were reported. Alterations in the blood–brain barrier (BBB) integrity resulting from distorted vascularization or inflammatory processes are yet another potential cause of the condition in its early stages. However, neuronal death could lead to enhanced ROS generation and the release of substantial amounts of iron (Andersen, 2004). This could occur regardless of the initial cause. Therefore, iron and oxidative stress caused by iron could be a shared mechanism that contributes to neurodegeneration (Ke and Qian, 2007).

According to this idea, therapy efforts should be focused on reducing the amount of iron found in the brain and suppressing the production of reactive oxygen species (ROS). Recent research has indicated that deferrioxamine, an iron chelator, is a crucial factor in the treatment of brain disorders (Liu et al., 2010). Utilizing the catechins found in green tea, particularly EGCG, as a potential nontoxic strategy with natural metal chelators is one possibility. This compound regulates amyloid precursor protein (APP) processing via a nonamyloidogenic pathway (Mandel et al., 2008). Animal models have provided evidence for it against Alzheimer's and Parkinson's disease attributed to its iron-chelating, antioxidant, and anti-inflammatory activities. Understanding the relationship between the scheduling of iron mismanagement and the advancement of neuronal loss would tell us a lot about how the disease starts. It would also make it possible to track changes in iron as a sign of how a disease is getting worse, and maybe even to do a preclinical diagnosis in cases where iron regulation goes wrong early on.

3.3.5 MUTAGENICITY AND CARCINOGENICITY

EGCG, EGC, and ECG applied topically inhibited tumorigenesis in mouse skin induced by several chemicals (Huang et al., 1992). This may have been accomplished by inhibiting ROS production and inflammation. Catechins found in green tea have been reported to inhibit carcinogenesis and repair DNA damage. Intake of green tea is linked to a lower chance of developing cancer according to research (Mu et al., 2003). EGCG exerts repressive effects on hepatocellular carcinoma, skin cancer, and duodenal cancer and also prevents metastasis of the melanoma cell line in lung cancer in mice. These effects may have been caused by blocking the communication between tumor promoters and membrane receptors. It considerably slowed down the formation of tumors of the RAP1-EIO, Namalwa, and HS-Sultan types that were implanted intraperitoneally in NOD/SCID mice (Bertolini et al., 2000). This was likely accomplished by inhibiting tumor invasion, preventing angiogenesis, and inducing cell death. EGCG reduced the activities of tyrosine kinase (TK) and mitogen-activated protein kinase (MAPK) in transformed NIH-pATMras fibroblasts (Wang and Bachrach, 2002). This caused a decline in the levels of ornithine decarboxylase (ODC), Ras, and Jun oncogenes.

3.4 THERAPEUTIC POTENTIAL OF EGCG

Cancer, heart disease, diabetes, neurological disorders, and obesity are just some of the illnesses that are on the rise in today's society, leading to a significant rise in the prevalence of the health crisis. Consequently, it is essential to make investments in products that improve overall health and wellness. Epigallocatechin gallate, often known as EGCG, is a flavonoid that can be found in a wide variety of plants, most notably tea. Multiple studies provide credence to the idea that EGCG has a variety of health benefits, including the ability to combat cancer, heart disease, diabetes, and obesity, amongst other conditions. Nevertheless, the inability of EGCG to be absorbed by the intestinal cells and its inherent volatility make it a less-than-ideal candidate for usage in either preventative or therapeutic applications. The encapsulation of EGCG within nanocarriers results in the compound's increased stability as well as increased therapeutic efficacy.

3.4.1 NANOCARRIERS FOR THE DELIVERY OF EGCG

Due to the high surface area-to-volume ratio that nanoparticles possess, they demonstrate properties distinct from those presented by traditional materials. Their malleability enables alteration of a variety of parameters, such as chemical composition and size, as well as manipulating the selection of ligands on the outer layer to assign specificity to particular structures (Sanvicens and Marco, 2008). In addition, the pharmacokinetics and stability of certain medications can be altered by the use of nanocarriers. This is especially true for EGCG, where nanotechnology has significantly improved the bioavailability of catechin (Huo et al., 2008). Nanosystems such as liposomes, lipid nanoparticles, inorganic nanocarriers, polymeric nanoparticles, gold nanoparticles, and peptide-based nanocarriers are all utilized in the process of EGCG distribution. The most common types of nanocarriers utilized for the transport of EGCG are lipid and polymeric nanocarriers. These nanocarriers have been described further below.

3.4.1.1 LIPID NANOPARTICLES

In the early 1990s, lipid nanoparticles were first developed; today, they are one of the nanosystems that are most frequently utilized for the delivery of drugs. These nanocarriers comprise a lipid matrix (Müller et al., 2000), and they have several benefits, such as high drug load, superior tolerability, controlled release qualities, and physical stability (Müller et al., 2000). The hydrophobic lipid phase, the hydrophilic aqueous phase, and one emulsifier are the minimum number of components necessary for their production. Solid lipid nanoparticles (SLNs) and nanostructured lipid carriers (NLCs) are the two most common varieties of lipid nanocarriers. SLNs are made up of solid lipids, whereas NLCs are formed from a mixture of liquid and solid lipids (Uner, 2006). The type of lipid that is utilized to make these two types of lipid nanocarriers differentiates them from one another. These nanocarriers exhibit distinctively varied patterns of encapsulation efficiency and release behavior, both of which can be attributed to the peculiar lipid crystalline structure that they possess. Since the lipid matrix of SLN is better ordered and has a fully crystalline structure when compared to NLC, SLN typically has a lower drug loading (Uner, 2006). This is because NLC has a less organized structure. Due to the crystalline rearrangement that occurs during long-term storage, it also has a tendency to expel the drug content. NLCs possess a greater ability for drug loading and storage stability when compared to SLNs. This is due to the fact that NLCs have a greater number of defects in the core, which are due to the occurrence of liquid lipid. The liquid lipid contributes to the formation of a more disorganized lipid matrix, possessing more cavities available to allocate the drug (Uner, 2006). The stability of EGCG in physiological conditions has been improved with the help of lipid nanoparticles, which have also been utilized to encourage the sustained release of a chemical and to enhance the oral bioavailability of the compound. The use of EGCG-loaded lipid nanocarriers is effective in treating a wide range of disorders, including atherosclerosis as well as neurodegenerative, skin, and eye conditions. Table 3.1 provides a summary of the most important findings concerning the use of lipid nanoparticles as carriers for EGCG.

TABLE 3.1 Lipid Nanoparticles Used as EGCG Carriers.

Particle	Size (nm)	Administration route	Results obtained	References
NLCs (glyceryl tridecanoate, soy lecithin, glyceryl tripalmitate, and chitosan Kolliphor HS15)	50	Oral	Strong resistance to degradation in alkaline as well as acidic environments. Studies conducted in vitro using macrophages derived from THP-1 showed that there was a reduction in inflammation as well as an accumulation of cholesterol.	Zhang et al., 2016
Phosphatidylcholine, phosphatidylinositol, phosphatidylethanolamine, and phosphatidic acid	30–80	Oral	Increased oral bioavailability of EGCG in neuronal cells in vivo, as well as induction of beta-secretase activity in neuronal cells in vitro.	Smith et al., 2010
NLCs (phosphatidylcholine, alpha-tocopherol acetate, and Kolliphor HS15)	108		Elevated levels of EGCG stability. A greater accumulation within the macrophages and a reduction in the production of MCP-1.	Zhang et al., 2016
NLCs (cetyl palmitate/ Phospholipon 80, Tween-80, and sesame oil)	126–167	Topical	EGCG undergoes photodegradation when exposed to UVA radiation.	Chen et al., 2017
Cationic lipid nanocarriers (Softisan® 100, glycerol, Poloxamer 188, CTAB/ DDAB, and Lipoid® S75)	~150	Ocular	Release of EGCG that is sustained in the biological medium. The cornea and sclera of a rabbit were both permeable.	Fangueiro et al., 2016
SLN (glycerol monostearate, soya lecithin, stearic acid, and pluronic F68)	157	N/A	Increased stability in the bodily fluids. Increased rates of cell death induction were observed in breast cancer cells (MDA-MB-231), as well as prostate cancer cells (DU-145).	Radhakrishnan et al., 2016

N/A: "not available" data.

Using natural lipids such as glyceryl tripalmitate and glyceryl tridecanoate, along with two surfactants, namely, soy lecithin and Kolliphor® HS15, chitosan-coated NLCs were created to prevent and reverse therosclerotic lesions by lowering the cholesterol content of macrophages (Zhang et al., 2013). The NLC formulation boosts the stability of EGCG and improves cell uptake, resulting in a 9-fold reduction in cholesterol buildup in macrophage cultures along with declining secretion of inflammatory factors (Zhang et al., 2013). This result was achieved by increasing cell uptake and EGCG stability. The researchers then synthesized a triglyceride-free formulation for EGCG encapsulation by exchanging triglyceride for alpha-tocopherol acetate, and they found results that were comparable to the previous findings. Nanovehicles were shown to improve the stability of EGCG as well as its concentration within the cytoplasm of macrophages (Zhang et al., 2016). This resulted in a decline in the production of the inflammatory cytokine MCP-1. Both sets of findings shed information on the possible role that nanocarriers loaded with EGCG could play in fighting against atherosclerosis.

When compared to free EGCG, the oral bioavailability of EGCG was greatly raised when nanolipidic particles were used, and their absorption into the systemic circulation was also boosted. This was demonstrated by Smith and colleagues. Nanocarriers loaded with EGCG were also able to stimulate the activity of the beta-secretase enzyme in neural cells. These findings point to the likelihood that EGCG could play a significant role in the treatment as well as the prevention of neurodegenerative disorders (Smith et al., 2010).

Recent research conducted by Chen et al. (2017) resulted in the development of lipid nanoparticles that are capable of encapsulating EGCG as well as other active chemicals for use in skincare products. Nanoparticles composed of lipids exhibited a high degree of homogeneity and demonstrated the ability to effectively encapsulate hydrophobic and hydrophilic substances, both on their own and in combination. After 168 h of exposure to UVA radiation, photostability tests showed that nanocarriers could not protect EGCG from photodegradation caused by light.

In order to improve the EGCG's stability and anticancer effects, Radhakrishnan et al. (2016) developed SLN for utilization as the delivery vehicle for the compound. SLNs successfully enhanced EGCG's stability in serum and under physiological settings. Additionally, it enabled continuous delivery of the molecule at a pH of 5. In addition, EGCG has been investigated as a potential treatment for ocular illnesses such as diabetic macular edema and glaucoma, both of which are linked to oxidative stress and the formation of ROS. Fangueiro et al. (2016) have only recently produced EGCG-loaded cationic lipid nanoparticles for ocular administration. These nanocarriers enabled EGCG penetration across the cornea and sclera of rabbits, and they were able to cause a prolonged release of EGCG in physiological media. In addition, it was discovered that formulations enriched with EGCG were not irritating and could be tolerated. These findings shed light on the fact that manufactured drug delivery vehicles have the ability to facilitate the topical administration of EGCG.

3.4.1.2 LIPOSOMES

Liposomes are comprised of phospholipids that are made of at least one lipid bilayer enclosing an aqueous environment. Their amphiphilic structure makes them adaptable nanocarriers for entrapping drugs that are hydrophilic, hydrophobic, or amphiphilic (Voinea and Simionescu, 2002). It is possible to finely control the size of liposomes and chemically modify the surface in order to target particular organs or escape the immune system. The sudden release of the liposomal contents can occur via membrane integrity interference by light, pH, temperature, and the presence of enzymes. This causes the lipid layer to be disrupted, which results in the immediate release of the drug amphiphilic (Voinea and Simionescu, 2002). Despite these encouraging findings, using them as carriers for EGCG in medicinal applications is still not well-documented.

Nanoliposomes loaded with EGCG synthesized from egg lecithin and cholesterol resulted in a significantly increased bactericidal effect against methicillin-resistant *Staphylococcus aureus* (MRSA) isolated from burn wound infections when compared to free EGCG (Gharib et al., 2013). Luo et al. (2014) synthesized liposomes from phosphatidylcholine (PhC)/cholesterol with the intention of preventing the development of cancer. The created liposome showed a high degree of stability under gastric conditions, with just 20% of its cargo being lost. The loss of cargo increases to 40% in the intestinal fluid. The formulation was also found to increase the inhibitory action of EGCG on the viability of tumor cells at greater concentrations. In order to increase the amount of EGCG that is absorbed by the mouth, liposomes with nonionic surfactants and cholesterol were synthesized (Song et al., 2014). The researchers also evaluated the permeability of Caco-2 cell monolayers to EGCG-entrapped liposomes and compared it to the permeability of free EGCG. The apparent permeability of EGCG was greatly improved because of the liposomes' ability to do so. When compared to the free drugs, the formulation showed significantly improved stability and significantly reduced toxicity (Song et al., 2014). These encouraging findings have prompted researchers to look into developing a nanoformulation based on liposomes that could boost the bioavailability of EGCG by improving the substance's intestinal permeability. Coloaded liposomes carrying EGCG and paclitaxel for the treatment of breast cancer intensify the synergistic impact of both chemicals in promoting MDA-MB-231 breast cancer cell death (Ramadass et al., 2015). They have only recently synthesized a liposome for the coloading of EGCG and paclitaxel for the treatment of breast cancer.

3.4.1.3 POLYMERIC NANOCARRIERS

Polymeric nanocarriers have the drug encapsulated within the polymer matrix, where it is shielded from the elements of the surrounding environment. The polymer may be natural or manmade. It is possible to functionalize the outer layer of the polymer by adding molecular markers in order to augment the pharmacokinetics of the drug or to target a particular tissue (Soppimath et al., 2001). Results obtained for the distribution of EGCG via polymeric nanocarriers both in vitro and in vivo have been promising.

The biocompatibility, low toxicity, and biodegradability of chitosan have encouraged its use in encapsulating EGCG (Delie and Blanco-Príeto, 2005). In addition to this, chitosan has mucoadhesive properties, which allow it to permeate enterocytes through the tight junctions (Delie and Blanco-Príeto, 2005). In vitro research conducted by Dube et al. (2010) demonstrated that the use of chitosan nanocarriers improved the absorption of EGCG via the enterocytes. Chitosan nanovesicles that were cross-linked with casein phosphopeptides were synthesized by Hu et al. (2012) in a manner that was analogous. The newly designed nanocarriers make EGCG more resistant to degradation in the digestive tract (Hu et al., 2012a). Additionally, the permeability of EGCG was found to be enhanced in the monolayers of Caco-2 cells (Hu et al., 2012b). Hong et al. (2014) synthesized EGCG-loaded nanocarriers that consisted of self-assembling chitosan and aspartic acid. After oral treatment of rabbits, these nanoformulations showed a considerable improvement in the antiatherosclerotic properties of EGCG (Hing et al., 2014). Khan et al. (2014) observed a dose-dependent reduction in the growth of the tumor in athymic mice that were implanted with prostate cancer cells and treated with EGCG-loaded chitosan nanocarriers. This was in comparison to the fact that both of the controls received either the nanocarriers or free EGCG. Similarly, chitosan tripolyphosphate (CS/TPP) nanocarriers modified with PEG and folic acid for EGCG encapsulation reduced the growth rates of MCF-7 breast cancer cells (Zeng et al., 2017). In addition, nanocarriers functionalized with folic acid induced better cellular uptake. In conclusion, the EGCG that had been encapsulated was able to produce larger degrees of regulation of the PI3K-Akt pathway and exhibit antiproliferative effects.

Recently, polylactic acid (PLA) and poly(lactide-co-glycolide) acid (PLGA) have been greatly researched due to their adaptability and high level of biocompatibility (Soppimath et al., 2001). These nanocarriers have an exterior layer that is easily modifiable with functional groups, which enables them to target particular cells specifically. The pace at which these nanocarriers degrade over time can be altered, and the nanocarriers themselves are synthesized to have high encapsulation rates and regulated release qualities (Soppimath et al., 2001).

In order to avoid damage to DNA, Srivastava et al. (2013) used PLGA nanocarriers that were loaded with EGCG. Prior to the infliction of DNA damage, mice in this study were given a topical treatment consisting of EGCG and PLGA EGCG nanocarriers. Free EGCG and EGCG-loaded nanocarrier pretreatment protect against DNA damage by 28% and 63%, respectively. In addition, EGCG-loaded nanocarriers demonstrated considerable stimulation of genes involved in DNA repair and suppression of genes involved in inflammation (Srivastava et al., 2013). The fact that PLA and PLGA polymers are unstable in acidic settings prevents them from being accepted for oral administration. This is despite the fact that both of these types of polymers have advantageous features. To increase the nanocarriers' stability in the digestive tract and to maximize the amount of loaded EGCG that was absorbed, Li and Gu (2014) used ovalbumin-dextran as a polymer. Furthermore, the formulation improved the apparent permeability coefficient of EGCG on Caco-2 monolayers in comparison with free EGCG. This led to an improvement in the absorption profile of EGCG (Li and Gu, 2014).

3.4.1.4 GOLD NANOCARRIERS

The core of these nanoparticles is comprised of gold and then a coating of functional molecules is deposited on top of it. They are capable of transporting complex compounds, such as medications that target specific cells (Hsieh et al., 2011). The ability of catechin to interact with metals and form complexes through the gallate ring makes it conceivable to synthesize gold nanocarriers that are coated with EGCG. Under acidic pH, gold EGCG complexes have a high degree of stability; nevertheless, in alkaline environments, they are unstable. In order to get around this drawback, Shukla et al. (2012) and Chen et al. (2014) came up with the idea of administering the drug directly into the tumor. The successful synthesis of radioactive gold nanocarriers coated with EGCG for the purpose of treating prostate cancer and other solid tumors was investigated (Shukla et al., 2012).

Chen et al. (2014) also produced nonradioactive gold nanocarriers coated with EGCG to suppress the emergence of tumors as well as their development. Utilizing a mouse melanoma cancer model, they reported that EGCG had a cytotoxic impact that showed promise both in vitro and in vivo. The nanocarriers promoted cytotoxic effects 4.91 times higher in murine melanoma cells than those achieved by treatment with free EGCG. This indicated that the nanocarriers had better anticancer activity. In order to improve EGCG's stability in the gastrointestinal tract, Hsieh et al. (2011) synthesized gold nanosystems that were stable in the gastrointestinal environment, with sustained release of EGCG over a period of 2 h. Additionally, the authors revealed that the formulation exhibited selective toxicity to malignant cells and suppressed the formation of implanted tumors in mice. These nanocarriers show promise as potential future nanoformulations for application in cancer therapy (Hsieh et al., 2012) due to their strong cytotoxicity toward malignant cells and their continuous release of the drug. Gold nanoparticles that have been coupled with EGCG have only very recently been used in the treatment of cardiovascular disorders. Khoobchandani et al. (2016) synthesized gold nanocarriers as a substitute for drug-coated stents. EGCG-Au nanocarriers prevented smooth muscle cells from migrating while keeping the viability and proliferation capacity of endothelial cells intact.

3.5 CONCLUSIONS

Data suggests that EGCG promotes the prevention and treatment of a variety of health issues, including Alzheimer's, Parkinson's, cancer, cardiovascular disorders, and obesity. This natural molecule is a popular choice for study as well as for the prevention and treatment of a number of ailments because EGCG is nontoxic and there are no recorded negative effects associated with its use. However, because of the limited bioavailability of this polyphenol molecule, a very high dose is required in order to achieve the therapeutic amounts that are desired. Nanocarriers have been utilized in several research studies to improve the bioavailability of EGCG as well as its stability. A wide variety of nanocarriers, such as liposomes, lipid nanoparticles, gold nanoparticles, polymeric nanoparticles, and other types of nanocarriers made of proteins and inorganic materials, have been utilized. Most of the research has been concentrated on lipid and polymeric nanocarriers, which may be because of the advantageous qualities that these nanocarriers possess, such as biocompatibility. On the other hand, there is still a lack of clarity on the safety of inorganic nanocarriers. However, the findings are quite encouraging, and the formulations using nanocarriers enhanced both the bioavailability and stability of EGCG. In addition, a number of studies demonstrated that the nanoformulations were able to significantly improve the intestinal barrier permeability when the particles were decorated with chitosan, causing the relaxation of enterocyte tight junctions. In addition, the inclusion of surface target ligands has the potential to improve the distribution of EGCG to aberrant cells, including cancer cells, which have been specifically targeted. In general, the use of nanocarriers has the potential to effectively augment the therapeutic effects of EGCG in the therapy of a wide variety of diseases, including cancer as well as neurological, skin, and eye conditions.

3.6 FUTURE DIRECTIONS

Since the expense of using nanotechnology is such a significant limitation, one of the most important things that have to be done is to bring down the cost/benefit ratio for the use of nanocarriers as drug delivery systems for both preventative and therapeutic purposes (Wang et al., 2014). In this scenario, lipid nanocarriers appear to have a lot of potential, given that they are not only affordable but also simple to scale up. The loading efficiency of these types of nanocarriers demonstrated outstanding results, which is vital for lowering both the prices and the toxicity associated with the excipients. Since this hydrophilic molecule is able to form complexes with the lipids, the great encapsulation efficiency that was achieved can be attributed to this property. Recent developments in EGCG nanodelivery systems have highlighted the significance of utilizing technology to enhance the therapeutic advantages of EGCG, which has excellent promise for potential future medical applications.

KEYWORDS

- **catechins**
- **EGCG**
- **green tea**
- **liposomes**
- **nanocarriers**

REFERENCES

Andersen J. K. Oxidative Stress in Neurodegeneration: Cause or Consequence? *Nat. Med.* **2004,** S18–S25.

Anderson, J. W.; Diwadkar, V. A.; Bridges, S. R. Selective Effects of Different Antioxidants on Oxidation of Lipoproteins from Rats. *Proc. Soc. Exp. Biol. Med* **1998,** *218* (4), 376–381.

Aucamp, J.; Gaspar, A.; Hara, Y.; Apostolides, Z. Inhibition of Xanthine Oxidase by Catechins from Tea (Camellia sinensis). *Anticancer Res.* **1997,** *17* (6D), 4381–4385.

Béliveau, R.; Gingras, D. Green Tea: Prevention and Treatment of Cancer by Nutraceuticals. *Lancet* **2004,** *364* (9439), 1021–1022.

Berletch, J. B.; Liu, C.; Love, W. K.; Andrews, L. G.; Katiyar, S. K.; Tollefsbol, T. O. Epigenetic and Genetic Mechanisms Contribute to Telomerase Inhibition by EGCG. *J. Cell. Biochem.* **2008,** *103* (2), 509–519.

Bertolini, F.; Fusetti, L.; Rabascio, C.; Cinieri, S.; Martinelli, G.; Pruneri, G. Inhibition of Angiogenesis and Induction of Endothelial and Tumor Cell Apoptosis by Green Tea in Animal Models of Human High-Grade Non-Hodgkin's Lymphoma. *Leukemia* **2000,** *14* (8), 1477–1482.

Bokuchava, M. A.; Skobeleva, N. I. The Biochemistry and Technology of Tea Manufacture. *Crit. Rev. Food Sci. Nutr.* **1980,** *12* (4), 303–370.

Chen, C. C.; Hsieh, D. S.; Huang, K. J.; Chan, Y. L.; Hong, P. D.; Yeh, M. K.; Wu, C. J. Improving Anticancer Efficacy of (-)-epigallocatechin-3-gallate Gold Nanoparticles in Murine B16F10 Melanoma Cells. *Drug Design Dev. Therapy* **2014,** *8*, 459–474.

Chen, L.; Lee, M. J.; Li, H.; Yang, C. S. Absorption, Distribution, Elimination of Tea Polyphenols in Rats. *Drug Metab. Dispos.* **1997,** *25* (9), 1045–1050.

Crespy, V.; Nancoz, N.; Oliveira, M.; Hau, J.; Courtet-Compondu, M. C.; Williamson, G. (2004). Glucuronidation of the Green Tea Catechins, (-)-epigallocatechin-3-gallate and (-)-epicatechin-3-gallate, by Rat Hepatic and Intestinal Microsomes. *Free Radic. Res.* **2004,** *38* (9), 1025–1031.

Delie, F.; Blanco-Príeto, M. J. Polymeric Particulates to Improve Oral Bioavailability of Peptide Drugs. *Molecules* **2005,** *10* (1), 65–80.

Dube, A.; Nicolazzo, J. A.; Larson, I. Chitosan Nanoparticles Enhance the Intestinal Absorption of the Green Tea Catechins (+)-Catechin and (-)-epigallocatechin Gallate. *Eur. J. Pharm. Sci* **2010,** *41* (2), 219–225.

Fangueiro, J. F.; Calpena, A. C.; Clares, B.; Andreani, T.; Egea, M. A.; Veiga, F. J.: Garcia, M. L.; Silva, A. M.; Souto, E. B. Biopharmaceutical Evaluation of Epigallocatechin Gallate-Loaded Cationic Lipid Nanoparticles (EGCG-LNs): In vivo, In Vitro and Ex Vivo Studies. *Int. J. Pharm.* **2016,** *502* (1-2), 161–169.

Fraga, C. G.; Oteiza, P. I. Iron Toxicity and Antioxidant Nutrients. *Toxicology* **2002,** *180* (1), 23–32.

Frank, J.; George, T. W.; Lodge, J. K.; Rodriguez-Mateos, A. M.; Spencer, J. P.; Minihane, A. M.; Rimbach, G. Daily Consumption of an Aqueous Green Tea Extract Supplement does not Impair Liver Function or Alter Cardiovascular Disease Risk Biomarkers in Healthy Men. *J. Nutr.* **2009,** *139* (1), 58–62.

Gharib, A.; Faezizadeh, Z.; Godarzee, M. Therapeutic Efficacy of Epigallocatechin Gallate-Loaded Nanoliposomes against Burn Wound Infection by Methicillin-Resistant Staphylococcus aureus. *Skin Pharmacol. Physiol.* **2013,** *26* (2), 68–75.

Graham H. N. Green Tea Composition, Consumption, and Polyphenol Chemistry. *Prev. Med.* **1992,** *21* (3), 334–350.

Guo, Q.; Zhao, B.; Li, M.; Shen, S.; Xin, W. Studies on Protective Mechanisms of Four Components of Green Tea Polyphenols against Lipid Peroxidation in Synaptosomes. *Biochim. Biophys. Acta* **1996,** *1304* (3), 210–222.

Halliwell B. Role of Free Radicals in the Neurodegenerative Diseases: Therapeutic Implications for Antioxidant Treatment. *Drugs Aging* **2001,** *18* (9), 685–716.

Henry, J. P.; Stephens-Larson, P. Reduction of Chronic Psychosocial Hypertension in Mice by Decaffeinated Tea. *Hypertension* **1984**, *6* (3), 437–444.

Higuchi, A.; Yonemitsu, K.; Koreeda, A.; Tsunenari, S. Inhibitory Activity of Epigallocatechin Gallate (EGCg) in Paraquat-Induced Microsomal Lipid Peroxidation--A Mechanism of Protective Effects of EGCg against Paraquat Toxicity. *Toxicology* **2003,** *183* (1-3), 143–149.

Hong, Z.; Xu, Y.; Yin, J. F.; Jin, J.; Jiang, Y.; Du, Q. Improving the Effectiveness of (-)-epigallocatechin gallate (EGCG) against Rabbit Atherosclerosis by EGCG-Loaded Nanoparticles Prepared from Chitosan and Polyaspartic Acid. *J. Agric. Food Chem.* **2014,** *62* (52), 12603–12609.

Hsieh, D. S.; Lu, H. C.; Chen, C. C.; Wu, C. J.; Yeh, M. K. The Preparation and Characterization of Gold-Conjugated Polyphenol Nanoparticles as a Novel Delivery System. *Int. J. Nanomed.* **2012,** *7*, 1623–1633.

Hsieh, D. S.; Wang, H.; Tan, S. W.; Huang, Y. H.; Tsai, C. Y.; Yeh, M. K.; Wu, C. J. The Treatment of Bladder Cancer in a Mouse Model by Epigallocatechin-3-gallate-gold Nanoparticles. *Biomaterials* **2011,** *32* (30), 7633–7640.

Hu, B.; Ting, Y.; Yang, X.; Tang, W.; Zeng, X.; Huang, Q. Nanochemoprevention by Encapsulation of (-)-epigallocatechin-3-gallate with Bioactive Peptides/Chitosan Nanoparticles for Enhancement of its Bioavailability. *Chem. Commun.* **2012a,** *48* (18), 2421–2423.

Hu, B.; Ting, Y.; Zeng, X.; Huang, Q. Cellular Uptake and Cytotoxicity of Chitosan-Caseinophosphopeptides Nanocomplexes Loaded with Epigallocatechin Gallate. *Carbohydr. Polym.* **2012b,** *89* (2), 362–370.

Huang, M. T.; Ho, C. T.; Wang, Z. Y.; Ferraro, T.; Finnegan-Olive, T.; Lou, Y. R.; Mitchell, J. M.; Laskin, J. D.; Newmark, H.; Yang, C. S. Inhibitory Effect of Topical Application of a Green Tea Polyphenol Fraction on Tumor Initiation and Promotion in Mouse Skin. *Carcinogenesis* **1992,** *13* (6), 947–954.

Hung, C. C.; Chiou, M. H.; Teng, Y. N.; Hsieh, Y. W.; Huang, C. L.; Lane, H. Y. Functional Impact of ABCB1 Variants on Interactions Between P-glycoprotein and Methadone. *PloS One* **2003,** *8* (3), e59419.

Huo, C.; Wan, S. B.; Lam, W. H.; Li, L.; Wang, Z.; Landis-Piwowar, K. R.; Chen, D.; Dou, Q. P.; Chan, T. H. The Challenge of Developing Green Tea Polyphenols as Therapeutic Agents. *Inflammopharmacology* **2008,** *16* (5), 248–252.

Ikeda, I.; Hamamoto, R.; Uzu, K.; Imaizumi, K.; Nagao, K.; Yanagita, T.; Suzuki, Y.; Kobayashi, M.; Kakuda, T. Dietary Gallate Esters of Tea Catechins Reduce Deposition of Visceral Fat, Hepatic Triacylglycerol, and Activities of Hepatic Enzymes Related to Fatty Acid Synthesis in Rats. *Biosci. Biotechnol. Biochem.* **2005,** *69* (5), 1049–1053.

Imai, K.; Nakachi, K. Cross Sectional Study of Effects of Drinking Green Tea on Cardiovascular and Liver Diseases. *BMJ* **1995,** *310* (6981), 693–696.

Ishii, T.; Minoda, K.; Bae, M. J.; Mori, T.; Uekusa, Y.; Ichikawa, T.; Aihara, Y.; Furuta, T.; Wakimoto, T.; Kan, T.; Nakayama, T. Binding Affinity of Tea Catechins for HSA: Characterization by High-Performance Affinity Chromatography with Immobilized Albumin Column. *Mol. Nutr. Food Res.* **2010,** *54* (6), 816–822.

Ke, Y.; Qian, Z. M. Brain Iron Metabolism: Neurobiology and Neurochemistry. *Progress Neurobiol.* **2007,** *83* (3), 149–173.

Kesharwani, R. K.; Misra, K. Prediction of Binding Site for Curcuminoids at Human Topoisomerase II α Protein; An in silico Approach. *Curr. Sci.* **2011,** 1060–1065.

Kesharwani, R. K.; Singh, D. B.; Singh, D. V.; Misra, K. Computational Study of Curcumin Analogues by Targeting DNA Topoisomerase II: A Structure-Based Drug Designing Approach. *Netw. Model. Anal. Health Inform. Bioinform.* **2018,** *7* (1), 1–7.

Kesharwani, R. K.; Srivastava, V.; Singh, P.; Rizvi, S. I.; Adeppa, K.; Misra, K. A Novel Approach for Overcoming Drug Resistance in Breast Cancer Chemotherapy by Targeting New Synthetic Curcumin Analogues against Aldehyde Dehydrogenase 1 (ALDH1A1) and Glycogen Synthase Kinase-3 β (GSK-3β). *Appl. Biochem. Biotechnol.* **2015,** *176* (7), 1996–2017.

Khan, N.; Bharali, D. J.; Adhami, V. M.; Siddiqui, I. A.; Cui, H.; Shabana, S. M.; Mousa, S. A.; Mukhtar, H. Oral Administration of Naturally Occurring Chitosan-Based Nanoformulated Green Tea Polyphenol EGCG Effectively Inhibits Prostate Cancer Cell Growth in a Xenograft Model. *Carcinogenesis* **2014,** *35* (2), 415–423.

Khoobchandani, M.; Katti, K.; Maxwell, A.; Fay, W. P.; Katti, K. V. Laminin Receptor-Avid Nanotherapeutic EGCg-AuNPs as a Potential Alternative Therapeutic Approach to Prevent Restenosis. *Int. J. Mol. Sci.* **2016,** *17* (3), 316.

Kim, S.; Lee, M. J.; Hong, J.; Li, C.; Smith, T. J.; Yang, G. Y.; Seril, D. N.; Yang, C. S. Plasma and Tissue Levels of Tea Catechins in Rats and Mice During Chronic Consumption of Green Tea Polyphenols. *Nutr. Cancer* **2000,** *37* (1), 41–48.

Kimura, M.; Umegaki, K.; Kasuya, Y.; Sugisawa, A.; Higuchi, M. The Relation between Single/Double or Repeated Tea Catechin Ingestions and Plasma Antioxidant Activity in Humans. *Euro. J. Clin. Nutr.* **2002,** *56* (12), 1186–1193.

Koo, S. I.; Noh, S. K. Green Tea as Inhibitor of the Intestinal Absorption of Lipids: Potential Mechanism for its Lipid-Lowering Effect. *J. Nutr. Biochem.* **2007,** *18* (3),

Lam, H.; Sakaguchi, K.; Ukeda, H.; Sawamura, M. Flow Injection Determination of Xanthine Oxidase Inhibitory Activity and Its Application to Food Samples. *Anal. Sci.* **2006,** *22* (1), 105–109.

Li, Z.; Gu, L. Fabrication of Self-Assembled (-)-epigallocatechin gallate (EGCG) Ovalbumin-Dextran Conjugate Nanoparticles and their Transport Across Monolayers of Human Intestinal Epithelial Caco-2 Cells. *J. Agric. Food Chem.* **2014,** *62* (6), 1301–1309.

Liu, Z.; Ma, L. P.; Zhou, B.; Yang, L.; Liu, Z. L. Antioxidative Effects of Green Tea Polyphenols on Free Radical Initiated and Photosensitized Peroxidation of Human Low Density Lipoprotein. *Chem. Phys. Lipids* **2000,** *106* (1), 53–63.

Liu, G.; Men, P.; Perry, G.; Smith, M. A. Nanoparticle and Iron Chelators as a Potential Novel Alzheimer Therapy. *Meth. Mol. Biol.* **2010**, *610*, 123–144.

Loktionov, A.; Bingham, S. A.; Vorster, H.; Jerling, J. C.; Runswick, S. A.; Cummings, J. H. Apolipoprotein E Genotype Modulates the Effect of Black Tea Drinking on Blood Lipids and Blood Coagulation Factors: A Pilot Study. *Br. J. Nutr.* **1998,** *79* (2), 133–139.

Luo, X.; Guan, R.; Chen, X.; Tao, M.; Ma, J.; Zhao, J. Optimization on Condition of Epigallocatechin-3-gallate (EGCG) Nanoliposomes by Response Surface Methodology and Cellular Uptake Studies in Caco-2 Cells. *Nanoscale Res. Lett.* **2014,** *9* (1), 291.

Mandel, S. A.; Amit, T.; Weinreb, O.; Reznichenko, L.; Youdim, M. B. Simultaneous Manipulation of Multiple Brain Targets by Green Tea Catechins: A Potential Neuroprotective Strategy for Alzheimer and Parkinson Diseases. *CNS Neurosci. Ther.* **2008,** *14* (4), 352–365.

Mishra, H.; Kesharwani, R. K.; Singh, D. B.; Tripathi, S.; Dubey, S. K.; Misra, K. Computational Simulation of Inhibitory Effects of Curcumin, Retinoic Acid and their Conjugates on GSK-3 Beta. *Netw. Model. Anal. Health Inform. Bioinform.* **2019,** *8* (1), 3.

Mu, L. N.; Zhou, X. F.; Ding, B. G.; Wang, R. H.; Zhang, Z. F.; Chen, C. W.; et al. A Case-control Study on Drinking Green Tea and Decreasing Risk of Cancers in the Alimentary Canal Among Cigarette Smokers and Alcohol Drinkers. *Zhonghua Liu Xing Bing Xue Za Zhi* **2003,** *24* (3), 192–195.

Mulder, T. P.; Rietveld, A. G.; van Amelsvoort, J. M. Consumption of Both Black Tea and Green Tea Results in an Increase in the Excretion of Hippuric Acid into Urine. *Am. J. Clin. Nutr.* **2005,** *81* (1 Suppl), 256S–260S.

Müller, R. H.; Mäder, K.; Gohla, S. Solid Lipid Nanoparticles (SLN) for Controlled Drug Delivery - A Review of the State of the art. *Euro. J. Pharm. Biopharm* **2000,** *50* (1), 161–177.

Nakagawa, K.; Miyazawa, T. Absorption and Distribution of Tea Catechin, (-)-epigallocatechin-3-gallate, in the Rat. *J. Nutr. Sci. Vitaminol.* **1997,** *43* (6), 679–684.

Nishimuta, H.; Ohtani, H.; Tsujimoto, M.; Ogura, K.; Hiratsuka, A.; Sawada, Y. Inhibitory Effects of Various Beverages on Human Recombinant Sulfotransferase Isoforms SULT1A1 and SULT1A3. *Biopharm. Drug Dispos.* **2007,** *28* (9), 491–500.

Okushio, K.; Matsumoto, N.; Kohri, T.; Suzuki, M.; Nanjo, F.; Hara, Y. Absorption of Tea Catechins into Rat Portal Vein. *Biol. Pharm. Bull.* **1996,** *19* (2), 326–329.

Otsuka, T.; Ogo, T.; Eto, T.; Asano, Y.; Suganuma, M.; Niho, Y. Growth Inhibition of Leukemic Cells by (-)-epigallocatechin gallate, The Main Constituent of Green Tea. *Life Sci.* **1998,** *63* (16), 1397–1403.

Ounjaijean, S.; Thephinlap, C.; Khansuwan, U.; Phisalapong, C.; Fucharoen, S.; Porter, J. B.; Srichairatanakool, S. Effect of Green Tea on Iron Status and Oxidative Stress in Iron-Loaded Rats. *Med. Chem.* **2008,** *4* (4), 365–370.

Rababah, T. M.; Hettiarachchy, N. S.; Horax, R. Total Phenolics and Antioxidant Activities of Fenugreek, Green Tea, Black Tea, Grape Seed, Ginger, Rosemary, Gotu Kola, and Ginkgo Extracts, Vitamin E, and Tert-butylhydroquinone. *J. Agric. Food Chem.* **2004,** *52* (16), 5183–5186.

Rachmilewitz, E. A.; Weizer-Stern, O.; Adamsky, K.; Amariglio, N.; Rechavi, G.; Breda, L.; Rivella, S.; Cabantchik, Z. I. Role of Iron in Inducing Oxidative Stress in Thalassemia: Can it be Prevented by Inhibition of Absorption and by Antioxidants? *Ann. N. Y. Acad. Sci.* **2005,** *1054*, 118–123.

Radhakrishnan, R.; Kulhari, H.; Pooja, D.; Gudem, S.; Bhargava, S.; Shukla, R.; Sistla, R. Encapsulation of Biophenolic Phytochemical EGCG Within Lipid Nanoparticles Enhances its Stability and Cytotoxicity Against Cancer. *Chem. Phys. Lipids* **2016,** *198*, 51–60.

Ramadass, S. K.; Anantharaman, N. V.; Subramanian, S.; Sivasubramanian, S.; Madhan, B. Paclitaxel/Epigallocatechin Gallate Coloaded Liposome: A Synergistic Delivery to Control the Invasiveness of MDA-MB-231 Breast Cancer Cells. *Coll. Surf. B Biointerfaces* **2015,** *125*, 65–72.

Raza, H.; John, A. In Vitro Protection of Reactive Oxygen Species-Induced Degradation of Lipids, Proteins and 2-Deoxyribose by Tea Catechins. *Food Chem. Toxicol* **2007,** *45* (10), 1814–1820.

Rund, D.; Rachmilewitz, E. Beta-Thalassemia. *N. Engl. J. Med.* **2005,** *353* (11), 1135–1146.

Salah, N.; Miller, N. J.; Paganga, G.; Tijburg, L.; Bolwell, G. P.; Rice-Evans, C. Polyphenolic Flavanols as Scavengers of Aqueous Phase Radicals and as Chain-Breaking Antioxidants. *Arch. Biochem. Biophys.* **1995,** *322* (2), 339–346.

Samman, S.; Sandström, B.; Toft, M. B.; Bukhave, K.; Jensen, M.; Sørensen, S. S.; Hansen, M. Green Tea or Rosemary Extract Added to Foods Reduces Nonheme-Iron Absorption. *Am. J. Clin. Nutr.* **2001,** *73* (3), 607–612.

Sanvicens, N.; Marco, M. P. Multifunctional Nanoparticles--Properties and Prospects for their use in Human Medicine. *Trends Biotechnol.* **2008,** *26* (8), 425–433.

Scalbert, A.; Williamson, G. Dietary Intake and Bioavailability of Polyphenols. *J. Nutr.* **2000,** *130* (8S Suppl), 2073S–2085S.

Shanafelt, T. D.; Call, T. G.; Zent, C. S.; Leis, J. F.; LaPlant, B.; Bowen, D. A.; Roos, M.; Laumann, K.; Ghosh, A. K.; Lesnick, C.; Lee, M. J.; Yang, C. S.; Jelinek, D. F.; Erlichman, C.; Kay, N. E. Phase 2 Trial of Daily, Oral Polyphenon E in Patients with Asymptomatic, Rai Stage 0 to II Chronic Lymphocytic Leukemia. *Cancer* **2013,** *119* (2), 363–370.

Shukla, R.; Chanda, N.; Zambre, A.; Upendran, A.; Katti, K.; Kulkarni, R. R.; Nune, S. K.; Casteel, S. W.; Smith, C. J.; Vimal, J.; Boote, E.; Robertson, J. D.; Kan, P.; Engelbrecht, H.; Watkinson, L. D.; Carmack, T. L.; Lever, J. R.; Cutler, C. S.; Caldwell, C.; Kannan, R.; ... Katti, K. V. Laminin Receptor Specific Therapeutic Gold Nanoparticles (198AuNP-EGCg) Show Efficacy in Treating Prostate Cancer. *Proc. Natl. Acad. Sci. U. S. A.* **2012,** *109* (31), 12426–12431.

Singh, D. V.; Agarwal, S.; Kesharwani, R. K.; Misra, K. 3D QSAR and Pharmacophore Study of Curcuminoids and Curcumin Analogs: Interaction with Thioredoxin Reductase. *Interdiscip. Sci.* **2013b,** *5* (4), 286–295.

Singh, D. B.; Gupta, M. K.; Kesharwani, R. K.; Misra, K. Comparative Docking and ADMET Study of Some Curcumin Derivatives and Herbal Congeners Targeting β-amyloid. *Netw. Model. Anal. Health Inform. Bioinform.* 2013a, *2* (1), 13–27.

Singh, P.; Kesharwani, R. K.; Keservani, R. K. Antioxidants and Vitamins: Roles in Cellular Function and Metabolism. In *Sustained Energy for Enhanced Human Functions and Activity*; Academic Press, 2017; pp 385–407. ISBN: 9780128054130.

Singh, P.; Kesharwani, R. K.; Misra, K.; Rizvi, S. I. The Modulation of Erythrocyte Na+/K+-ATPase Activity by Curcumin. *J. Adv. Res.* **2015,** *6* (6), 1023–1030.

Singh, P.; Kesharwani, R. K.; Misra, K.; Rizvi, S. I. Modulation of Erythrocyte Plasma Membrane Redox System Activity by Curcumin. *Biochem. Res. Int.* **2016,** 702039.

Smith, A.; Giunta, B.; Bickford, P. C.; Fountain, M.; Tan, J.; Shytle, R. D. Nanolipidic Particles Improve the Bioavailability and Alpha-Secretase Inducing Ability of Epigallocatechin-3-gallate (EGCG) for the Treatment of Alzheimer's Disease. *Int. J. Pharm.* **2010,** *389* (1-2), 207–212.

Snyder, A. M.; Connor, J. R. Iron, the Substantia Nigra and Related Neurological Disorders. *Biochim. Biophys. Acta* **2009,** *1790* (7), 606–614.

Song, Q.; Li, D.; Zhou, Y.; Yang, J.; Yang, W.; Zhou, G.; Wen, J. Enhanced Uptake and Transport of (+)-catechin and (-)-epigallocatechin Gallate in Niosomal Formulation by Human Intestinal Caco-2 Cells. *Int. J. Nanomed.* **2014,** *9*, 2157–2165.

Soppimath, K. S.; Aminabhavi, T. M.; Kulkarni, A. R.; Rudzinski, W. E. Biodegradable Polymeric Nanoparticles as Drug Delivery Devices. *J. Control. Release* **2001,** *70* (1-2), 1–20.

Srivastava, A. K.; Bhatnagar, P.; Singh, M.; Mishra, S.; Kumar, P.; Shukla, Y.; Gupta, K. C. Synthesis of PLGA Nanoparticles of Tea Polyphenols and their Strong in vivo Protective Effect Against Chemically Induced DNA Damage. *Int. J. Nanomed.* **2013,** *8*, 1451–1462.

Surh, Y. Molecular Mechanisms of Chemopreventive Effects of Selected Dietary and Medicinal Phenolic Substances. *Mutat. Res.* **1999,** *428* (1-2), 305–327.

Tesoriere, L.; D'Arpa, D.; Butera, D.; Allegra, M.; Renda, D.; Maggio, A.; Bongiorno, A.; Livrea, M. A. Oral Supplements of Vitamin E Improve Measures of Oxidative Stress in Plasma and Reduce Oxidative Damage to LDL and Erythrocytes in Beta-thalassemia Intermedia Patients. *Free Radic. Res.* **2001,** *34* (5), 529–540.

Uner, M. Preparation, Characterization and Physico-Chemical Properties of Solid Lipid Nanoparticles (SLN) and Nanostructured Lipid Carriers (NLC): Their Benefits as Colloidal Drug Carrier Systems. *Die Pharmazie* **2006,** *61* (5), 375–386.

Upadhyaya, J.; Kesharwani, R. K.; Misra, K. Metabolism, Pharmacokinetics and Bioavailability of Ascorbic Acid; Synergistic Effect with Tocopherols and Curcumin. *J. Comput. Intell. Bioinform.* **2009,** *2* (1), 77–84.

Valcic, S.; Burr, J. A.; Timmermann, B. N.; Liebler, D. C. Antioxidant Chemistry of Green Tea Catechins. New Oxidation Products of (-)-Epigallocatechin Gallate and (-)-epigallocatechin from their Reactions with Peroxyl Radicals. *Chem. Res. Toxicol.* **2000,** *13* (9), 801–810.

Voinea, M.; Simionescu, M. Designing of 'Intelligent' Liposomes for Efficient Delivery of Drugs. *J. Cell. Mol. Med.* **2002,** *6* (4), 465–474.

Vyas, N.; Keservani, R. K.; Nayak, A.; Jain, S.; Singhal, M. Effect of Tamarindus Indica and Curcuma Longa on Stress Induced Alopecia. *Pharmacologyonline* **2010,** *1*, 377–384.

Wang, Y. C.; Bachrach, U. The Specific Anti-Cancer Activity of Green Tea (-)-epigallocatechin-3-gallate (EGCG). *Amino acids* **2002,** *22* (2), 131–143.

Wang, Z. Y.; Huang, M. T.; Lou, Y. R.; Xie, J. G.; Reuhl, K. R.; Newmark, H. L.; Ho, C. T.; Yang, C. S.; Conney, A. H. Inhibitory Effects of Black Tea, Green Tea, Decaffeinated Black Tea, and Decaffeinated Green Tea on Ultraviolet B Light-Induced Skin Carcinogenesis in 7,12-dimethylbenz[a]anthracene-initiated SKH-1 Mice. *Cancer Res.* **1994,** *54* (13), 3428–3435.

Wang, S.; Su, R.; Nie, S.; Sun, M.; Zhang, J.; Wu, D.; Moustaid-Moussa, N. Application of Nanotechnology in Improving Bioavailability and Bioactivity of Diet-Derived Phytochemicals. *J. Nutr. Biochem.* **2014,** *25* (4), 363–376.

Wang, X.; Tian, W. Green Tea Epigallocatechin Gallate: A Natural Inhibitor of Fatty-Acid Synthase. *Biochem. Biophys. Res. Commun.* **2001,** 288(5), 1200–1206.

Yang, T. T.; Koo, M. W. Hypocholesterolemic Effects of Chinese Tea. *Pharmacol. Res.* **1997,** *35* (6), 505–512.

Yang, T. T.; Koo, M. W. Chinese Green Tea Lowers Cholesterol Level Through an Increase in Fecal Lipid Excretion. *Life Sci.* **2000,** *66* (5), 411–423.

Zecca, L.; Youdim, M. B.; Riederer, P.; Connor, J. R.; Crichton, R. R. Iron, Brain Ageing and Neurodegenerative Disorders. *Nat. Rev. Neurosci.* **2004,** *5* (11), 863–873.

Zeng, L.; Yan, J.; Luo, L.; Ma, M.; Zhu, H. Preparation and Characterization of (-)-Epigallocatechin-3-gallate (EGCG)-Loaded Nanoparticles and their Inhibitory Effects on Human Breast Cancer MCF-7 Cells. *Sci. Rep.* **2017,** *7*, 45521.

Zhang, J.; Nie, S.; Martinez-Zaguilan, R.; Sennoune, S. R.; Wang, S. Formulation, Characteristics and Antiatherogenic Bioactivities of CD36-targeted Epigallocatechin Gallate (EGCG)-Loaded Nanoparticles. *J. Nutr. Biochem.* **2016,** *30*, 14–23.

Zhang, J.; Nie, S.; Wang, S. Nanoencapsulation Enhances Epigallocatechin-3-gallate Stability and its Antiatherogenic Bioactivities in Macrophages. *J. Agric. Food Chem.* **2013,** *61* (38), 9200–9209.

Zhang, A.; Zhu, Q. Y.; Luk, Y. S.; Ho, K. Y.; Fung, K. P.; Chen, Z. Y. Inhibitory Effects of Jasmine Green Tea Epicatechin Isomers on Free Radical-Induced Lysis of Red Blood Cells. *Life Sci.* **1997,** *61* (4), 383–394.

Zhou, B.; Wu, L. M.; Yang, L.; Liu, Z. L. Evidence for Alpha-Tocopherol Regeneration Reaction of Green Tea Polyphenols in SDS Micelles. *Free Radic. Biol. Med.* **2005,** *38* (1), 78–84.

CHAPTER 4

IMMUNOMODULATION PROPERTY OF ANTIOXIDANTS

KIRAN PATIL[1], SOPAN NANGARE[2], MEGHANATH SHETE[3], MADHAV SHELKE[4], MATIN SHAIKH[5], MRUGENDRA POTDAR[1], VINIT AGNIHOTRI[1], AND YOGEETA GOYAL[1]

[1]Department of Pharmaceutics, SVKM Institute of Pharmacy, Dhule, India

[2]Department of Pharmaceutics, H. R. Patel Institute of Pharmaceutical Education and Research, Shirpur, India

[3]Department of Pharmaceutics, R. C. Patel Institute of Pharmaceutical Education and Research, Shirpur, India

[4]Department of Pharmaceutical Quality Assurance, SVKM Institute of Pharmacy, Dhule, India

[5]Department of Pharmaceutical Chemistry, H. R. Patel Institute of Pharmaceutical Education and Research, Shirpur, India

ABSTRACT

Modification in the immune response consisting of induction, expression, amplification, or inhibition of any portion/phase of the immune response is referred to as immune system modulation. Immunomodulators are biological/synthetic compounds that can activate, inhibit, or regulate any element of the immune system, encompassing both the adaptive and innate arms. Antioxidants can defend against the injury created by diverse free radicals at several scales. It has been reported that the utilization of antioxidants diminishes the oxidative stress related to cancer, atherosclerosis,

Antioxidants as Nutraceuticals. Nayan A. Gujarathi, Raj K. Keservani, Rajesh K. Kesharwani, Bhushan R. Rane, Yogeeta Sameer Goyal (Eds.)

neurodegenerative diseases, inflammation, etc., which results in the shielding of immune cells. Accordingly, it gained special consideration from research scholars to evaluate the immunomodulatory function of antioxidants. In this book chapter, the existing scientific knowledge on the immunomodulation properties of antioxidants has been reviewed. At first, a brief illustration related to the immune system, classification of the immunomodulating agent, need for immunomodulators, and merits and demerits of immunomodulators have been added. Next, the defense by antioxidants and the significance of antioxidants toward the disease have been discussed. The application of antioxidants as immunomodulators has been elaborated with special emphasis on different antioxidant defenses for immunomodulation. Moreover, the update in antioxidants as immunomodulators is also summarized. Finally, the present problems and future possibilities of antioxidant immunomodulation properties have been explored. In the future, this book chapter may help academic and industry researchers investigate the immunomodulation properties of naturally present antioxidants.

4.1 INTRODUCTION

4.1.1 FREE RADICALS IN DISEASES

Free radicals are species that have one or more unpaired electrons in their molecular structure (Lobo et al., 2010). Hence, they are always in search of other free radicals or molecules for pairing and stabilization. It makes them highly reactive species that could affect numerous things in their own way (Phaniendra et al., 2015). The importance of free radicals in medical science has increased in the last decade, and it is also an area of interest for chemists and biochemists (Alkadi, 2020). The potential of free radicals to cause various degenerative diseases and reperfusion injuries can be well-justified by researchers worldwide (Di Meo and Venditti, 2020; Kehrer and Klotz, 2015; Neha et al., 2019). Many chronic diseases, such as cancer, asthma, allergy, aging, cirrhosis, cataracts, hypertension, and atherosclerosis, are some of the examples mainly caused due to free radicals (Dröge, 2002; Kehrer and Klotz, 2015; Sharma et al., 2018). Free radicals are reactive oxygen species with unpaired electrons, and their reactivity depends on the nature of oxygen (Florence, 1995). Some of the reactive oxygen species are mentioned in Table 4.1.

TABLE 4.1 Types of Reactive Oxygen Species.

Reactive oxygen species	Molecular formula
Molecular oxygen	O_2
Hydroxyl radical	$OH\bullet$
Superoxide radical	$O_2\bullet$
Singlet oxygen	$^1O_2$
Hydrogen peroxide	H_2O_2
Lipid peroxide	LOOH
Alkoxyl radical	$RO\bullet$
Peroxyl radical	$ROO\bullet$
Semiquinone radical	$Q^{-}\bullet$

4.1.2 IMMUNE SYSTEM

The immune system comprises special organs, cells, and chemicals that protect the body from harmful substances, germs, and cellular changes. White blood cells, antibodies, complement system, lymphatic system, spleen, thymus, and bone marrow are the main components of the immune system (2022). In memory cells, the immune system records everything it has ever defeated to fight faster in the future. Many things activate the immune system that the body does not recognize as its own, called antigens, including the proteins on the surfaces of bacteria, fungi, and viruses ([CSL STYLE ERROR: reference with no printed form.]). The immune system comprises an innate immune response (nonspecific) and an adaptive immune response (specific) (Fig. 4.1) (Jantan et al., 2015).

When a harmful substance or germ triggers an immune response, these systems are closely linked and work together. An innate immune system provides a general defense against harmful substances and germs. It involves a combination of physical, chemical, and cellular responses against pathogens. Its primary function is to protect the body from the spread and movement of foreign pathogens. It fights mainly using immune cells such as natural killer cells, macrophages, neutrophils, dendritic cells, mast cells, basophils, and eosinophils. Adaptive immunity is the second line of defense against nonself-pathogens (Jantan et al., 2015). The adaptive immune system makes antibodies to combat specific pathogens that it has previously encountered; therefore, it is also known as a specific or acquired immune response. It is mediated through T and B lymphocytes (Marshall et al., 2018). The adaptive immune response is meant to attack nonself-pathogens but can sometimes

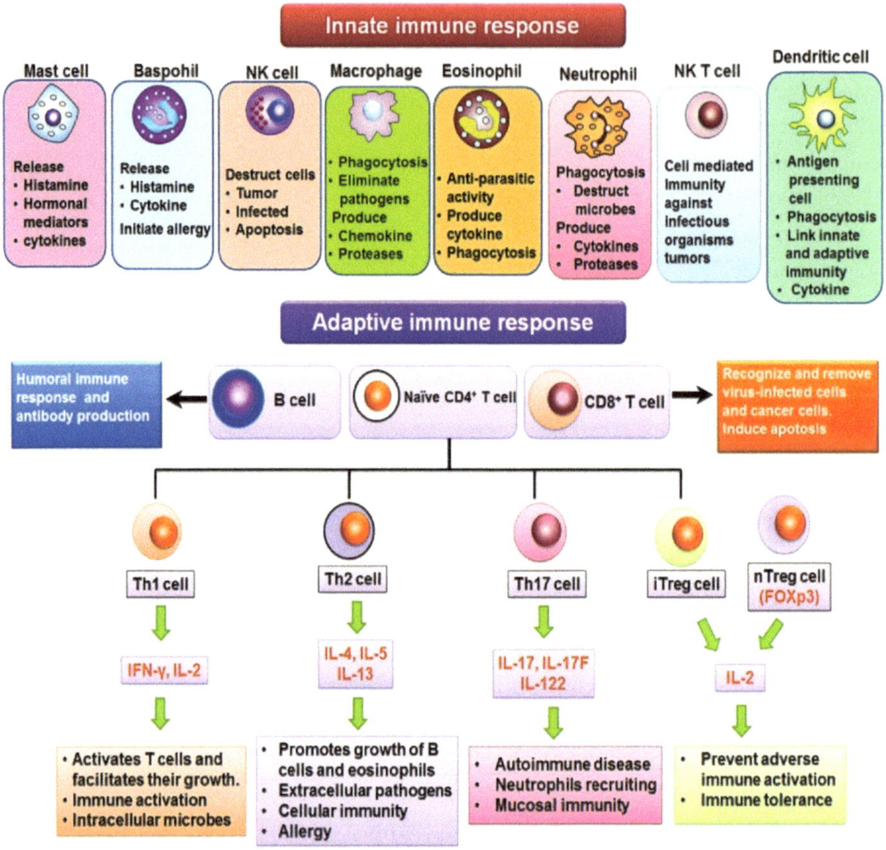

FIGURE 4.1 Cells of innate and adaptive immune responses.

Source: Reprinted from Jantan et al., 2015. Copyright © 2015 Jantan, Ahmad and Bukhari. https://creativecommons.org/licenses/by/4.0/

make errors and attack itself, also known as autoimmune diseases (e.g., lupus, rheumatoid arthritis). An innate immune response happens immediately, whereas an adaptive immune response takes time. However, the effects of adaptive immunity are long-lasting, highly specific, and sustained by memory T cells over their whole lives (Netea et al., 2020).

4.1.3 IMMUNOMODULATING AGENTS

An immunomodulator is an agent that stimulates, suppresses, or modulates the immune system, both adaptive and innate. Immunomodulators can be categorized clinically as immunosuppressants and immunostimulants

(Fig. 4.2) (Kumar et al., 2012). Immunostimulants are nonspecific as they are used to enhance a body's ability to resist infection and act through innate and adaptive immune responses. Immunostimulants serve both as prophylactics and immunopotentiators by enhancing immunity in healthy individuals. An immunoadjuvant is a nonspecific substance acting to enhance the immune response to an antigen with which it is administered such as vaccines (Agarwal and Singh, 1999). An immunosuppressive agent suppresses the immune system and reduces the risk of autoimmune diseases and foreign body rejection, such as an organ transplant (Kumar et al., 2012; Zdanowicz, 2009).

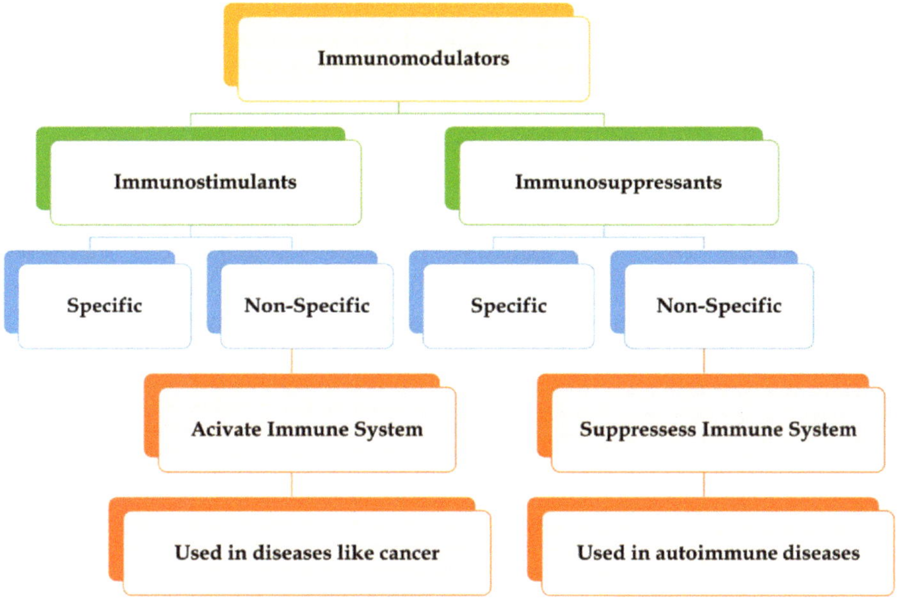

FIGURE 4.2 Classification of immunomodulators.

4.1.4 NEED FOR IMMUNOMODULATORS

The immune system regulates body homeostasis in healthy organisms (Taniguchi et al., 2009). The immune system is constantly manipulated by various exogenous and endogenous factors, either directly or invisibly. Daily and occasional exposure to these factors affects our health by suppressing or stimulating our defenses. This could either make us susceptible to disease or protect us from it. The body is constantly bombarded with these animate and inanimate objects throughout our lives, from waking up in the morning to slipping into bed at night. Therefore, no living thing can escape its beneficial or harmful effects. Moreover, the coexistence of human and animal pathogens results in new diseases and exacerbates existing ones with changing global scenarios. Immunomodulation is being used to combat a wide range of human and animal diseases, including incurable diseases such as viral diseases, cancers, and autoimmune diseases (Mahima et al., 2013). Our immune system is influenced by both animal and nonanimal factors around us. The immune system alone cannot protect us from external factors in all circumstances. As a primary defense system, immunity must be strong enough to combat all factors. Therefore, there is a need for immunomodulatory therapy, which can normalize or modulate pathophysiological processes. The best way to boost immunity is through a healthy diet, regular exercise, adequate sleep, and a stress-free life. An ideal diet should contain essential elements, such as carbohydrates, vitamins, and trace minerals. A deficiency of these components results in disease because they play specific roles in immunity, from its development to its active role (Maggini et al., 2018). Hence, the foods that we consume daily, such as vegetables, spices, herbs, fruits, etc., can also positively or negatively manipulate our immune system (Ülger et al., 2018). For proper therapy, there is a great need to understand the defense mechanisms of immunomodulating agents. Presently, antioxidants are extensively reported for different diseases/disorders as immunomodulating agents. Therefore, in the next section, we will describe the importance of antioxidants and their defense mechanisms.

4.2 ANTIOXIDANTS AND DEFENSE

In recent days, there has been a lot of interest in free radicals and related species. Principally, reactive oxygen species are mostly made up of reactive oxygen species and nitrogen species. They are produced in our bodies by a variety of endogenous systems. In addition, exposure to assorted physicochemical circumstances or pathophysiological states can also result in the production of reactive free-radical species. It has been revealed that the free radicals may damage lipids, proteins, and other biomolecules. Finally, it has been linked to aging and a variety of human illnesses (Aher et al., 2011). Therefore, there is a prerequisite for restricting the impact of free radicals on the body. Since its inception, plenty of scientists have reported the new door for efficient management of such issues. In this case, the utilization of antioxidants for the treatment of such ailments is the attention-grabbing arena. Mainly, antioxidants are substances that can modify the oxidant–antioxidant makeup of the body via neutralizing pro-oxidant agents (Ajith et al., 2017). Immunomodulators, which enhance or decrease the host's defensive response, can be employed as preventatives or treatments. In this vein, natural compounds having immunomodulatory and antioxidant properties are extensively utilized in the cure of a variety of illnesses (Liu et al., 2020). In this section, we have summarized the defense of antioxidants and the significance of antioxidants in disease. Even though it is clear from the interactions of oxygen that it is harmful, exclusively aerobes tolerate its existence, owing to inherent antioxidant defense (Aher et al., 2011). Significantly, antioxidant defense relies on different mechanisms that mainly include the removal of free radicals as well as other reactive species through catalysis. The protection of biomolecules using proteins (heat shock proteins) against oxidative harm can also be one of the defenses provided by antioxidants. Likewise, substances with a low molecular weight can also help reduce free radicals and other active species. Moreover, the use of proteins reduces the peroxidase presence (Halliwell and Gutteridge, 2015). It has been divulged that the reported antioxidants may induce substantial immunomodulatory processes in animals, resulting in an improved oxidant–antioxidant balance (Ajith et al., 2017). It has been mentioned that the utilization of antioxidants can help to prevent the disease or modulate the state of a particular disease (Knight, 2000). In this streak, plenty of investigation has revealed that the use of antioxidants has an inverse effect on several diseases. Additionally, the combination of different antioxidants has demonstrated better results for diverse applications, such as disease or disorder treatment, in contrast to a single antioxidant (Vivekananthan et al., 2003). Concisely, existing studies, mainly preclinical studies as well as epidemiological studies related to antioxidants, conclude that they must be utilized on a daily basis (Aher et al., 2011). Owing to nutritional differences in Western countries, the call for antioxidants is varied as compared to India. In this line, there is continuous development related to the investigation of antioxidant efficacy. Devasagayam et al. enlisted potent antioxidants that include vanillin, chlorogenic acid, gingerol, withaferin, picrolive, dehydrozingerone, pedunculagin, emblicanin, glycyrrhizin, glabridin, vicenin, orientin, curcumin, caffeine, etc. (Devasagayam et al., 2004). It acts through different mechanisms to treat the disease with no toxic effects. For example, the use of oil-soluble vitamin E facilitates the breaking of the chain during the lipid peroxidation process in the body's cell membranes. In addition, it acts as a chain breaker in low-density lipids (Kagan et al., 2002). In another case, vitamin E is used in the treatment of alcoholics due to its ability to boost the immune response and host defense (Wang and Watson, 1994). Moreover, the utilization of aqueous soluble vitamin C has demonstrated excellent free-radical scavenging activity. Besides this, lutein, lycopene, and carotenoids prove the potential of quenching $^1O_2$ and ROO* (Devasagayam et al., 2004; Kagan et al., 2002). In 2020, it was stated that endoplasmic reticulum stress resulted in a number of pathological conditions such as kidney, liver, and heart diseases. In this condition, the selection of natural antioxidants for the treatment of the abovementioned diseases can also provide better relief. Therefore, it will be an innovative approach to mitigate life-threatening diseases (Reyes-Fermín et al., 2020). Recently published work reported that the plant derivative silymarin (an antioxidant) shows immunomodulatory activity via inhibition of T-lymphocyte function (lower dose) or stimulation of the inflammatory response (higher dose). Interestingly, silymarin immunomodulatory response depends on dose as well as time (Esmaeil et al., 2017). Taken as a whole, natural antioxidants exhibit immune system modulation abilities that may be due to their impact on immune cells, mainly natural killer cells, macrophages, granulocytes, etc. (Nair et al., 2019). Figure 4.3 depicts the immunomodulation scheme of antioxidants.

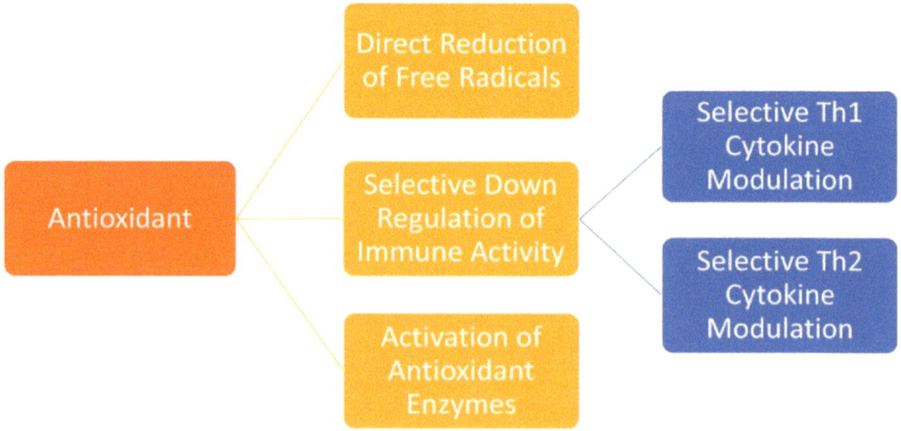

FIGURE 4.3 Different immunomodulation schemes by antioxidants.

4.3 APPLICATIONS OF ANTIOXIDANTS AS IMMUNOMODULATORS

The chemicals/substances that can be used to support immune functions by increasing or decreasing specific activity and helping to respond to threats are known as immunomodulators. Immunomodulators may work in various ways, like decreasing inflammation, preventing nerve damage, blocking the activity of interleukin, stopping or slowing down the growth of cancer cells, etc. Free radicals are formed as a byproduct during the metabolism process in the human body. These electrically charged molecules sensitize the cell for oxidation, which is collectively known as oxidative stress. Moreover, the increased oxidative stress may cause chronic inflammation and damage healthy cells. The dysfunction in the immune system is accountable for various diseases like asthma, arthritis, allergies, ulcerative colitis, parasitic diseases, infectious diseases, cancer, and many more. The class of chemicals derived from a plant that is used for immunomodulatory action is glycosides, flavonoids (Keservani and Sharma, 2014; Keservani et al., 2016a, 2016b), coumarins, sapogenins, alkaloids, thiosulfinates, volatile oils, terpenoids, phenolics, polyphenols, polysaccharides, steroids, etc. It has been observed that the plants mentioned in Ayurveda and used for the preparation of 'Rasayanas' possess strong antioxidant activity. Moreover, these preparations have been preferably used to counteract the effects of aging, diabetes, atherosclerosis, cancer, rheumatoid arthritis, autoimmune disease, Parkinson's disease, etc. Moreover, they show different activities like immunostimulant, immunoadjuvant, immunosuppressant, etc., and these activities occur via phagocytosis stimulation, macrophage activation, lymphoid cell stimulation, immunostimulatory effect on peritoneal macrophages, cellular immune function enhancement and nonspecific cellular immune system effect, increased nonspecific immunity mediators and natural killer cell numbers, antigen-specific immunoglobulin production increase, reducing chemotherapy induces leukopenia, and increasing the interleukin-2 and circulating total white cell counts (Kumar et al., 2012). The human body has a natural mechanism to create antioxidants, but during aging, it has been observed that this mechanism gets affected, so there is a need for an external supply of antioxidants. To build innate immunity in aging people, the use of natural products with antioxidant activity may perform better with increased immunity (Pathak et al., 2020). Moreover, it has been hypothesized that immune cells such as macrophages recruit inflammatory monocytes in the alveolar cells and allow the production of large amounts of cytokines in the alveoli, leading to a hyperinflammatory response in severely ill patients with

COVID-19. Morbidity and mortality in severe COVID-19 are associated with hyperinflammation and interference with cytokine signaling. Moreover, it has been observed that medical practitioners often prescribe immunomodulators to enhance the immune response against infectious diseases. The overall effect may significantly reduce hyperinflammation in these patients (Rizk et al., 2020). Therefore, in this section, we have discussed the different examples of antioxidants and their applications in immunomodulating a list of health issues.

The various fruits contain antioxidants, and the same are responsible for immunomodulatory properties. Some of the antioxidants present in various fruits that were used as immunomodulatory action to treat the disease conditions were discussed. Vitamin C (ascorbic acid), which is present in most of the fruits, scavenges ROS produced due to cellular metabolism. Furthermore, the antioxidants present in fruit inhibit the cells from oxidative damage, inflammatory dysfunction, and neurodegenerative disorders. A literature survey revealed that vitamin C is one of the most popular and effective antioxidants. Researchers proved that it enhances immune function in different diseases. Furthermore, the effect on various immune cells has been shown using in vivo models and humans. It mimics the proliferation process of lymphocytes, the activity of natural killer cells, and chemotaxis. Moreover, vitamin C plays a vital role in protecting the intestinal cells from inflammatory stimuli. The natural sources of vitamin C, including citrus, kiwi, mango, papaya, tomato, broccoli, green leafy vegetables, etc., fulfill the human need for 100–200 mg per day via diet. Therefore, it will be helpful for the immune system of a healthy human to maintain its integrity (Mousavi et al., 2019). Vitamin E, which is a very well-known antioxidant and is also found in all plasma lipoproteins and cell membranes, has strong chain-breaking antioxidant properties. In humans, it prevents oxidative stress in DNA, low-density lipoproteins, and polyunsaturated fatty acids. The said properties were used in various diseases as immunomodulators. Polyphenols present in various fruits, such as epigallocatechin-3-gallate, epigallocatechin, or epicatechin-3-gallate, primarily enhance the generation of interleukin by human white blood cells. Thus, they are responsible for declining the activity of proinflammatory cytokines secreted by macrophages and enhancing the anti-inflammatory cytokines. Moreover, the intake of polyphenols such as flavones, flavanones, flavone-3-ols, catechins, procyanidins, resveratrol, and anthocyanidins supports the maintenance of a proper balance of Th1/Th2 and obstructs the production of immunoglobulin E (IgE). This mechanism is applicable to the management of allergies. Flavonoids such as skaempferol, quercetin, myricetin, and cyaniding inhibit the ROS and reactive nitrogen species, which helps in the management of allergy, inflammation, and viral–microbial infection. Overall, these chemical constituents, which have antioxidant properties, neutralize the ROS and result in various immunomodulatory activities.

Curcumin crude extract and the active principle of the plant have anti-inflammatory, antitumor, and antibacterial activity (Catanzaro et al., 2018). Moreover, it affects innate and adaptive immunity by modulating immune cell function including T and B cells (Boroumand et al., 2018). It has been reported that curcumin shows hepatoprotective, antiviral, antifungal, and antileishmanial activities. Furthermore, curcumin inhibits NO production, cyclooxygenase 2 (COX 2), nuclear factor-kappa B (NK kB), lipoxygenase in NK cells, and IFN-γ, which results in a declined inflammatory response (Jantan et al., 2015). Tulsi (*Ocimum sanctum*) is one of the very popular plants that is used since ancient times to cure various disorders. It contains essential oils, for instance, eugenol, carvacrol, apigenin flavonoids, anthocyanins, and many more, which contribute to the immunomodulatory properties. Moreover, the herb of Tulsi is widely used in wound healing and infection (Hemalatha et al., 2011). One of the studies reported that a significant increase was observed in bone marrow cellularity along with total white blood cell count and hemoglobin concentration after the treatment of *Ocimum sanctum*. Parts of *Ocimum sanctum*, as well as hot or cold extract, can be used in the management of bronchitis, bronchial asthma, dysentery, diarrhea, malaria, skin diseases, chronic fever, painful eye diseases, insect bites, etc. Moreover, the uses of Tulsi in various disorders are explained in traditional medicine. Furthermore, numerous researchers reported the different activities of *Ocimum sanctum*, like antimicrobial, antifungal, antidiabetic, antifertility, anticancer, hepatoprotective, cardioprotective, analgesic, antispasmodic, antiemetic, and many more (P. Prakash, 2005). *Asparagus racemosus* is known as Shatavari, which has been used since ancient times, and Ayurveda mentions its numerous uses in various disorders. Moreover, the steroidal saponins present in Shatavari are widely used. It has multiple applications or activities, like immunomodulatory, antitussive, antiulcer, galactagogue, anticarcinogen, adaptogen, antidiarrheal, antioxidant, etc. The root extract of the wild form of Asparagus racemosus is eminent for its immunomodulatory properties. Numerous researchers have reported the immunomodulatory properties of Asparagus racemosus, viz., that it modulates macrophase activation, restores neutrophil and lymphocyte counts, and delays the progress of tumors in experimental animals (Pise et al., 2015). *Allium sativum* (Lasun) contains organosulfur compounds, which have been proven to be responsible for inhibiting the growth of tumors and modulating the activity of diverse chemical carcinogens (Schäfer and Kaschula, 2014). Furthermore, garlic extract enhances the cytotoxicity of peripheral blood lymphocytes and protects them from UV-induced suppression of contact hypersensitivity (Foroutan-Rad et al., 2017). It was found that the aged garlic extract contains S-allylcysteine and S-allylmercapto-L-cysteine, which exhibit radical scavenger activity. In addition to it, organosulfur compounds, including S-allyl cysteine, have been found to retard the growth of chemically induced and transplantable tumors in several animal models. Therefore, the consumption of garlic may provide some kind of protection from cancer development (Londhe et al., 2011). *Aloe vera* is known for its anti-inflammatory, specific antibody production, wound healing, dermal ischemia properties, and many more (Sandner et al., 2020). Moreover, it was proven that contracting wound area and collagen synthesis show wound healing properties. The reduction of leukocyte adhesion, as well as proinflammatory cytokines, inhibits the inflammatory process following burn injury. It was demonstrated that after the administration of aloe vera, there was a marked increase in the phagocytic and proliferative activity of the reticuloendothelial system. Aloe vera gel contains anthraquinones and chromones in the inner gel. It can directly inhibit the cyclooxygenase pathway and reduce prostaglandin E2 production, which possesses strong anti-inflammatory effects. It contains anthraquinones (aloin) and chromone (aloesin) components, and *it* has a pharmacological activity to alleviate inflammatory responses in inflammatory bowel disease (Radha and Laxmipriya, 2015). *Azadirachta indica (Neem)*: the rich chemical constituent of neem is azadirachtin, and other constituents are nimbolinin, nimbin, nimbidin, nimbidol, sodium nimbinate, salannin, gedunin, and quercetin. It has a rich source of antioxidants, so it acts as a free-radical scavenger. Azadirachtin and nimbolide showed concentration-dependent antiradical scavenging activity and reductive potential as per the order: nimbolide > azadirachtin > ascorbate. The neem ingredient shows an effective role in the management of cancer through the regulation of cell-signaling pathways. Neem modulates the activity of various tumor suppressor genes, angiogenesis, transcription factors, and apoptosis. Neem also plays a role as an anti-inflammatory via the regulation of proinflammatory enzyme activities, including the cyclooxygenase (COX) and lipoxygenase (LOX) enzymes. Neem has numerous properties, including antibacterial, antiviral, antidandruff, antidiabetic, neuroprotective, antifungal, antimalarial, antinephrotoxic, and anticancer activity (Alzohairy, 2016; Supriyanto et al., 2021). Eucalyptus, 1,8-cineole, Eucalyptus, α-pinene, linalool, and citronellal are the volatile compounds present in Eucalyptus in high amounts. It has a very long history of being used in the management of cold, cough, influenza, and other respiratory infections. The main component of Eucalyptus, 1,8-cineole, has a pungent and sharp scent, and it has anti-inflammatory and analgesic properties (Sandner et al., 2020). *Camella sinensis* L. (*Theaceae*) tea is a regular refreshment drink for Indians and worldwide. The leaves contain a high amount of quercetin, gallic acid, epigallocatechin gallate, caffeine, and its intermediate, theophylline. These constituents have strong antioxidant properties and they can modulate the immune properties too. In the last few decades, the number of green tea consumers has drastically increased due to its remarkable results. The chemical constituents in tea derived from the catechins have antioxidant properties for the human body. These constituents modulate cardiovascular health. Furthermore, it was demonstrated that green tea extract regulates the secretion of the anti-inflammatory cytokine TGF-β. Moreover, it inhibits the lipopolysaccharide-induced NO production, which results in the anti-inflammatory and immunomodulatory properties of green tea extract on cells of the innate immune system (Rahayu et al., 2018a). Citrus fruit juices contain a wide range of micronutrients (vitamins and minerals) and bioactive compounds. Several of these micronutrients are important for immune function support, and citrus fruit juice is a particularly good source of two of them, vitamin C and folate. In addition to micronutrients, citrus fruit juices contain a number of polyphenolic flavonoid compounds of relevance to the immune system. These micronutrients play roles in supporting the immune response, controlling inflammation, and preventing or controlling oxidative stress, which promotes inflammation and harms the immune response (Miles and Calder, 2021). *Terminalia chebula* contains potent antioxidant components such as chebulagic acid, ellagic acid, and gallic acid. They counteract ROS and scavenge free radicals. Moreover, these antioxidants reveal immunosuppressive properties, which are responsible for the inhibition of cytokines such as interleukin-1, TNF-alpha, and TNF beta, which results in anti-inflammatory activity. *Citrullus lanatus* (watermelon) contains beta-carotene, lycopene, which have antioxidant properties. Furthermore, they play a significant part in the management of cancer and cardiovascular complications. Moreover, the literature states that the chemical constituents of *Citrullus lanatus* are responsible for analgesic and anti-inflammatory, antiulcer, laxative, hepatoprotective, and antimicrobial properties.

Stephania tetrandra S. contains alkaloids, namely, tetrandrine, which shows immunomodulation potential. According to the literature, tetrandrine inhibits the production of P-glycoprotein. Therefore, it efficiently controls the translocation of the nuclear glucocorticoid receptor in selected MOLT-4T cells (Xu et al., 2020). A literature survey suggested that curcumin is utilized as an adjuvant to improve the immunological response of many vaccinations, in addition to its immunostimulatory properties. In a recent survey, curcumin nanoparticles were administered as an adjunct to the Bacillus Calmette–Guérin (BCG) vaccination. As a result, curcumin improved antigen-presenting cell activity as well as inflammatory cytokine production. Therefore, it demonstrated a long-term defense against tuberculosis (Ahmad et al., 2019). Another study recently claimed that curcumin has a neuroprotective impact via different mechanisms. Principally, it includes the activation of microglia migration. In addition, it resulted in a reduction of miR-155, stimulation of phagocytosis of amyloid plaques, and reduced CD33 expression. Accordingly, it boosted TREM2, which actively participated in the microglial cell recruitment. Therefore, curcumin can be used as an anti-Aβ vaccine immunoadjuvant (Teter et al., 2019). Currently, different antioxidants have been reported as immunoadjuvants for different vaccines. Out of plenty of antioxidants, resveratrol has been preferred as an immunomodulatory agent in the treatment of different health issues. Principally, it can be preferred as an immunoadjuvant in the case of the pseudorabies virus vaccine. The combination of resveratrol and the vaccine resulted in the induction of T-lymphocytes, as well as high antibody and cytokine production. Accordingly, there is effective relief from the rabies virus as compared to the bare vaccine (Chen et al., 2019). *Quillaja saponaria* containing QS-21 has been reported as an immunoadjuvant for cancer vaccines. As per the literature, it shows the good potential of an immunoadjuvant because it boosts the antibodies to kill the cancer antigens (Ragupathi et al., 2010). It has been revealed that the administration of curcumin with the Listereaat-Mage-B vaccine for the treatment of metastasis resulted in improved efficacy of the vaccine. Principally, it is because of the rising cell response, mainly CD^{4+} cells and CD^{8+} cells. Moreover, TNBC model 4 T1 shows a decrease in IL-6 levels. Overall, it assured the immunoadjuvant role of the Listereaat-Mage-B vaccine for the effective treatment of metastasis (Singh et al., 2013). Colchicine is derived from plants of the Colchicum (genus), notably *C. autumnale* (*autumn crocus*). As per the literature, colchicine is one of the earliest herbs, having been employed for decades to cure gout. Moreover, it has been reported for plenty of diseases and disorders. Mainly, it blocks the IL-1β maturation, whereas it impedes the activation of the NALP3 inflammasome that is produced by a crystal of monosodium urate (Martinon et al., 2006). In addition, the use of colchicine boosted the activation of nuclear factor-kappa B and dendritic cells that affect the cellular immune response in the body (Mizumoto et al., 2005). It has been disclosed that resveratrol can be used as a potential immunomodulatory agent in the management of several illnesses. The use of resveratrol increases T-lymphocyte proliferation. In addition, it boosted the attenuated cytokines in stimulated spleen cells, resulting in immunomodulatory effects (Feng et al., 2002). Despite this, the incorporation of resveratrol resulted in the protection of STAT3 and ICAM-1 phosphorylation stimulated by IL-6 (Wung et al., 2005). In addition to this, resveratrol preference in the treatment of disease resulted in the suppression of lymphocyte adhesion because of the prevention of nuclear factor-kappa B-containing p65 subunit translocation (Park et al., 2009). Therefore, resveratrol will open a new door for the treatment of immune-related health concerns. Quercetin shows antioxidant potential and is widely utilized in the management of several health issues including cancer, metabolic diseases, inflammation, etc. (Batiha et al., 2020). As per published literature, the use of quercetin demonstrates the suppression of CRP, COX-2, and iNOS in the liver. Principally, it may be because of inhibition of nuclear factor-kappa B activation (García-Mediavilla et al., 2007). In another study, it shows the potential for the regulation of cell-centered immunity. Possibly, it is because of the stimulation of IFN-γ phenotype expression. In addition, it shows the inhibition of Th2-based production of the cytokine IL4 from peripheral blood mononuclear cells (PBMCs) (Nair et al., 2002). Interestingly, lycopene is a carotenoid that is plentiful in plants and fruits. A literature survey reported that lycopene has strong antioxidant capabilities, and because of this, it has been preferred for a variety of medical uses. Mainly, the administration of lycopene works by lowering the levels of IL-6 and IL-8. Moreover, in the case of rhinovirus-induced airway inflammation, lycopene decreases the levels of interferon-gamma-inducible protein and nuclear factor-kappa B (Saedisomeolia et al., 2009). Curcumin has been demonstrated to have a variety of biological functions. It comprises immunomodulatory, antidiabetic, anti-inflammatory, and anticancer properties. It has been confirmed that the application of curcumin mainly influences the development of nonalcoholic fatty liver disease. Herein, curcumin helps modulate the expression of proinflammatory cytokines. It includes the modulation of expressions of tumor necrosis factor-alpha (TNF-α) and interferon γ (IFN-γ) induced by leptin (Inzaugarat et al., 2017). Genistein is identified to be naturally found in soybeans. As per published data, genistein demonstrates chemoprotective ability, whereas it can be used as an antiangiogenic agent. It contains the potential for antityrosine kinase protein properties. It helps to control the regulation of inflammatory markers that resulted in the monitoring of neuroinflammation and high-fat diet-induced gut dysbiosis. Accordingly, it provides better control over cognitive functions (López et al., 2018). In 2014, Li and coauthors divulged the use of alkaloidal drugs, namely, berberine, for a variety of applications. Importantly, berberine provides broad-spectrum action because of nuclear factor-kappa B phosphorylation inhibition and activation of the NRLP3 inflammasome (Mai et al., 2020). Interestingly, in the case of type 1 diabetes, the use of berberine offers the inhibition of lipopolysaccharide-induced inflammation in β-cells. In addition, it significantly reduces the Th1 and Th17-associated cytokines (Li et al., 2014). Yet another investigation confirmed the applicability of berberine in metabolic syndrome. In this case, the utilization of berberine resulted in the modification of inflammatory protein responses. Therefore, it provides relief to patients from several metabolic health issues (Cao and Su, 2019). Since its inception, the use of ginseng has been reported for immune-related health issues as well as it has been widely utilized for cancer treatment, intestinal dysfunction, etc. As per published literature, the use of ginseng offers a boost in splenocyte proliferation. In addition, the action of ginseng resulted in the stimulation of the production of Th1/Th2 cytokines and IgG2a/IgG1. Overall, ginseng shows such changes in a system that might be because of its immunoadjuvant potential (Sun et al., 2007). In 1996, it was reported as an immunoadjuvant for the polyvalent influenza vaccine. Herein, it reduces the chances of infection with the influenza virus based on increasing the capability of a vaccine (Scaglione et al., 1996). It is worthy to mention that the use of ginseng in autoimmune diabetic adults offers better outcomes. Mainly, the use of ginseng with a combination of other naturally obtained actives resulted in the enhanced pancreatic β-cell function. In addition to this, it helps modulate the T-lymphocytes, which offers benefits for the management of autoimmune diabetic conditions (Xu and Zhang, 2008). Overall, the use of plenty of antioxidants has immunosuppressant and immunoadjuvant applications in the biomedical field, as given in Table 4.2.

TABLE 4.2 List of Some Plant-Derived Antioxidants and Their Immunomodulatory Mechanisms.

Sr. no.	Source	Common name	Active constituent	Immune potentiating mechanism	Ref.
1	*Ocimum sanctum Linn. (Labiateae)*	Tulsi	Eugenol	↑IFN-Y, ↑IL-4, ↑Th cells, and ↑NK cells	(Mondal et al., 2011)
2	*Aloe vera Tourn.ex Linn. (Liliaceae)*	Kumaari	Polysaccharides (Acemannan)	↑ of the induction of maturation in immature DCs, ↑mixed lymphocyte reaction, and ↑IL-12	(Lee et al., 2001)
				↑ IL-6, ↑ TNF-γ, ↑surface antigen expression, and ↑IFN- γ	(Zhang and Tizard, 1996)
				↑Scavenge free radicals' survival, ↑mitogenic activity, ↑hematopoiesis, ↑activation of MAPK survival, ↑peripheral lymphocytes, ↑TNF-γ, and ↑IL-1	(Kumar and Kumar, 2019)
3	*Andrographis paniculata Nees (Acanthaceae)*	Kaalmegha	Andrographolide	↑ Proliferation of lymphocytes, ↑ IL-2, ↓TNF-α, ↓IL-β, IL-6, ↓IL-12, ↓IL-18, ↓IL-23, ↑Th-1, ↓Th-2 results in ↓IL-4, and ↓IL-13 with reduced antibody response and inhibition of MHC-1, CD40, CD80, CD86, and manose receptor	(Mishra et al., 2021; Rajagopal et al., 2003)
4	*Asparagus racemosus Wild. (Liliaceae)*	Shatavari	Fructo-oligosaccharides (FOS)	FOS-rich polysaccharide fraction ↑ natural killer cell activity	(Thakur et al., 2012)
5	*Tinospora cordifolia Miers. (Menispermiaceae)*	Amrita, guduuchii	Arabinogalactan	↑production of NO by stimulating splenocytes and macrophages and ↑cytokinenin mediators	(Upadhyaya et al., 2011)
	Panax ginseng Wall. (Araliaceae)	Ninjin	Ginsenosides (Protopanaxidiol)	↑TNF-γ, ↑IL-6, ↑CD29, CD43, ↑CD80, CD86, ↑CD43, CD69, ↑CD80, CD86 ↑TNF-a	(Kim et al., 2019; Shin et al., 2018)
			protopanaxatriol	↑CD3, CD28, and CD69 ↑IL-6, ↑ IL-4	(Lee et al., 2004; Wang et al., 2014)

TABLE 4.2 *(Continued)*

Sr. no.	Source	Common name	Active constituent	Immune potentiating mechanism	Ref.
7	*Achillea millefolium C. Koch (Compositae)*	Yarrow	Essential oils of Achillea millefolium C. Koch	Modulate macrophage production by ↑ NO, ↑H_2O_2, and ↑TNF-α	(Lopes et al., 2003, 2005)
8	*Murraya koenigii (L) Spreng. (Rutaceae)*	Surabhini-nimba	Plant	↑ NO	(Shah et al., 2008)
9	*Lagenaria siceraria Mol. (Cucurbitaceae)*	Katu-tumbi	*p*-hydroxybenzoic acid, gallic acid	↑% Neutrophils	(Mohan and Sanjay, 2014)
10	*Gymnema sylvestre R.Br. (Asclepiadaceae)*	Gurmaar	Methanolic extract of the plant	↑ Phagocytic action by ↑NO, ↑ROS	(Singh et al., 2015)
11	*Heracleum persicum Desf. (Apiaceae)*	Golpar	plant	↑ Th cells, ↑IL-2, ↑INF-γ, and ↑ macrophage	(Atefeh et al., 2010)
12	*Theobroma cacao L.*	Cocoa	Catechin and epicatechin content	↑IFN-γ, ↑IL-2	(Barth et al., 2003; Romagnani, 2004)
13	*Crocus sativus L. (C. sativus)*	Safron	Safranal, Crocin, and Crocetin	↓TNF-α, ↓8-iso-PGF2a, and ↓SP-100 β ↓TNF-α level in diazinon-treated groups, blocking TNF-α-induced Bcl-XS, and caspase-3 mRNA expression	(Hariri et al., 2010; Soeda et al., 2001)
14	*Silybum marianum L. Gaertn.*	Silymarin	Silibin	↑TNF, ↑ iNOS, ↑ IL-1, and ↑IL-6 mRNA ↓IL-2, ↓IL-4	(Johnson et al., 2003)
15	*Spirulina platensis*	Spirulina	plant	↑IL-8, ↑IL-1 β, ↑IL-2, ↑TNF-α, ↑NF-kB, ↑MCP-1, ↑MiP-1α, ↑MiP-1β, ↑IP-10, ↑enzyme cyclo-oxygenase-2, and ↑THP-1	(Maddaly, 2010)

TABLE 4.2 *(Continued)*

Sr. no.	Source	Common name	Active constituent	Immune potentiating mechanism	Ref.
16	*Camellia sinensis L. (Theaceae)*	Tea/Green Tea	Polyphenols	↑IL-17A, ↑IL-8, and ↑HBD-2	(Rahayu et al., 2018b)
17	*Leptospermum scoparium*	Manuka Honey	Quercetin	↓ERK, ↓MAPK, ↓TNF-α, ↓IL-1β, and ↓IL-6	(Cho et al., 2003; Wadsworth et al., 2001)
				↑ IFN-γ, ↓IL-4	(Nair et al., 2002)
			Apigenin	inhibit IFN-γ-mediated STAT1 activation, ↓PD-L1	(Xu et al., 2018)
			Luteolin	↓ERK and p38, ↓TNF-α in LPS-induced murine macrophages, ↓TNF-α, and ↓IFN-γ	(García-Lafuente et al., 2009; Xagorari et al., 2002; Xia et al., 2016)
			Chrysin	↓IL-2, ↓IL-1β, ↓IL-12, ↓IFN-γ, ↓TNF-α, ↓IL-6, and ↓IL-1β	(Shin et al., 2009; Xiao et al., 2014)
			Genistein	↓PD-L1	(Xu et al., 2018)
18	*Turmeric*	Haldi	Curcumin	↓IL-8, ↓MIP-1a, ↓MCP-1, ↓IL-1b, ↓TNF-α, ↓Th-1, and IL-12	(Abe et al., 1999; Kang et al., 1999)
19	*Nigella sativa*	black cumin	Thymoquinone	↓IL-4,↑IFN-γ	(Keyhanmanesh et al., 2010)
20	*Berberis vulgaris*	Common barberry	Berberine	↓ TNF-α, ↓IL-2, ↓ IL-4, and ↓ IL-10	(Lin and Lin, 2011)
				↓ IL-4, ↑ IL-12, and ↑ IFN-γ	(Kim et al., 2003)
21	*Emblica officinalis*	Amla	Vitamin C	↓IL-4, ↓IL-10, ↓TGF-β, ↑IgM, ↑IgY, and ↑IgA	(Shojadoost et al., 2021)

TABLE 4.2 *(Continued)*

Sr. no.	Source	Common name	Active constituent	Immune potentiating mechanism	Ref.
22	*Piper longum*	Indian long pepper	Piperine	↓CD40, ↓CD86, ↓MHC-II, ↓CCR7, ↑CCR5, ↓IL-6, ↓TNF, ↓MCP-1, ↓IFN-γ, ↓IL-4, ↓IL-17, and ↓IL-2.	(Rodgers et al., 2009)
23	*Syzygium aromaticum*	Clove	Eugenol	↓NO, ↓TNF α, and ↑IL-6	(Dibazar et al., 2015)
24	*Vitis vinifera (Vitaceae)*	Grapes	Resveratrol	↓TGF-β, ↓ IFN-γ, ↓IL-12, ↓IL-10, ↓IL-6, ↓pSTAT-3, and NF-kB	
	Vaccinium corym-bosum (Ericaceae)	Blueberries			(Davoodvandi et al., 2020; Fei et al., 2018; Zhang et al., 2020, 2019)
	Rubus idaeus (Rosaceae)	Raspberries			
	Morus alba (Moraceae)	Mulberries			
25	*Arachis hypogaea (Fabaceae)*	Peanuts	Resveratrol	↓TGF-β, ↓ IFN-γ, ↓IL-12, ↓IL-10, ↓IL-6, ↓pSTAT-3, and NF-kB	(Jeong et al., 2012)

Abbreviations: IL: interleukin, ERKs: extracellular signal-regulated kinases, MAPKs: mitogen-activated protein kinases, IFN-γ: interferon gamma, PD-L1: programed death-ligand 1, Th cells: T helper cells, NK cells: Natural killer cells, TNF: Tumor Necrosis Factor, MHC-1: Major histocompatibility complex, NO: Nitrous Oxide, H2O2: Hydrogen Peroxide, ROS: Reactive oxygen species, THP-1: spontaneously immortalized monocyte-like cell line 1, hBD-2: Human beta-defensin-2, STAT: Signal Transducer and Activator of Transcription, NF-kB: Nuclear factor kappa B, TGF: Transforming growth factor, Ig: Immunoglobin, ↑: Upregulation, ↓: Downregulation

4.4 CURRENT CHALLENGES AND FUTURE PROSPECTS

It is crystal clear that the existence of free radicals and associated species has gained huge consideration from researchers. Particularly, the origin of such species is nitrogen and oxygen-derived. It is revealed that the pathophysiological conditions, physiochemical alternation, etc. are the endogenous systems that resulted in the generation of free radicals. As a result, it affects the nature of proteins, DNA, lipids, etc., and finally, it is converted into a disease state. Immunomodulation has risen to prominence across the globe as people recognized the significance of the immune system in maintaining a disease-free state. Immune system modification depicts the alteration of the immune response that includes induction, expression, and amplification of the immune response phase. For example, immune response stimulation is important in immunocompromised patients. Besides this, immune response suppression is a leading need in the case of several autoimmune diseases, allergic conditions, etc. In these cases, the antioxidant offers plenty of benefits for modulating the immune response related to their needs. Despite their plentiful benefits, the negative effects of antioxidants could be ascribed to the incorrect assortment of antioxidants. Importantly, it may be because we do not take into account the immunological foundation of the disease. Additionally, the immunological dynamics of the pharmacological agents containing antioxidant activity also need to be authenticated. Ultimately, treatment must be selected depending on the immunopharmacology of the antioxidant medication as well as the immunological foundation of the illness. As a result, it is proposed that future antioxidant research should concentrate on immuno-oxidative pathobiology to truly comprehend its therapeutic potential and efficacy, as well as economical clinical care. With a phase of investigation on oxidants and antioxidants, it is appropriate to focus specifically on the domains. In this vein, more solid evidence is needed to validate the hypothesis that the majority (if not all) of illnesses are caused by radical damage. Importantly, the belief that antioxidants may prevent or treat a variety of pathological conditions has to be reconsidered as well. The comparatively new finding that compounds with high antioxidant activity (by in vitro study) might well have nonantioxidant impacts on cells and tissues, which must encourage, rather than deter, more study in this area. Many investigations reveal that the use of a single antioxidant may not be that beneficial for the management of different chronic diseases. In this regard, there is a necessity to use a combination of two or more antioxidants for modulation of the immune response. Herein, the optimization of the concentration of antioxidants is a crucial step for researchers. Despite abundant development in research of different natural antioxidants for modulation of the immune response, there is a prime urge to complete preclinical and clinical investigations for further potential applications. Hence, it will open a fresh era for researchers to investigate the combination of antioxidants for the effective management of severe health issues.

4.5 CONCLUSIONS

Antioxidants show the ability to defend against the severe harm caused by the existence of plenty of free radicals and other reactive species at various levels. Particularly, the link involving free radicals, antioxidants, and the functioning of numerous organs/organ systems is extremely complicated. Herein, the revelation of redox signaling represents a watershed moment in this critical relationship. Emphasis is being placed on several techniques for protecting vital tissues and organs from oxidative damage caused by free radicals. Many innovative techniques have been developed by scientific fraternities. Additionally, major discoveries have been achieved in recent years. In this book chapter, we have illustrated the immunomodulation properties of antioxidants, which include the basics of immunomodulation, antioxidant defenses, and the application of plenty of antioxidants in immunomodulation. Moreover, the current updates in antioxidants as immunomodulators have reflected significant advancements. It is crystal clear that the antioxidant exhibited immunomodulatory properties that may vary with dose and time, which necessitates confirmation before treatment of any illness. Despite this, the negative results of antioxidants could be ascribed to the erroneous assortment of respective antioxidants. Especially, it may be because of the lack of accountability for the immunological foundation of disease. In the future, this book chapter will unlock an innovative window for academicians and industry researchers to investigate the immunomodulation properties of naturally present antioxidants.

CONFLICT OF INTEREST

None to declare

ACKNOWLEDGMENT

The authors are grateful to the management and principal of the SVKM Institute of Pharmacy, Dhule, for allowing them to accomplish the task efficiently.

KEYWORDS

- **antioxidant**
- **immunomodulator**
- **immune system**
- **free radicals**
- **antioxidant defense**

REFERENCES

Abe, Y.; Hashimoto, S.; Horie, T. Curcumin Inhibition of Inflammatory Cytokine Production by Human Peripheral Blood Monocytes and Alveolar Macrophages. *Pharmacol. Res.* **1999,** *39,* 41–47.

Agarwal, S.; Singh, V. Immunomodulators: A Review of Studies on Indian Medicinal Plants and Synthetic Peptides. Part - I: Medicinal Plants. *Proc. Indian Nat. Sci. Acad. - Part B: Biol. Sci.* **1999,** *B65,* 179–204.

Aher, V. D.; Wahi, A.; Pawdey, A. M.; Sonawane, A. Antioxidants as Immunomodulator: An Expanding Research Avenue. *Int. J. Curr. Pharm. Res.* **2011,** *3,* 8–10.

Ahmad, S.; Bhattacharya, D.; Kar, S.; Ranganathan, A.; Van Kaer, L.; Das, G. Curcumin Nanoparticles Enhance Mycobacterium bovis BCG Vaccine Efficacy by Modulating Host Immune Responses. *Infect. Immun.* **2019,** 87.

Ajith, Y.; Dimri, U.; Dixit, S. K.; Singh, S. K.; Gopalakrishnan, A.; Madhesh, E.; Rajesh, J. B.; Sangeetha, S. G. Immunomodulatory Basis of Antioxidant Therapy and Its Future Prospects: An Appraisal. *Inflammopharmacology* **2017,** *25,* 487–498.

Alkadi, H. A Review on Free Radicals and Antioxidants. *Infec. Disord. - Drug Targets* **2020,** *20,* 16–26.

Alzohairy, M. A. Therapeutics Role of Azadirachta indica (Neem) and Their Active Constituents in Diseases Prevention and Treatment. *Evid-Based Complement. Altern. Med. : ECAM.* **2016,** 2016.

Atefeh, H.; Azamia, M.; Abdolhamid-Angaj, S. Medicinal Effects of Heracleum Persicum (Golpar). *Middle-East J. Sci. Res.* **2010,** *5,* 174–176.

Barth, H.; Berg, P. A.; Klein, R. Methods for the In Vitro Determination of An Individual Disposition Towards TH1- or TH2-Reactivity by the Application of Appropriate Stimulatory Antigens. *Clin. Exp. Immunol.* **2003,** *134,* 78–85.

Batiha, G. E.-S.; Beshbishy, A. M.; Ikram, M.; Mulla, Z. S.; El-Hack, M. E. A.; Taha, A. E.; Algammal, A. M.; Elewa, Y. H. A. The Pharmacological Activity, Biochemical Properties, and Pharmacokinetics of the Major Natural Polyphenolic Flavonoid: Quercetin. *Foods.* **2020,** *9,* 374.

Boroumand, N.; Samarghandian, S.; Hashemy, S. I. Immunomodulatory, anti-inflammatory, and antioxidant effects of curcumin. *J. Herbmed Pharmacol.* **2018,** *7,* 211–219.

Cao, C.; Su, M. Effects of Berberine on Glucose-Lipid Metabolism, Inflammatory Factors and Insulin Resistance in Patients with Metabolic Syndrome. *Exp. Ther. Med.* 2019.

Catanzaro, M.; Corsini, E.; Rosini, M.; Racchi, M.; Lanni, C. Immunomodulators Inspired by Nature: A Review on Curcumin and Echinacea. *Molecules.* **2018,** *23,* 2778.

Chen, M.; Chen, X.; Song, X.; Muhammad, A.; Jia, R.; Zou, Y.; Yin, L.; Li, L.; He, C.; Ye, G.; et al. The Immune-Adjuvant Activity and the Mechanism of Resveratrol on Pseudorabies Virus Vaccine in a Mouse Model. *Int. Immunopharmacol.* **2019,** *76,* 105876.

Cho, S.-Y.; Park, S.-J.; Kwon, M.-J.; Jeong, T.-S.; Bok, S.-H.; Choi, W.-Y.; Jeong, W.-I.; Ryu, S.-Y.; Do, S.-H.; Lee, C.-S.; et al. Quercetin Suppresses Proinflammatory Cytokines Production Through MAP Kinases and NF-κB Pathway in Lipopolysaccharide-Stimulated Macrophage. *Mol. Cell. Biochem.* **2003,** *243,* 153–160.

Davoodvandi, A.; Darvish, M.; Borran, S.; Nejati, M.; Mazaheri, S.; Reza Tamtaji, O.; Hamblin, M. R.; Masoudian, N.; Mirzaei, H. The Therapeutic Potential of Resveratrol in a Mouse Model of Melanoma Lung Metastasis. *Int. Immunopharmacol.* **2020,** *88,* 106905.

Devasagayam, T. P. A.; Tilak, J. C.; Boloor, K. K.; Sane, K. S.; Ghaskadbi, S. S.; Lele, R. D. Free Radicals and Antioxidants in Human Health: Current Status and Future Prospects. *J. Assoc. Physicians. India* **2004,** *52,* 4.

Dibazar, S. P.; Fateh, S.; Daneshmandi, S. Immunomodulatory Effects of Clove (Syzygium aromaticum) Constituents on Macrophages: In Vitro Evaluations of Aqueous and Ethanolic Components. *J. Immunotoxicol.* **2015,** *12,* 124–131.

Dröge, W. Free Radicals in the Physiological Control of Cell Function. *Physiol. Rev.* **2002,** *82,* 47–95.

Esmaeil, N.; Anaraki, S. B.; Gharagozloo, M.; Moayedi, B. Silymarin Impacts on Immune System as an Immunomodulator: One Key for Many Locks. *Int. Immunopharmacol.* **2017,** *50,* 194–201.

Fei, X.; Wang, A.; Wang, D.; Meng, X.; Ma, J.; Hong, L.; Qin, R.; Wang, A.; Dong, J.; Huang, Q.; et al. Establishment of Malignantly Transformed Dendritic Cell Line SU3-ihDCTC Induced by Glioma Stem Cells and Study on Its Sensitivity to Resveratrol. *BMC Immunol.* **2018,** *19,* 7.

Feng, Y.-H.; Zhou, W.-L.; Wu, Q.-L.; Li, X.-Y.; Zhao, W.-M.; Zou, J.-P. Low Dose of Resveratrol Enhanced Immune Response of Mice. *Acta Pharmacol. Sinica.* **2002,** *23,* 893–897.

Florence, T. M. The Role of Free Radicals in Disease. *Aust. New Z. J. Ophthalmol.* **1995,** *23,* 3–7.

Foroutan-Rad, M.; Tappeh, K. H.; Khademvatan, S. Antileishmanial and Immunomodulatory Activity of Allium sativum (Garlic). *J. Evid. Based Complementary Altern. Med.* **2017,** *22,* 141–155.

García-Lafuente, A.; Guillamón, E.; Villares, A.; Rostagno, M. A.; Martínez, J. A. Flavonoids as Anti-Inflammatory Agents: Implications in Cancer and Cardiovascular Disease. *Inflamm. Res.* **2009,** *58,* 537–552.

García-Mediavilla, V.; Crespo, I.; Collado, P. S.; Esteller, A.; Sánchez-Campos, S.; Tuñón, M. J.; González-Gallego, J. The Anti-Inflammatory Flavones Quercetin and Kaempferol Cause Inhibition of Inducible Nitric Oxide Synthase, Cyclooxygenase-2 and Reactive C-protein, and down-Regulation of the Nuclear Factor kappaB Pathway in Chang Liver cells. *Eur. J. Pharm.* **2007,** *557,* 221–229.

Halliwell, B.; Gutteridge, J. M. C. *Free Radicals in Biology and Medicine*; Oxford University Press: USA.

Hariri, A. T.; Moallem, S. A.; Mahmoudi, M.; Memar, B.; Hosseinzadeh, H. Sub-Acute Effects of Diazinon on Biochemical Indices and Specific Biomarkers in Rats: Protective Effects of Crocin and Safranal. *Food Chem. Toxicol.* **2010,** *48,* 2803–2808.

Hemalatha, R.; Babu, K. N.; Karthik, M.; Ramesh, R.; Kumar, B. D.; Kumar, P. U. Immunomodulatory Activity and Th1/Th2 Cytokine Response of Ocimum sanctum in Myelosuppressed Swiss Albino Mice. *Trends Med. Res.* **2011,** *6,* 23–31.

Inzaugarat, M. E.; De Matteo, E.; Baz, P.; Lucero, D.; García, C. C.; Gonzalez Ballerga, E.; Daruich, J.; Sorda, J. A.; Wald, M. R.; Cherñavsky, A. C. New Evidence for the Therapeutic Potential of Curcumin to Treat Nonalcoholic Fatty Liver Disease in Humans. *PLoS One.* **2017,** *12,* e0172900.

Jantan, I.; Ahmad, W.; Bukhari, S. N. A. Plant-derived Immunomodulators: An Insight on Their Preclinical Evaluation and Clinical Trials. *Front. Plant Sci..* **2015,** 6,.

Jeong, M. H.; Yang, K. M.; Choi, Y. J.; Kim, S. D.; Yoo, Y. H.; Seo, S. Y.; Lee, S. H.; Ryu, S. R.; Lee, C. M.; Suh, H. suk; et al. Resveratrol Analog, HS-1793 Enhance Anti-Tumor Immunity by Reducing the CD4+CD25+ Regulatory T Cells in FM3A Tumor Bearing Mice. *Int. Immunopharmacol.* **2012,** *14,* 328–333.

Johnson, V.; He, Q.; Osuchowski, M.; Sharma, R. Physiological Responses of a Natural Antioxidant Flavonoid Mixture, Silymarin, in BALB/c Mice. *Planta Med.* **2003,** *69,* 44–49.

Kagan, V. E.; Kisin, E. R.; Kawai, K.; Serinkan, B. F.; Osipov, A. N.; Serbinova, E. A.; Wolinsky, I.; Shvedova, A. A. Toward Mechanism-based Antioxidant Interventions. *Ann. N. Y. Acad. Sci.* **2002,** *959,* 188–198.

Kang, B. Y.; Song, Y. J.; Kim, K.-M.; Choe, Y. K.; Hwang, S. Y.; Kim, T. S. Curcumin Inhibits Th1 Cytokine Profile in CD4 + T cells by Suppressing Interleukin-12 Production in Macrophages. *Br. J. Pharm.* **1999,** *128,* 380–384.

Kehrer, J. P.; Klotz, L.-O. Free Radicals and Related Reactive Species as Mediators of Tissue Injury and Disease: Implications for Health. *Crit. Rev. Toxicol.* **2015,** *45,* 765–798.

Keservani, R. K.; Sharma, A. K. Flavonoids: Emerging Trends and Potential Health Benefits. *J. Chin. Pharm. Sci.* **2014,** *23* (12), 815.

Keservani, R. K.; Sharma, A. K.; Kesharwani, R. K. Nutraceutical and Functional Foods for Cardiovascular Health. In *Food Process Engineering (pp. 291–312)*; Apple Academic Press, CRC Press, 2016a; pp 257–278.

Keservani, R. K.; Sharma, A. K.; Kesharwani, R. K. Medicinal Effect of Nutraceutical Fruits for the Cognition and Brain Health. *Scientifica* **2016b;** *2016,* 3109254. DOI: 10.1155/2016/3109254.

Keyhanmanesh, R.; Boskabady, M. H.; Khamneh, S.; Doostar, Y. Effect of Thymoquinone on the Lung Pathology and Cytokine Levels of Ovalbumin-Sensitized Guinea Pigs. *Pharmacol. Rep.* **2010,** *62,* 910–916.

Kim; Doo; Jeong; Kim; Lee; Yang; Lee; Kim; Lee; Huh; et al. Enhancing Immunomodulatory Function of Red Ginseng Through Fermentation Using Bifidobacterium Animalis Subsp. lactis LT 19-2. *Nutrients.* **2019,** *11,* 1481.

Kim, T. S.; Kang, B. Y.; Cho, D.; Kim, S. H. Induction of Interleukin-12 Production in Mouse Macrophages by Berberine, A Benzodioxoloquinolizine Alkaloid, Deviates CD4+ T Cells from a Th2 to a Th1 Response. *Immunology*. **2003,** *109,* 407–414.

Knight, J. A. Free Radicals, Antioxidants, and the Immune System. *Ann. Clin. Lab. Sci.* **2000,** *30,* 145–158.

Kumar, D.; Arya, V.; Kaur, R.; Bhat, Z. A.; Gupta, V. K.; Kumar, V. A Review of Immunomodulators in the Indian Traditional Health Care System. *J. Microbiol. Immunol. Infec.* **2012,** *45,* 165–184.

Kumar, S.; Kumar, R. Role of Acemannan O-acetyl Group in Murine Radioprotection. *Carbohydr. Polym.* **2019,** *207,* 460–470.

Lee, E.; Ko, E.; Lee, J.; Rho, S.; Ko, S.; Shin, M.-K.; Min, B.; Hong, M.-C.; Kim, S.; Bae, H. Ginsenoside Rg1 Enhances CD4+ T-cell Activities and Modulates Th1/Th2 Differentiation. *Int. Immunopharmacol.* **2004,** *4,* 235–244.

Lee, J. K.; Lee, M. K.; Yun, Y.-P.; Kim, Y.; Kim, J. S.; Kim, Y. S.; Kim, K.; Han, S. S.; Lee, C.-K. Acemannan Purified from Aloe Vera Induces Phenotypic and Functional Maturation of Immature Dendritic Cells. *Int. Immunopharmacol.* **2001,** *1,* 1275–1284.

Li, Z.; Geng, Y.-N.; Jiang, J.-D.; Kong, W.-J. Antioxidant and Anti-Inflammatory Activities of Berberine in the Treatment of Diabetes Mellitus. *J. Evid. Based Complementary Altern. Med.* **2014,** *2014,* 1–12.

Lin, W.-C.; Lin, J.-Y. Berberine Down-Regulates the Th1/Th2 Cytokine Gene Expression Ratio in Mouse Primary Splenocytes in the Absence or Presence of Lipopolysaccharide in a Preventive Manner. *Int. Immunopharmacol.* **2011,** *11,* 1984–1990.

Liu, S.; Wang, L.; Ren, Q.; Wang, J.; Li, Y.; Wang, G.; Gao, H.; Du, R.; Qin, W. Immunomodulatory and Antioxidant Activities of a Polysaccharide from Ligustrum vicaryi L. Fruit. *J. Evid. Based Complementary Altern. Med.* **2020,** *2020,* 1–10.

Lobo, V.; Patil, A.; Phatak, A.; Chandra, N. Free Radicals, Antioxidants and Functional Foods: Impact on Human Health. *Pharmacogn. Rev.* **2010,** *4,* 118.

Londhe, V. P.; Gavasane A T; Nipate S S; Bandawane D D; Chaudhari P D Role of Garlic (Allium Sativum) In Various Diseases: An Overview. *J. Pharm. Res. Opin.* **2011,** *1,* 129–134.

Lopes, F. C. M.; Benzatti, F. P.; Jordão Junior, C. M.; Moreira, R. R. D.; Carlos, I. Z. Effect of the Essential oil of Achillea Millefolium L. in the Production of Hydrogen Peroxide and Tumor Necrosis Factor-Alpha in Murine Macrophages. *Rev. Bras. Clienc. Farm.* **2005,** *41,* 401–405.

Lopes, F. C. M.; Placeres, M. P.; Moreira, R. R. D.; Santos, L. E. dos; Carlos, I. Z. Avaliação da Atividade imunológica de Achillea Millefolium L. ('mil-folhas'). *Rev. Bras. Farmacogn.*. **2003,** *13,* 11–13.

López, P.; Sánchez, M.; Perez-Cruz, C.; Velázquez-Villegas, L. A.; Syeda, T.; Aguilar-López, M.; Rocha-Viggiano, A. K.; del Carmen Silva-Lucero, M.; Torre-Villalvazo, I.; Noriega, L. G.; et al. Long-Term Genistein Consumption Modifies Gut Microbiota, Improving Glucose Metabolism, Metabolic Endotoxemia, and Cognitive Function in Mice Fed a High-Fat Diet. *Mol. Nutr. Food Res.* **2018,** *62,* 1800313.

Maddaly, R. The Beneficial Effects of Spirulina Focusing on its Immunomodulatory and Antioxidant properties. *Nutr. Diet. Suppl.* **2010,** 73.

Maggini, S.; Pierre, A.; Calder, P. Immune Function and Micronutrient Requirements Change over the Life Course. *Nutrients* **2018,** *10,* 1531.

Mahima; M. Ingle, A.; Verma, A. K.; Tiwari, R.; Karthik, K.; Chakrabort, S.; Deb, R.; Rajagunala, S.; Rathore, R.; Dhama, K. Immunomodulators in Day to Day Life: A Review. *Pak. J. Biol. Sci.* **2013,** *16,* 826–843.

Mai, W.; Xu, Y.; Xu, J.; Zhao, D.; Ye, L.; Yu, G.; Wang, Z.; Lu, Q.; Lin, J.; Yang, T.; et al. Berberine Inhibits Nod-Like Receptor Family Pyrin Domain Containing 3 Inflammasome Activation and Pyroptosis in Nonalcoholic Steatohepatitis via the ROS/TXNIP Axis. *Front. Pharmacol.* **2020,** 11.

Marshall, J. S.; Warrington, R.; Watson, W.; Kim, H. L. An Introduction to Immunology and Immunopathology. *Allergy, Asthma Clin. Immunol.* **2018,** *14,* 49.

Martinon, F.; Pétrilli, V.; Mayor, A.; Tardivel, A.; Tschopp, J. Gout-Associated Uric Acid Crystals Activate the NALP3 Inflammasome. *Nature* **2006,** *440,* 237–241.

Di Meo, S.; Venditti, P. Evolution of the Knowledge of Free Radicals and Other Oxidants. *Oxid. Med. Cell. Longev.* **2020,** *2020,* 1–32.

Miles, E. A.; Calder, P. C. Effects of Citrus Fruit Juices and Their Bioactive Components on Inflammation and Immunity: A Narrative Review. *Front. Immunol.* **2021,** *12,* 2558.

Mishra, A.; Shaik, H. A.; Sinha, R. K.; Shah, B. R. Andrographolide: A Herbal-Chemosynthetic Approach for Enhancing Immunity, Combating Viral Infections, and Its Implication on Human Health. *Molecules* **2021,** *26,* 7036.

Mizumoto, N.; Gao, J.; Matsushima, H.; Ogawa, Y.; Tanaka, H.; Takashima, A. Discovery of Novel Immunostimulants by Dendritic-Cell–Based Functional Screening. *Blood.* **2005,** *106,* 3082–3089.

Mohan, G. K.; Sanjay, J. S. Free Radical Scavenging, Immunomodulatory Activity and Chemical Composition of Luffa Acutangula Var: Amara (Cucurbitaceae) Pericarp. *J. Chil. Chem. Soc.* **2014,** *59,* 2299–2302.

Mondal, S.; Varma, S.; Bamola, V. D.; Naik, S. N.; Mirdha, B. R.; Padhi, M. M.; Mehta, N.; Mahapatra, S. C. Double-Blinded Randomized Controlled Trial for Immunomodulatory Effects of Tulsi (Ocimum sanctum Linn.) Leaf Extract on Healthy Volunteers. *J. Ethnopharmacol.* **2011,** *136,* 452–456.

Mousavi, S.; Bereswill, S.; Heimesaat, M. M. Immunomodulatory and Antimicrobial Effects of Vitamin C. *Eur. J. Microbiol. Immunol.* **2019,** *9,* 73–79.

Nair, A.; Chattopadhyay, D.; Saha, B. Plant-Derived Immunomodulators. In *New Look to Phytomedicine*; Elsevier, 2019; pp 435–499.

Nair, M. P.; Kandaswami, C.; Mahajan, S.; Chadha, K. C.; Chawda, R.; Nair, H.; Kumar, N.; Nair, R. E.; Schwartz, S. A. The Flavonoid, Quercetin, Differentially Regulates Th-1 (IFNγ) and Th-2 (IL4) Cytokine Gene Expression by Normal Peripheral Blood Mononuclear Cells. *Biochim. Biophys. Acta.* **2002,** *1593,* 29–36.

Neha, K.; Haider, M. R.; Pathak, A.; Yar, M. S. Medicinal Prospects of Antioxidants: A Review. *Eur. J. Med. Chem.* **2019,** *178,* 687–704.

Netea, M. G.; Domínguez-Andrés, J.; Barreiro, L. B.; Chavakis, T.; Divangahi, M.; Fuchs, E.; Joosten, L. A. B.; van der Meer, J. W. M.; Mhlanga, M. M.; Mulder, W. J. M.; et al. Defining Trained Immunity and its Role in Health and Disease. *Nat. Rev. Immunol.* **2020,** *20,* 375–388.

P Prakash, N. G. Therapeutic uses of Ocimum Sanctum Linn (Tulsi) with a Note on Eugenol and its Pharmacological Actions: A Short Review. *Indian J. Physiol. Pharmacol.* **2005,** *49,* 125–131.

Park, H.-J.; Jeong, S.-K.; Kim, S.-R.; Bae, S.-K.; Kim, W.-S.; Jin, S.-D.; Koo, T. H.; Jang, H.-O.; Yun, I.; Kim, K.-W.; et al. Resveratrol Inhibits Porphyromonas Gingivalis

Lipopolysaccharide-Induced Endothelial Adhesion Molecule Expression by Suppressing NF-κB Activation. *Arch. Pharm. Res.* **2009,** *32,* 583–591.

Pathak, S.; Fillah Fithria, R.; Hariyadi, D. M.; Pathak, Y. Immunomodulation Using Natural Products To Provide Innate Immunity To Ageing Populations As Preventive Measure For Covid-19. *Curr. Trends Pharm. Res.* **2020,** 7.

Phaniendra, A.; Jestadi, D. B.; Periyasamy, L. Free Radicals: Properties, Sources, Targets, and Their Implication in Various Diseases. *Indian J. Clin. Biochem.* **2015,** *30,* 11–26.

Pise, M. V.; Rudra, J. A.; Upadhyay, A. Immunomodulatory Potential of Shatavarins Produced from Asparagus Racemosus Tissue Cultures. *J. Nat. Sci. Biol. Med.* **2015,** *6,* 415–420.

Radha, M. H.; Laxmipriya, N. P. Evaluation of Biological Properties and Clinical Effectiveness of Aloe Vera: A Systematic Review. *J. Tradit. Complement. Med.* **2015,** *5,* 21–26.

Ragupathi, G.; Damani, P.; Deng, K.; Adams, M. M.; Hang, J.; George, C.; Livingston, P. O.; Gin, D. Y. Preclinical Evaluation of the Synthetic Adjuvant SQS-21 and its Constituent Isomeric Saponins. *Vaccine* **2010,** *28,* 4260–4267.

Rahayu, R. P.; Prasetyo, R. A.; Purwanto, D. A.; Kresnoadi, U.; Iskandar, R. P. D.; Rubianto, M. The Immunomodulatory Effect of Green Tea (Camellia sinensis) Leaves Extract on Immunocompromised Wistar Rats Infected by Candida Albicans. *Vet. World.* **2018a**, *11,* 765–770.

Rahayu, R. P.; Prasetyo, R. A.; Purwanto, D. A.; Kresnoadi, U.; Iskandar, R. P. D.; Rubianto, M. The Immunomodulatory Effect of Green Tea (Camellia sinensis) Leaves Extract on Immunocompromised Wistar Rats Infected by Candida albicans. *Vet. World.* **2018b**, *11,* 765–770.

Rajagopal, S.; Kumar, R. A.; Deevi, D. S.; Satyanarayana, C.; Rajagopalan, R. Andrographolide, a Potential Cancer Therapeutic Agent Isolated from Andrographis Paniculata. *J. Exp. Ther. Oncol.* **2003,** *3,* 147–158.

Reyes-Fermín, L. M.; Aparicio-Trejo, O. E.; Avila-Rojas, S. H.; Gómez-Sierra, T.; Martínez-Klimova, E.; Pedraza-Chaverri, J. Natural Antioxidants' Effects on Endoplasmic Reticulum Stress-Related Diseases. *Food Chem. Toxicol.* **2020,** *138,* 111229.

Rizk, J. G.; Kalantar-Zadeh, K.; Mehra, M. R.; Lavie, C. J.; Rizk, Y.; Forthal, D. N. Pharmaco-Immunomodulatory Therapy in COVID-19. *Drugs 2020 80:13.* **2020,** *80,* 1267–1292.

Rodgers, G.; Doucette, C. D.; Spurrell, D. R.; Hoskin, D. W.; West, K. A.; Liwski, R. S. Immunomodulatory Effects of Piperine on Dendritic Cell Function (50.36). *J. Immunol.* **2009,** *182,* 50.36 LP-50.36.

Romagnani, S. Immunologic Influences on Allergy and the TH1/TH2 Balance. *J. Allergy Clin. Immunol.* **2004,** *113,* 395–400.

Saedisomeolia, A.; Wood, L. G.; Garg, M. L.; Gibson, P. G.; Wark, P. A. B. Lycopene Enrichment of Cultured Airway Epithelial Cells Decreases the Inflammation Induced by Rhinovirus Infection and Lipopolysaccharide. *J. Nutr. Biochem.* **2009,** *20,* 577–585.

Sandner, G.; Heckmann, M.; Weghuber, J. Immunomodulatory Activities of Selected Essential Oils. *Biomolecules* **2020,** *10,* 1139.

Scaglione, F.; Cattaneo, G.; Alessandria, M.; Cogo, R. Efficacy and Safety of the Standardised Ginseng Extract G115 for Potentiating Vaccination Against the Influenza Syndrome and Protection against the common cold [corrected]. *Drugs under Exp. Clin. Res.* **1996,** *22,* 65–72.

Schäfer, G.; Kaschula, C. The Immunomodulation and Anti-Inflammatory Effects of Garlic Organosulfur Compounds in Cancer Chemoprevention. *Rev. Bras. Farmacogn.* **2014,** *14,* 233–240.

Shah, A. S.; Wakade, A. S.; Juvekar, A. R. Immunomodulatory Activity of Methanolic Extract of Murraya Koenigii (L) Spreng. Leaves. *Indian J. Exp. Biol.* **2008,** *46,* 505–509.

Sharma, G. N.; Gupta, G.; Sharma, P. A Comprehensive Review of Free Radicals, Antioxidants, and Their Relationship with Human Ailments. *Crit. Rev. Eukar. Gene Expression* **2018,** *28,* 139–154.

Shin, E. K.; Kwon, H.-S.; Kim, Y. H.; Shin, H.-K.; Kim, J.-K. Chrysin, A Natural Flavone, Improves Murine Inflammatory Bowel Diseases. *Biochem. Biophys. Res. Commun.* **2009,** *381,* 502–507.

Shin, M.-S.; Song, J. H.; Choi, P.; Lee, J. H.; Kim, S.-Y.; Shin, K.-S.; Ham, J.; Kang, K. S. Stimulation of Innate Immune Function by Panax Ginseng after Heat Processing. *J. Agric. Food Chem.* **2018,** *66,* 4652–4659.

Shojadoost, B.; Yitbarek, A.; Alizadeh, M.; Kulkarni, R. R.; Astill, J.; Boodhoo, N.; Sharif, S. Centennial Review: Effects of Vitamins A, D, E, and C on the Chicken Immune System. *Poult. Sci.* **2021,** *100,* 100930.

Singh, M.; Ramos, I.; Asafu-Adjei, D.; Quispe-Tintaya, W.; Chandra, D.; Jahangir, A.; Zang, X.; Aggarwal, B. B.; Gravekamp, C. Curcumin Improves the Therapeutic Efficacy of Listeria-Mage-b Vaccine in Correlation with Improved T-cell Responses in Blood of a Triple-Negative Breast Cancer Model 4T1. *Cancer Med.* **2013,** *2,* 571–582.

Singh, V. K.; Dwivedi, P.; Chaudhary, B. R.; Singh, R. Immunomodulatory Effect of Gymnema sylvestre (R.Br.) Leaf Extract: An In Vitro Study in Rat Model. *PlOS ONE.* **2015,** *10,* e0139631.

Soeda, S.; Ochiai, T.; Paopong, L.; Tanaka, H.; Shoyama, Y.; Shimeno, H. Crocin Suppresses Tumor Necrosis Factor-α-induced Cell Death of Neuronally differentiated PC-12 cells. *Life Sci.* **2001,** *69,* 2887–2898.

Sun, J.; Hu, S.; Song, X. Adjuvant Effects of Protopanaxadiol and Protopanaxatriol Saponins from Ginseng Roots on the Immune Responses to Ovalbumin in Mice. *Vaccine.* **2007,** *25,* 1114–1120.

Supriyanto, S.; Widjanarko, S. B.; Rifa'i, M.; Yunianta, Y. Immunomodulatory Activity of Methanol Leaf Extract of Neem (*Azadirachta indica* Juss) Against Suppressor and Proinflammatory Molecules. *J. Trop. Life Sci.* **2021,** *11,* 309–315.

Taniguchi, Y.; Yoshioka, N.; Nakata, K.; Nishizawa, T.; Inagawa, H.; Kohchi, C.; Soma, G. I. Mechanism for Maintaining Homeostasis in the Immune System of the Intestine. *Anticancer Res.* **2009,** *29,* 4855–4860.

Teter, B.; Morihara, T.; Lim, G. P.; Chu, T.; Jones, M. R.; Zuo, X.; Paul, R. M.; Frautschy, S. A.; Cole, G. M. Curcumin Restores Innate Immune Alzheimer's Disease Risk Gene Expression to Ameliorate Alzheimer Pathogenesis. *Neurobiol. Dis.* **2019,** *127,* 432–448.

Thakur, M.; Connellan, P.; Deseo, M. A.; Morris, C.; Praznik, W.; Loeppert, R.; Dixit, V. K. Characterization and in Vitro Immunomodulatory Screening of Fructo-Oligosaccharides of Asparagus Racemosus Willd. *Int. J. Biol. Macromol.* **2012,** *50,* 77–81.

Ülger, T. G.; Songur, A. N.; Çırak, O.; Çakıroğlu, F. P. Role of Vegetables in Human Nutrition and Disease Prevention. In *Vegetables—Importance of Quality Vegetables to Human Health*; InTech, 2018; p.

Upadhyaya R.; Pandey R. P.; Sharma V. V. A. K. Assessment of the Multifaceted Immunomodulatory Potential of the Aqueous Extract of Tinospora Cordifolia. *Res. J. Chem. Sci.* **2011,** *1,* 71–79.

Vivekananthan, D. P.; Penn, M. S.; Sapp, S. K.; Hsu, A.; Topol, E. J. Use of Antioxidant Vitamins for the Prevention of Cardiovascular Disease: Meta-Analysis of Randomised Trials. *Lancet.* **2003,** *361,* 2017–2023.

Wadsworth, T. L.; McDonald, T. L.; Koop, D. R. Effects of Ginkgo Biloba Extract (EGb 761) and Quercetin on Lipopolysaccharide-Induced Signaling Pathways Involved in the Release of Tumor Necrosis Factor-α 1 1Abbreviations: EGb 761, Ginkgo Biloba Extract; LPS, Lipopolysaccharide; ROIs, Reactive Oxygen i. *Biochem. Pharmacol.* **2001,** *62,* 963–974.

Wang, Y.; Liu, Y.; Zhang, X.-Y.; Xu, L.-H.; Ouyang, D.-Y.; Liu, K.-P.; Pan, H.; He, J.; He, X.-H. Ginsenoside Rg1 Regulates Innate Immune Responses in Macrophages Through Differentially Modulating the NF-κB and PI3K/Akt/mTOR Pathways. *Int. Immunopharmacol.* **2014,** *23,* 77–84.

Wang, Y.; Watson, R. R. Ethanol, Immune Responses, and Murine AIDS: The Role of Vitamin E as an Immunostimulant and Antioxidant. *Alcohol* **1994,** *11,* 75–84.

Wung, B. S.; Hsu, M. C.; Wu, C. C.; Hsieh, C. W. Resveratrol Suppresses IL-6-induced ICAM-1 Gene Expression in Endothelial Cells: Effects on the Inhibition of STAT3 phosphorylation. *Life Sci.* **2005,** *78,* 389–397.

Xagorari, A.; Roussos, C.; Papapetropoulos, A. Inhibition of LPS-Stimulated Pathways in Macrophages by the Flavonoid Luteolin. *Br. J. Pharm.* **2002,** *136,* 1058–1064.

Xia, N.; Chen, G.; Liu, M.; Ye, X.; Pan, Y.; Ge, J.; Mao, Y.; Wang, H.; Wang, J.; Xie, S. Anti-Inflammatory Effects of luteolin on Experimental Autoimmune Thyroiditis in Mice. *Exp. Ther. Med.* **2016,** *12,* 4049–4054.

Xiao, J.; Zhai, H.; Yao, Y.; Wang, C.; Jiang, W.; Zhang, C.; Simard, A. R.; Zhang, R.; Hao, J. Chrysin Attenuates Experimental Autoimmune Neuritis by Suppressing Immuno-Inflammatory Responses. *Neuroscience* **2014,** *262,* 156–164.

Xu, L.; Zhang, Y.; Tian, K.; Chen, X.; Zhang, R.; Mu, X.; Wu, Y.; Wang, D.; Wang, S.; Liu, F.; et al. Apigenin Suppresses PD-L1 Expression in Melanoma and Host Dendritic Cells to Elicit Synergistic Therapeutic Effects. *J. Exp. Clin. Cancer Res.* **2018,** *37,* 261.

Xu, W.; Wang, X.; Chen, S.; Wu, H.; Tanaka, S.; Onda, K.; Sugiyama, K.; Yamada, H.; Hirano, T. Tetrandrine Enhances Glucocorticoid Receptor Translocation Possibly Via Inhibition of P-Glycoprotein in Daunorubicin-Resistant Human T Lymphoblastoid Leukemia Cells. *Eur. J. Pharm.* **2020,** *881,* 173232.

Xu, X.-W.; Zhang, D.-X. Effect of Tangyikang in Improving the Function of Pancreatic Islet Beta Cells in Patients with Latent Autoimmune Diabetes Mellitus in Adults. *Chin. J. Integr. Traditional Western Med.* **2008,** *28,* 882–885.

Zdanowicz, M. M. The Pharmacology of Immunosuppression. *Am. J. Pharm. Educ.* **2009,** *73,* 144.

Zhang, L.; Tizard, I. R. Activation of a Mouse Macrophage Cell Line by Acemannan: The Major Carbohydrate Fraction from Aloe vera gel. *Immunopharmacology* **1996,** *35,* 119–128.

Zhang, Q.; Huang, H.; Zheng, F.; Liu, H.; Qiu, F.; Chen, Y.; Liang, C.-L.; Dai, Z. Resveratrol exerts antitumor effects by downregulating CD8 + CD122 + Tregs in Murine Hepatocellular Carcinoma. *OncoImmunology* **2020,** 9.

Zhang, Y.; Yang, S.; Yang, Y.; Liu, T. Resveratrol Induces Immunogenic Cell Death of Human and Murine Ovarian Carcinoma Cells. *Infect. Agents Cancer* **2019,** *14,* 27.

PART II

NOVEL STRATEGIES OF ANTIOXIDANTS IN THE TREATMENT OF CHRONIC DISEASES

CHAPTER 5

ANTIOXIDANTS AS NUTRACEUTICALS IN THE PREVENTION AND TREATMENT OF CARDIOVASCULAR DISEASE

AMEY SUKHIA[1], NAYAN A. GUJARATHI[2], TULSHIDAS S. PATIL[2], ABHIJEET AHER[2], BHUSHAN RANE[3], and RAJ K. KESERVANI[4]

[1]*Department of Pharmacy Sciences, Creighton University, Omaha, Nebraska, USA*

[2]*Shri Vile Parle Kelavani Mandal's Institute of Pharmacy, Dhule, Maharashtra, India*

[3]*Shri D.D. Vispute College of Pharmacy and Research Center, New Panvel, Maharashtra, India*

[4]*Faculty of B. Pharmacy, CSM Group of Institutions, Prayagraj, Uttar Pradesh, India*

ABSTRACT

Cardiovascular diseases (CVDs) are the most common cause of mortality all over the globe. There are various etiological factors behind the initiation of CVD. Among these, one of the significant factors is oxidative stress, primarily cellular stress that arises due to various free radicle species. These free radicles stimulate and initiate various pathways or help to oxidize various components. Which eventually imbalance the cell by an overburden of the reactive species inside the cell and the inability of the cellular component to detoxify them. To mitigate these species, antioxidants are the potential solution to the problem by scavenging and quenching these species. Therefore, the use of antioxidants, which are therapeutic activities with the most negligible

Antioxidants as Nutraceuticals. Nayan A. Gujarathi, Raj K. Keservani, Rajesh K. Kesharwani, Bhushan R. Rane, Yogeeta Sameer Goyal (Eds.)

side effects, would be the logical solution to resolve the imbalance in the cell, thereby using nutraceuticals to prevent and treat various pathologies initiated by oxidative stress in CVD can be mitigated. This chapter discusses the role of reactive species in the etiology of various heart-related diseases, and further, the chapter discusses various nutraceuticals with antioxidant properties.

5.1 INTRODUCTION

Cardiovascular disease (CVD) is a common cause of mortality and morbidity in developed and developing countries. There are primary risk factors that initiate CVD, and they are categorized as follows. Lifestyle risk factors mainly include smoking, unhealthy diet, and lethargic lifestyle, underlying disease factors include hypertension, obesity, hyperlipidemia, and diabetes mellitus, whereas nonmodifiable factors such as age, family history, or any genetic disorder. Furthermore, dietary factors are the most contributing factors that majorly initiate CVD and various underlying diseases related to CVD. Diet plays a significant contributing factor directly or indirectly through risk factors including hypertension, dyslipidemia, and diabetes mellitus, and ameliorating these risk factors helps to decrease the mortality and morbidity related to CVD (Piepoli et al., 2016). Also, several studies mentioned the protective effects of various food and food supplements on CVD prevention and treatment, and the role of food supplements with some medicinal values comes into the picture, that is, nutraceuticals, also known as pharmaceutical food. Nutraceuticals are all-natural compounds obtained from natural sources with some therapeutic value, and they are used in various diseases like diabetes mellitus, obesity, osteoporosis, CVD. Mainly nutraceuticals are classified according to their functions, such as dietary fibers, probiotics, prebiotics, antioxidants (Ghani et al., 2019; Keservani et al., 2010a, 2010b, 2017, 2020). As the chapter is mainly concerned with antioxidants, we will further discuss the potential use of antioxidants as a nutraceutical. Over the years, much scientific evidence has shown antioxidants' effective and preventive role in CVD.

Furthermore, it is known that alteration in the oxidative status is associated with various CVDs. Alteration in the oxygen (O_2) status has a potential role with alteration in the protective mechanism of the cells and therefore damages the cell and impair their normal function, which is commonly known as oxidative stress. Additionally, oxidative stress is any condition in which oxidant metabolite has a detrimental effect on the local or systemic environment (Rane et al., 2012). Moreover, oxidative stress leads to the production of reactive oxygen species (ROS), and a high level of ROS acts as the main contributing factor in the activation of the immune cells, which eventually leads to local and systemic inflammation (Mangge et al., 2014).

As CVD is a multifactor etiological factor, the symptoms become challenging to recognize early. However, inflammation caused by oxidative stress can help detect the disease early as inflammation leads to the initiation and progression of various CVD (Libby et al., 2002). Therefore, looking for the inflammation site can help to get pathological information. Moreover, the role of ROS in the development of atherosclerosis can be understood by the increased level of endothelium ROS, which eventually causes endothelial dysfunction and causes inflammation (Mangge et al., 2014). Furthermore, some other scientific evidence mentioned that the increased level of ROS has a close association with impairment of the mitochondrial respiratory system, and this impaired condition might be the cause or the consequence of oxidative stress (Di Meo et al., 2016).

Additionally, in normal cellular functioning, free radicals are generated, which are mitigated by the endogenous antioxidants, but in patients with oxidative stress conditions, the ROS overburden the endogenous antioxidant, and it was observed that patients majorly lack antioxidants. In this condition, it is mainly encouraged to take exogenous antioxidants through supplements, which interfere with the disease-related inflammation and pacify the oxidative stress condition. Therefore, the potential role of nutraceuticals becomes of utmost importance in the diet to compete with the underlying heart condition (Mangge et al., 2014).

Before diving into the role of nutraceutical antioxidants in CVD (CVD) and various food supplements used in CVD, it is essential to discuss the oxidative and nitrosative stress(the free radicle having reactive nitrogen element) physiopathological implications on various CVDs. There are various sources of ROS that can hamper the cell and cause damage to it. The various sources of ROS are mentioned below, which can help understand the mechanism clearly regarding various disease states and their correlation with ROS. As mentioned before, in any metabolic reaction, ROS generation takes place, but antioxidants alleviate them and maintain normal physiology. Various cell organelles play an essential role in ROS production, which generally help carry out the body signaling a normal functionality, majorly endoplasmic reticulum and mitochondria, and play a potential role in producing the ROS in the cell. Furthermore, there are various reasons for the overproduction of ROS and its possible implication for initiation of the CVD.

5.1.1 ROS PRODUCTION IN CYTOSOL

Various cell components have a significant contribution to the production of intracellular ROS, that is there are various soluble intracellular components including hydroquinone, flavins, and catecholamines that can undergo redox reaction and lead to ROS production. Moreover, specific enzymes can produce ROS, such as xanthine oxidase (XO). The XO is oxidized to uric acid in normal healthy conditions, mainly regulated by xanthine dehydrogenase, which utilizes nicotinamide adenine dinucleotide phosphate ($NADP^+$) as an electron acceptor. However, in the injured cell, the dehydrogenase form is converted to the oxidase form, leading to superoxide radical production during xanthine oxidation to uric acid (Di Meo et al., 2016).

5.1.2 ROS PRODUCTION IN MITOCHONDRIA

Mitochondria are a significant source of ROS in most mammalian cells. The mitochondria take up most of the O_2 to produce energy in adenosine triphosphate (ATP), mainly through the electron transport chain (ETC). The production of ROS in mitochondria mainly takes place in the mitochondrial matrix majorly. Hydrogen peroxide (H_2O_2), a non-radical ROS, produced in mitochondria in the abnormal condition mainly in the absence of the electron acceptor coenzyme Q (Zorov et al., 2014). It diffused out from the mitochondria to cytosol, and as the concentration of the ROS in the cytosol increases it induces the cell dysfunction which eventually cause cell apoptosis (Di Meo et al., 2016).

There are other sources of ROS production in the cell, such as peroxisomes, endoplasmic reticulum, and plasma membrane, that generate various kinds of reactive species such as H• hydrogen atom, CCl_3• trichloromethyl; a carbon-centered radical, O_2^-• superoxide; an O_2-centered radical, OH• hydroxyl are some of the ROS produced inside the cell but as mentioned before it has a detrimental effect when not detoxified or mitigated by antioxidants (Di Meo et al., 2016). Furthermore, enzymes in cytosols primarily thiols and flavins undergo a redox reaction, which is stimulated by native low-density lipoproteins (LDL) and which initiates ROS production. Moreover, various environmental factors such as toxic chemicals, smoke, and convert the toxic metabolite into ROS (Mügge, 1998).

Besides, the ROS reactive nitrogen species (RNS) can induce stress, which is termed nitrosative stress. The stress is induced by free radicals with the reactive nitrogen element, with a major association with nitric oxide (NO•), nitrogen dioxide (NO_2), and peroxynitrite ($ONOO^-$)—which are produced or regulated by enzymes such as nitric oxide synthase (NOS)—by-products from abnormal mitochondrial electron chain (Gorecki et al., 2018). Stimulants for the production of reactive species are mentioned in Table 5.1.

TABLE 5.1 Stimulants for ROS Production.

Intracellular stimulant	Extracellular stimulant
Endoplasmatic reticulum	Environmental factors
Cytochrome P450 family	Toxic chemicals, smoke high energy irradiation
Plasma membrane	Mechanical stress
Lipoxygenase, cyclooxygenase, NADPH oxidase, NO synthase	
Soluble enzymes	Cytokines
XO	Lipopolysaccharide
Small molecules	Catalytic metal ions
Thiols, flavins, catecholamines.	
Peroxisomes	Angiotensin II
Oxidases, flavoproteins	Native LDL

NO• is a free radical that contains free electrons and is mainly synthesized by tissues by utilizing NOS, L-arginine, and citrulline in the presence of NOS and O_2 with NADPH as a cosubstrate leads in the formation of NO• (Kurutas, 2016), (NO•) also has a potential role in the regulation of cardiovascular motor tone, attuning the myocardial contractility, also controlling cell proliferation and platelet aggregation and activation (Napoli et al., 2013). Therefore, the significant contribution to the production of RNS is ROS enzymes. Mainly there are three types of NOS enzymes found in the human body, neuronal nitric oxide synthetase (NNOS), endothelial nitric oxide synthetase (ENOS), which has a role in maintaining vascular homeostasis, and inducible nitric oxide synthetase (INOS it is mainly located in myocytes, macrophages and stimulated by inflammatory response). Furthermore, in infectious conditions or in the condition of septic, INOS and NNOS are taken up by the endothelial and muscle cells, respectively, leading to the over-production of ROS and causing vascular and arteriolar dysfunction (Gorecki et al., 2018).

From the NOS, as mentioned above, endothelial NOS has a specialized role in regulating cardiovascular functions, utilizing calcium which helps bind calmodulin to enzyme ENOS maintain cardiac homeostasis, and control the involvement of genes in atherogenesis. Furthermore, as a quencher for O_2 in the blood, INOS can produce substantial NO levels. A potent oxidant, $ONOO^-$, can be formed when NO and O_2 combine to produce an oxidant. While neither NO nor O_2 can attack a wide range of biological targets, $ONOO^-$ can attack various biological components that can interact with it and impart its effects. $ONOO^-$ also involves NO signaling mechanisms that entail protein modifications (Förstermann and Sessa, 2012).

Discussing the ROS/RNS role and its importance in homeostasis, the further section deals with the potential role of reactive species in various CVDs.

5.2 ROLE OF ROS/RNS IN CVD

5.2.1 HYPERTENSION

Hypertension is a condition with complex etiological causes, and in most cases, it is hard to interpret the significant cause of the disorder. Further, oxidative and nitrosative stress appeared to play a potential role in hypertension and was highlighted as a common factor in the disorder (Doughan et al., 2008). Additionally, several in vitro, in vivo studies suggest evidence of ROS/RNS stimulation and activation of specific molecular mechanisms, which increase the blood pressure (Ward et al., 2005).

A variety of methods can cause oxidative stress-induced hypertension. Mechanisms of ROS-induced endothelium and vascular smooth muscle cell dysfunction in hypertension are discussed future; mainly, shear stress and high blood pressure are two examples of the many variables that can activate the NADPH oxidase enzyme and produce ROS. Endothelial nitric oxide synthase (ENOS) is uncoupled from NO production when the redox state changes (NO). Vascular remodeling and endothelial dysfunction are caused by increased amounts of intracellular ROS, which alter redox-sensitive signaling pathways that lead to contraction of blood vessels, structural remodeling, fibrosis, and inflammation. ROS most likely has the most significant impact on blood pressure regulation at the level of the vasculature (Briones and Touyz, 2010). As vascular cells, primarily endothelial cells, and smooth muscles, can produce ROS, some other sources of ROS production are induced through angiotensin II, which has an activation effect on mitochondrial NADPH oxidase and other oxidases that eventually induce hypertension (Briones and Touyz, 2010). Figure 5.1 represents the prognosis of hypertension condition by reactive species. A series of studies confirm the reactive species' involvement in hypertension. XO activity in the mesenteric microcirculation of spontaneously hypertensive rats (SHR) is enhanced, accompanied by an increase in arteriolar tone (Viel et al., 2008). Mervaala et al. confirm the increase in XO level with transgenic rats having overexpression of renin and angiotensin II (Mervaala et al., 2001).

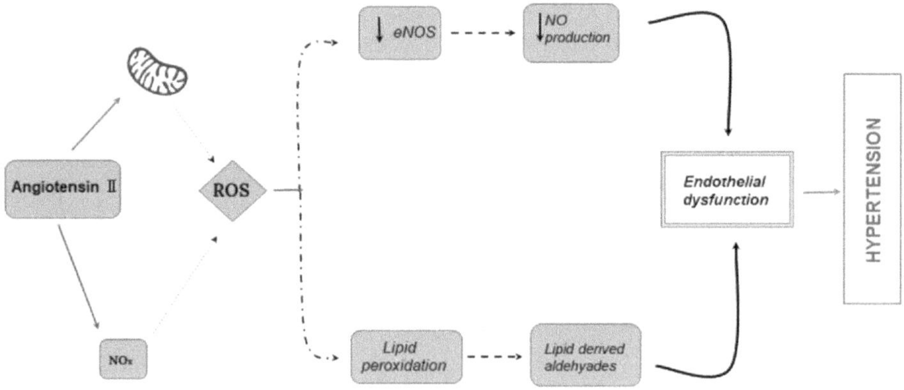

FIGURE 5.1 Prognosis of hypertension by reactive species.

Furthermore, as we have discussed earlier, the nitrosative stress increases the production of $ONOO^-$, a potent oxidant that oxidizes the essential NO synthase cofactor, and induces the increase in the production of superoxide, which induces the stress condition and causes dysfunction. Additionally ROS-induced lipid peroxidation, leads in the generation of secondary products (lipid-derived aldehydes) that causes endothelial dysfunction and hypertension (Sorriento et al., 2018). The further confirmation regarding the correlation of angiotensin II, ROS, and oxidative was bolstered by the in vivo studies in some hypertensive human patients Increases in ROS-related characteristics were found in smooth muscle cells from the arteries of hypertension patients after treatment with angiotensin II (Touyz and Schiffrin, 2004). Furthermore, in hypertension patients, higher oxidative stress indicators such as malondialdehyde, F2-isoprostanes, GSSG, and the DNA oxidation marker 8-oxo-7,8-dihydro-2′-deoxyguanosine(8-oxo-dG) have a strong correlation with blood pressure (Rodrigo et al., 2007).

5.2.2 ATHEROSCLEROSIS

CVD is thought to be exacerbated by atherosclerosis, an inflammatory disease that affects both large and medium-sized arteries. Cholesterol metabolism and transport, as well as influx and efflux within cells, are closely regulated in healthy conditions. When these homeostatic systems become imbalanced in favor of either increased cholesterol influx or decreased efflux, the development of atherosclerosis can occur. There are numerous lipoproteins in the bloodstream, each of which performs a different function in the transportation of lipids. LDL is one of the most significant lipoproteins found in the bloodstream, and its role is to transport cholesterol from the liver to the tissues of the body (McLaren et al., 2011). Endocytic of LDL particles is usually facilitated by the LDL receptor (LDLr). As part of its role in cholesterol metabolism, HDL (high-density lipoproteins) transports extra cholesterol from peripheral tissues back to the liver, where it is eliminated through the bile. Reverse cholesterol transportation is the term for this process. This is true even though the small intestine retains 95% of biliary cholesterol that is excreted in the feces. Because poorer endothelial function has been linked to both high LDL cholesterol and low HDL cholesterol, it has been proposed that raising LDL cholesterol and HDL cholesterol is both pro- and antiatherogenic (Moss and Ramji, 2016). As fatty deposits and plaques accumulate in the walls of large and medium arteries, an immunological response to the fatty deposit accumulation is prevalent in atherosclerosis, which can lead to heart disease. ApoB-(apolipoprotein-B) containing lipoproteins, such as LDL and other lipoprotein residues, make up the initial fatty deposit in the intima of arteries, known as a fatty streak. Oxidation of the oxidized LDL (oxLDL) can be caused by the confined LDL. Endothelial cells near the oxLDL-rich intima of an artery begin secreting inflammatory cytokines and chemokines because of this inflammatory response. The inflammatory response circulating monocytes are then drawn to the oxidized LDL buildup and move into the intima, where they develop into macrophages. After migrating into the artery intima, monocytes are exposed to macrophage colony-stimulating factor and develop into macrophages, a process linked with enhanced expression of scavenger receptors (SRs) on their cell surface once they have been introduced to the arterial walls. Thereafter, foam cells loaded with lipid aggregate and create an early lesion, which eventually matures and develops into an atherosclerotic plaque (Moss and Ramji, 2016). Figure 5.2 depicts the atherosclerosis process by initiation with reactive free radicle species.

Furthermore, it is oxidized LDL that stimulates vascular ROS production, by activating NOX and uncoupling endothelial nitric oxide synthase (NOS), both of which lead to vascular endothelial dysfunction. Moreover, ROS helps to convert macrophages to foam cells which eventually leads to the formation of plaque (Sorriento et al., 2018).

Therefore, we can conclude that reactive species have a potential role in CVD and has to be checked. Here the role of antioxidants takes place, the further section deals with the antioxidant's role and functions in inhibiting and controlling reactive species.

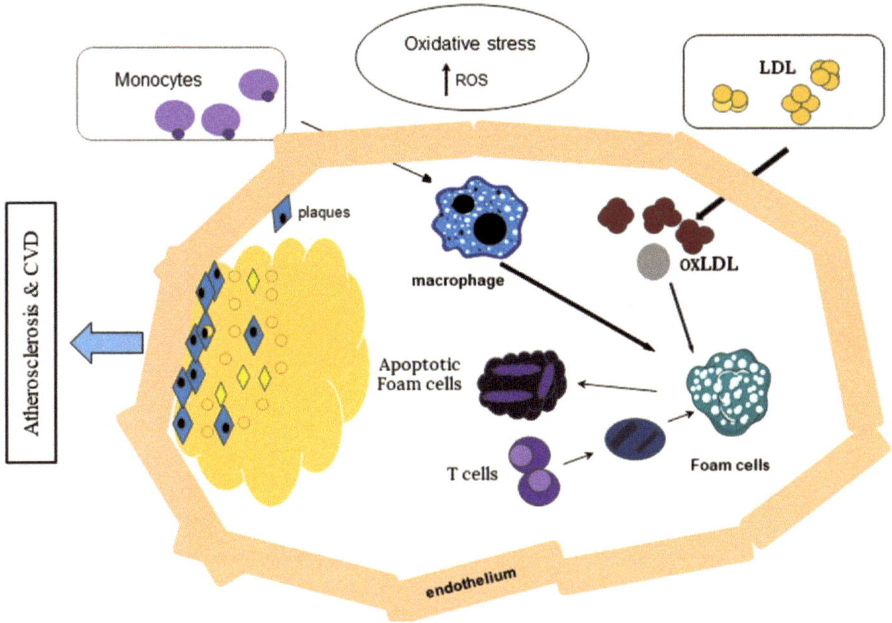

FIGURE 5.2 Reactive free radicle species causing atherosclerosis.

5.3 ANTIOXIDANT DEFENSE MECHANISM

Oxidative stress alters the cellular constituents of our bodies, resulting in a variety of diseases. Heart disease has been linked to a lack of antioxidants in the body. Antioxidants boost the body's natural defenses against free radicals and are an excellent way to combat oxidative stress. ROS/RNS are countered in vivo by a complex antioxidant defense network that works in unison. Antioxidants with and without enzymes are necessary to control ROS/RNS levels and repair oxidative cellular damage. Antioxidant enzymes lower lipid hydroperoxide and H_2O_2 levels, making them crucial in preventing lipid peroxidation and preserving the integrity and function of cell membranes (Gorecki et al., 2018).

The primary enzymes that neutralize ROS/RNS are superoxide dismutase (SOD), catalase (CAT), and glutathione peroxidase (GPx), where SOD is the primary enzyme present mainly in cytoplasm and mitochondria which accelerated the process of converting superoxide to neutral element as superoxide act as a strong reducing agent and SOD as strong electron accepting or oxidizing agent. SOD is present majorly in every aerobic cell and extracellular fluids. Moreover, other enzymes such as CAT, a peroxisomal enzyme found solely in most tissues, are responsible for converting H_2O_2 into water and O_2. The selenoprotein GPx enzymes, on the contrary, are the most essential H_2O_2-removing enzymes in the body. GPx enzymes remove H_2O_2 from the environment by utilizing it to oxidize reduced glutathione (GSH) to oxidized glutathione (GSSG) (Bahoran et al., 2006).

However, the endogenous antioxidants can defend the ROS/RNS in normal conditions; eventually, in oxidative or nitrosative stress, the overproduction of the ROS/RNS hampers the ability of antioxidants; therefore, the requirement for exogenous antioxidants is needed. So antioxidants, in terms of supplements or nutrients, are required to be taken externally to overcome the stress condition.

5.4 NUTRACEUTICALS USED IN CVD

Given the above-discussed involvement of oxidative and nitrosative stress in the etiology and pathogenesis of various CVDs, antioxidant therapy seems to be a valuable strategy to restore the impaired balance between oxidants and antioxidants. Most nutraceutical antioxidants can show a beneficial effect in CVS diseases. The various antioxidants are discussed thoroughly, with their potential benefits in a further section.

5.4.1 SELENIUM

The essential trace element, selenium (Se), is present in various naturally available food materials and dietary supplements. Se is present in many different chemical forms in organic such as selenomethionine and dimethyl selenide, and inorganic forms such as selenites and selenates. Selenomethionine, a significant source of dietary Se in humans, is also extensively employed in clinical trials as a chemical form of Se supplementation. It has been estimated that about 25 selenoproteins in humans have a crucial role in several bodily functions due to nutritional value as well as involvement in various pathophysiological functions, including thyroid hormone metabolism, the adaptive and acquired immune system, and prevention of certain cancers, DNA synthesis, and protection from oxidative damage and infection (Benstoem et al., 2015). Also, evidence suggests that Se also has a crucial role in the ideal functioning of the cardiovascular system. Therefore, Se is recommended as an essential nutrient in dietary or food supplements. While balanced Se levels are required for various biological functions in the human body, extremely low or extremely high Se intake might have adverse effects; daily Se intake is determined by the Se level of the soil on which crops grow (Tinggi, 2008). A chronic Se deficit was initially reported in a northwestern Chinese region (Yang et al., 1988). Patients had fast-progressing cardiomyopathy that resulted in severe fibrosis and degenerative alterations, which is now referred to as Keshan disease after the Chinese region (MacFarquhar et al., 2010). In contrast to Se deficiency, Se poisoning occurs less frequently and is caused by inadvertent/suicidal intake or in most instances oversupplementation of Se in the daily diet comprising of high Se levels. Selenosis (acute Se overdose) also causes nausea, dizziness, and edema in the pulmonary region; other symptoms are brittle nails and hair in patients (MacFarquhar et al., 2010).

Selenoenzymes are the enzymes present in the body that serve to have crucial to the induction of an antioxidant defense mechanism. There are various selenoenzymes in the body, mainly GPx's and Thioredoxin reductases (TrxR) enzymes, whereas GPx protects cells from lipoprotein or DNA damage. In humans, six GPx family selenoenzymes are present—GPx1, GPx3, GPx4, GPx5, and GPx6 with high antioxidant activity. In addition to shielding cells from oxidative damage caused by ROS and RNS, these GPx play a crucial role in protecting cells from the oxidative damage caused by superoxide, hydrogen peroxide, hydroxyl radicals, NO, and $ONOO^-$ (Benstoem et al., 2015).

Furthermore, the second enzyme, TrxR, is present in humans and found in different body regions, mainly in the cytosol and in the cell's mitochondria. The function of neutralizing intracellular hydrogen peroxide regenerates thioredoxin to restore the cell's redox balance by impacting the inflammatory signaling pathways that modify ROS by inhibiting nuclear factor-kappa B (McKenzie et al., 1998). Increasing evidence points to the role of selenoenzyme in antioxidant defense against damaging ROS and RNS attacks(Arbogast and Ferreiro, 2010). Therefore, it is common to utilize blood Se levels to diagnose oxidative stress-related diseases.

5.4.1.1 THE ROLE OF SELENIUM AND SELENOPROTEINS AND SELENOENZYMES ON THE HUMAN HEART

Se is a crucial element in the body's antioxidant defense mechanism. Selenoproteins have been identified that play diverse roles in regulating cellular redox processes. As a result of an imbalance in the Se concentration, which eventually increases ROS generation, the physiological system may experience oxidative stress, damaging cell membranes, proteins, and DNA. Human disorders, particularly heart disease, have been related to ROS damage. When ROS are present, they can trigger the oxidation of LDL, which is linked with the onset of atherogenesis in the heart (Flores-Mateo et al., 2006). Several investigations have studied serum Se levels as a risk factor for CVD. One hypothesis is that high Se as antioxidant selenoenzymes and selenoproteins may help reduce the production of oxidized LDL thereby reducing the incidence of heart diseases (Rees et al., 2013). In vivo studies show that Se deficiency downregulate the LDL receptor, which is essential for an optimum regulation of the cholesterol level in plasma (Loscalzo, 2014). The presence of selenoproteins P, which is found mainly in plasma, may significantly regulate the plasma cholesterol level by protecting LDL oxidation from ROS. This study provides further evidence that selenoprotein P plays an essential antioxidative role in protecting LDL from oxidation and preventing atherosclerosis. It has also been reported that by increasing the NO bioavailability, which eventually decreases oxidative stress, TrxR plays a significant role in preventing the development of atherosclerosis (Benstoem et al., 2015).

The antioxidative actions of GPx and TrxR in myocardial ischemia-reperfusion (I/R) injury have piqued researchers' interest due to evidence from epidemiological studies that Se has a role in heart disorders. In a population with low Se serum concentration. I/R injury has been shown to cause ROS generation, which has to be detrimental to tissue. A high Se diet can mitigate reperfusion's effects, while a Se shortage can damage the intrinsic myocardial tolerance to ischemic shock (Lim et al., 2009). A recent study showed that adding sodium selenite to reperfusion solutions at specific doses helped rats recover from ischemia reperfusion-induced heart damage (MacFarquhar et al., 2010). Additional research has shown in a rat model that Se deprivation leads to enhanced myocardial damage with elevated protein and lipid peroxidation during myocardial I/R by Venardos and coworkers (Venardos et al., 2004). It was further bolstered by Tanguy and coworkers' findings in which experiments on rats were performed with Se shortage demonstrated enhanced myocardial damage and an altered recovery of cardiac function following myocardial I/R. The reason for these findings was due to a decreased GPx activity in the blood and cardiomyocytes (Tanguy et al., 2003).

Furthermore, synthetic Se compounds and their biological activities that imitate selenoprotein antioxidant action have been synthesized and investigated (Benstoem et al., 2015). Ebselen has exhibited a weak GPx-like activity in vivo and could be a promising cardioprotective agent for myocardial I/R injury. In animal studies, ebselen can have cardioprotective effects when administered orally before ischemic reperfusion, and this may involve the induction of stress protein HSP27 and the preservation of GSH. The effectiveness of ebselen as an antioxidant is not only for its ability to mimic the GPx, but it is also an excellent substrate for mammalian TrxR for the catalysis of hydrogen peroxide reduction via the Trx/TrxR system (Azad and Tomar, 2014).

So far, over 25 selenoproteins found and expressed in various tissues and cells and exhibit numerous functions. Figure 5.3 depicts the selenoproteins essentially showing antioxidant properties. GPx detoxifies intracellular hydrogen peroxide, thus protecting the cell from lipoprotein and DNA damage while TrxR regenerates thioredoxin and thereby balances the redox status of the cell. Moreover, as a member of the Msr family of antioxidant enzymes, SelR is often referred to as methionine-sulfoxide reductase B1 (MsrB1). The Msr family also contains the MsrA, B2, and B3 nonselenoprotein enzymes. On proteins, SelR diminishes the oxidized methionine residues. A reversible reaction between ROS and SelR converts methionine to methionine-sulfoxides, which can afterward be reduced back to methionine. A key regulator of the action of signaling molecules, this reversible oxidation and reduction regulates cellular redox activities. In addition, ROS is consumed throughout these cycles, increasing protein oxidation resistance (Lee et al., 2013).

Selenoprotein showing antioxidant properties
Glutathione peroxidase 1 (GPx1)
Glutathione peroxidase 2 (GPx2)
Glutathione peroxidase 3 (GPx3)
Glutathione peroxidase 4 (GPx4)
Glutathione peroxidase 5 (GPx5)
Glutathione peroxidase 6 (GPx6)
Selenium K (SelK)
Selenium R (SelR)
Selenium W (SelW)

FIGURE 5.3 Selenoproteins showing antioxidant properties.

Additionally, SelR is the only enzyme in the Msr family that is majorly upregulated in cardiac hypertrophy and I/R models suggesting the importance of Selr during cardiac arrest (Kim and Gladyshev, 2004). SelR expression may be increased by ROS-induced methionine sulfoxide production, reducing damage to stressed cardiomyocytes. Additionally, SelR is involved in the dynamic remodeling of actin in response to cardiac stress (Lee et al., 2013). One subfamily, including Selk, SelW, SelT, and SelH, forms mixed disulfides with substrate proteins and binds DNA in a redox-sensitive manner. SelW is primarily found in the cytoplasm of cells, with a miniscule fraction also found on the cell membrane. Early investigations revealed that SelW may have antioxidant properties because of its strong affinity for glutathione binding.

Moreover, researchers discovered that SelK is present in various organs and tissues outside the heart and skeletal muscle, including the pancreas, liver, and even the placenta. Cardiomyocytes were protected from external oxidative stress by overexpression of SelK, which lowered intracellular ROS levels. According to these findings, SelK may serve as an antioxidant in the heart (Croft et al., 2007). Therefore, thoroughly discussing the role of Se on the human heart and its potential role as an antioxidant, it can be anticipated to prevent and treat CVDs.

5.4.2 VITAMIN E

Vitamin E, also known as tocopherols, is a lipid-soluble vitamin that has numerous stereoisomers, of which the α-tocopherol is the most pharmacologically active isomer. Vitamin E is also considered the primary antioxidant source in lipoproteins and plasma. Vitamin E's antioxidant properties stem from its lipophilic properties and its characteristic in preventing lipid peroxidation (Plantinga et al., 2007). Various research supports the tocopherol cardioprotective, antioxidant, and anti-inflammatory property (Noguchi et al., 2001). Moreover, certain in-line evidence supports the potential role of vitamin E in treating and prophylaxis for many CVDs; also, various in vivo, clinical, and observational studies indicate the beneficial effects of vitamin E on cardiovascular health. In fact, certain other studies show the harmful effects that the heart might have when an individual is vitamin E deficient (Riemersma et al., 1989).

Furthermore, there is evidence of vitamin E supplement utilization in atherosclerosis. LDL oxidation is a critical component of atherosclerosis and plays a role in its pathogenesis through a vast range of mechanisms. Oxidized LDL stimulates the endothelial cells to release inflammatory stimulants such as cell adhesion molecules and macrophage colony-stimulating factors. These inflammatory indicators are responsible for the recruitment and penetration of monocytes into the artery wall, as well as the proliferation and differentiation of macrophages/monocytes; the macrophages detect further oxidation of LDL through the scavenger's receptor present on the macrophage, which initiates the phagocytosis of oxidized LDL which eventually results in the production of foam cells. Other putative atherogenic features of oxidized LDL include their cytotoxic effects on cultured endothelial cells (Saremi and Arora, 2010).

Additionally, various in vivo evidence supports the claim of vitamin E's role in atherosclerosis. Ferre et al. evaluated the effect of apolipoprotein E-deficient mice with antiatherogenic diets on hepatic lipid peroxidation and aortic atherosclerosis. They divided apolipoprotein E-deficient mice into five groups based on feeding—they received standard chow, chow with palm, chow with coconut, chow with sunflower-seed oil, or chow with olive oil. Further, the mouse livers were removed and analyzed for lipid peroxidation, α-tocopherol content, and oxidative enzyme activity. The size of atherosclerotic plaques in the mouse aortas was also measured; diets high in vitamin E (olive or sunflower oil-supplemented diets) were found to protect against hepatic lipid peroxidation. Furthermore, they discovered that diets supplemented with olive, palm, or sunflower oil, which has a potential source of vitamin E, have smaller aortic atherosclerotic lesions (Ferré et al., 2001).

Moreover, another study conducted by Thomas et al. evaluated the anti-atherogenic effects of vitamin E and coenzyme Q10 (CoQ10). Mice were divided into groups and fed high-fat diets containing either vitamin E or CoQ10 or vitamin E plus CoQ10 for 24 weeks. Mice were given vitamin E, and CoQ10 showed a considerable reduction in tissue lipid hydroperoxides. When compared to control mice, all treatment groups had considerably lower aortic cholesterol. Aortic root, arch, and descending thoracic aorta atherosclerosis were reduced in mice given vitamin E + CoQ10. Plasma from mice fed CoQ10 or vitamin E plus CoQ10 was found to be more resistant to ex vivo lipid peroxidation than control animals, The aortic root atherosclerosis in mice given only vitamin E was reduced (Thomas et al., 2001).

Additionally, to support the claim of the active role of antioxidants on CVDs, there are certain clinical trial studies that demonstrate using vitamin E as an antioxidant. Stephens's et al. performed a randomized controlled trial of coronary disease patients with vitamin E; the study enrolled 2002 individuals with angiographically confirmed coronary artery disease and followed them for 510 days. A total of 1035 patients were given α-tocopherol capsules divided into two different doses, 800 and 400 IU, while 967 were given placebo capsules. Cardiovascular death and nonfatal MI, as well as nonfatal Ml alone, were the primary outcomes. The outcomes of the study have found increase concentration of serum α-tocopherol concentration in patients who were actively administered vitamin E capsules and no change was observed in patients with a placebo. The author concluded that patients with α-tocopherol administration significantly decreased the risk of nonfatal myocardial infarction (MI)—in the individuals with angiographically established symptomatic coronary atherosclerosis—with the advantageous effect till 1 year after the treatment (Stephens et al., 1996). Additionally, Boaz et al. demonstrated a randomized placebo-controlled trial with hemodialysis patients as patients with hemodialysis have greater oxidative stress conditions; therefore, the role of vitamin E as a potential antioxidant was investigated with 196 patients with preexisting CVDs aged between 40–75 and received 800 IU/day vitamin E or similar placebo, patients were followed for 519 days with the major outcome endpoint as a myocardial infraction (no fatal or fatal), ischemic stroke, unstable angina, and peripheral vascular diseases. Secondary outcome or minor outcome as total mortality and cardiovascular-disease mortality. Findings from the study mentioned a total of 16% of vitamin E patients and 33% of placebo patients have primary endpoints, respectively. 5.1% of vitamin E patients and 17% of placebo patients had a myocardial infarction, respectively. The author concluded that vitamin E reduces CVD and myocardial infarction (Boaz et al., 2000).

Furthermore, certain observational studies investigated vitamin E-rich diet's correlation with an incidence of coronary heart disease; the Health Professionals Follow-up Study by Rimm et al. comprised 39,910 healthy male health professionals in the USA, with the age range from 40–75 years. The participants filled out extensive food questionnaires and were tracked for 4 years, during when coronary heart disease outcomes were recorded. Those who ingested more than 60 IU vitamin E daily had a considerably decreased risk of coronary heart disease than men who consumed less than 7.5 IU daily (Rimm et al., 1993).

Thoroughly discussing in vitro, in vivo, clinical, and observational studies related to the beneficial effects of vitamin E as an antioxidant on atherosclerosis and various CVD supplementation of vitamin E, and including vitamin E in diet would potentially decrease the incidence of fatal effects related to heart disease.

5.4.3 VITAMIN C

Vitamin C is a water-soluble substance. Because humans cannot synthesize ascorbic acid from scratch, body concentrations are maintained through vitamin C ingestion. When vitamin C is oxidized, it creates dihydroxy ascorbic acid, which is transported into our cells via glucose transporters and subsequently restored to ascorbic acid for cellular usage (Subramani et al., 2014). Vitamin C is an electron donor and acts as a reducing agent. Most of the known biochemical and physiological actions of vitamin C are mainly owing to its action as an electron donor. Vitamin C also has an antioxidant property because, by donating its electrons, it prevents other compounds from being oxidized. However, vitamin C gets oxidized in the process. Furthermore, vitamin C is a reducing property and can oxidize itself by many species, inside the body, and have greater potential to induce various diseases. Additionally, vitamin C can reduce both the reactive species with free radicals, as well as the reactive species without free radicals, thereby increases the range of vitamin C effect. One example related to CVDs is the reduction of many ROS which has an atherogenic effect on atherosclerosis; vitamin C prevents the initiation of atherosclerosis by reactive species by reducing most of the species. Moreover, when reactive species reacts and induces lipid peroxidation that eventually reacts with DNA and subsequently induces mutation and cell damage. Therefore, ascorbate as an antioxidant prevents the formation of some reactive O_2 and RNS which can induce lipid peroxidation and thereby decrease the chances of DNA damage and prevent cell damage (Padayatty et al., 2003).

There are various conditions caused by deficiency related to vitamin C the most common one is scurvy, a pathological condition characterized by joint pains, bleeding, poor wound healing, bone fragility, tooth, and hair loss. Although scurvy is a fatal disease, many other diseases are directly or indirectly related to the deficiency of vitamin C, such as endothelial dysfunction, hypertension, stroke, and atherosclerosis. Besides that, vitamin C's role in vascular and cardiac protection and the amelioration of diseases related to CVD has been studied in several preclinical research (Padayatty et al., 2003). Heller et al. have investigated the potential of vitamin C in enhancing and protecting NO from free radicals as these reactive species cause the inactivation of NO, which has a potential role in the mechanism of myogenic tone (vasoconstriction), coagulation, and atherosclerosis. The researchers conducted the study using human endothelial cells and investigated the role of added L-ascorbic acid on cellular NO synthesis; the results were in line with the beneficial role of Vitamin C in the form of ascorbic acid has a crucial role in NO synthesis and can be used as a supplement for protective vascular effects (Heller et al., 1999).

Besides the preclinical studies, specific clinical and observational studies have investigated the correlation between vitamin C and CVD and their association with other cardiac events. Guan et al. analyzed the effect of vitamin C supplements on systolic (SBP) and diastolic (DBP) blood pressure in hypertensive patients; 614 patients were analyzed before and after supplementation with vitamin C and the result suggested that vitamin C supplement has a significant role in reducing blood pressure (Guan et al., 2020). Furthermore, Ashor and others conducted a meta-analysis study where they pooled the data of 44 clinical trial results and concluded that vitamin C has a significantly improved effect on endothelial function and therefore it can lower various underlying pathological conditions related to endothelial dysfunction (Ashor et al., 2014). However, some studies are in contrast with the above studies; for instance, Rimm et al. conducted an observational study with 39,910 US male health professionals aged 45–75 years who have an underlying disease condition related to the heart. The patients were given a high intake of vitamin C. The author concluded the result by mentioning no beneficial relationship between the vitamin C supplement and a heart condition (Rimm et al., 1993).

Taken together, all the studies both in preclinical and clinical studies suggested the use of vitamin C has a beneficial effect on CVD. However, certain observation studies specifically conducted by Rimm et al. have shown no vitamin C effect on CVD. Moreover, most studies have variable doses of vitamin C and cannot be compared in the commonplace. Therefore, there is a need to conduct a specific randomized trial with a predetermined and specific dose range that can help bolster the claim of vitamin C's role in CVD.

5.4.4 LYCOPENE

Lycopene is the fat-soluble pigment hydrocarbon compound, also known as a type of carotenoid mainly present in guava, tomatoes, and other foods with red color. Lycopene has many conjugated double bonds. Because of the abundance of the conjugated double bonds, there are many different isomeric forms of lycopene, but only some are found in natural food items; all the *trans* configurations are usually present in naturally available lycopene sources. Moreover, because the abundance of the double bonds makes lycopene a potential antioxidant agent, it was lately attracted for its potential as an antioxidant in involvement in preventing CVDs (Arab and Steck, 2000). The study also suggested that lycopene has a greater affinity toward the singlet O_2 and has the most substantial quenching capacity than other carotenoids (Di Mascio et al., 1989). Therefore, they have the potential to be utilized as a potent antioxidizing agent.

Earlier studies also suggested the claim that dietary supplementation of lycopene can attenuate atherogenesis by mitigating oxidative stress also lipid lowering capability is majorly due to an increase in NO level. Furthermore, certain clinical studies also indicated that lycopene supplementation could benefit endothelial function, lipid peroxidation, increase in SOD, and reduce blood pressure (Ghaffari and Roshanravan, 2020).

It is noteworthy that lycopene can reduce cholesterol by preventing LDL oxidation; both in vitro and in vivo suggested the same claim (Napolitano et al., 2007). In brief, the researchers conducted the study on six healthy individuals for 3 months and gave the supplementation of 60 mg/day of lycopene, and the result concluded that there was a significant drop in plasma LDL concentration and no effect on HDL concentration. In the same study, the author conducted a study investigating the hypocholesterolemia effect in vitro, the author conducted a study by incubating macrophage cells and their results show that there is a decrease in the concentration of cholesterol synthesis (Fuhrman et al., 1997). Moreover, investigating lycopene concentration in adipose tissue can be better than measuring the concentration of lycopene in plasma and serum because the major storage site of lycopene in the body is adipose tissue and is supposed to be the better investigational site than plasma and serum (Kohlmeier and Kohlmeier, 1995).

Many studies show the relationship between lycopene and CVD, including some clinical trials. Rissanen et al. conducted a prospective population-based study in which they compared the men's lycopene serum concentration and concluded that the men with low lycopene concentration had 10 times increased acute coronary attack (Rissanen et al., 2001). Furthermore, the case–control study included 531 patients diagnosed with MI and controlled patients adjusted for smoking and age. The subjects were compared for lycopene plasma concentration. Overall, the study did not show any significant result of lycopene as a potent antioxidant (Hak et al., 2003).

Lastly, arterial stiffness and endothelial dysfunction are the early signs of atherosclerosis. The study suggested using brachial–ankle pulse wave velocity (BaPWV) as a biomarker for arterial stiffness and inflammation. The study was conducted by Kim and others, including 264 healthy women patients, and measured for BaPWV. The result provides the inverse relationship between BaPWV and lycopene, and the author concluded that BaPWV could be used as an early marker for early atherosclerosis changes (Kim et al., 2010).

The potential role of lycopene in protecting various CVDs from the studies mentioned above; lycopene can be attributed as an antioxidant agent. However, its utilization as a supplement is still in question because of the limited number of studies; the results are not comparable because it lacks generalization due to the limited number of samples; some confounding factors can also hamper the results. Therefore, it is suggested to develop a study that could help to translate results easily and help to get a concrete conclusion regarding the supplementation role of lycopene from the study.

5.4.5 FLAVONOIDS

Flavonoids (Keservani and Sharma, 2014; Keservani et al., 2016a; Keservani et al., 2016b) are phenolic metabolites with anticarcinogenic, anti-inflammatory, cardioprotective, antioxidative, and antimutagenic effects. Catechins in green and black tea, anthocyanins and resveratrol in grapes, and soy isoflavones are the well-researched flavonoids in the therapy of hypertension (Ghaffari and Roshanravan, 2020). Flavonoids are an important family of natural compounds, containing polyphenolic structures, therefore they are also termed polyphenols (Ciumărnean et al., 2020).

Flavonoids are present in many vegetables and fruits, and at the plant level, flavonoids have the function of combating oxidative stress; also, they filter ultraviolet radiation and prevent plants from abiotic and biotic stress. Moreover, certain studies suggested the antioxidant role of flavonoids in pathologies such as atherosclerosis, Alzheimer's, hypertension, etc. Considering the role of flavonoids, they find usage in numerous nutritional, medical, pharmacological, and cosmetic applications. The amount and content of polyphenols in plants are variable based on the species, section of the plant, age, storage, geographical distribution, and mode of cultivation (Rees et al., 2018).

The antioxidant property of the flavonoids is carried out by three primary mechanisms: (1) inhibiting the production of ROS, (2) quenching or eliminating ROS, or (3) increasing or boosting the antioxidant system. Single or multiple pathways can achieve antioxidant effects. Additionally, some of the flavonoids can act on the enzymes responsible for the production of ROS such as XO, which is responsible for reactive species production (Sánchez et al., 2019). Mainly the aglycone part of the flavonoids is the deciding factor for the antioxidant capacity, the stronger the aglycone part, the better the antioxidizing capacity; and as the glycone moieties increase, the antioxidizing capacity decreases (Arts et al., 2004).

It is well known that NO in the endothelium plays a vital role in regulating blood pressure and vascular tone, as we know that NO is mainly concerned with the vasodilation of the blood vessels. The vasodilation effect on blood vessels by NO is primarily initiated by the activation of the cyclic guanosine monophosphate (cGMP)-protein kinase cascade in vessels which results in the stimulation of potassium channel and eventually leads to a hyperpolarized state that inhibits the calcium influx, which leads to vasodilation. In simpler words, NO acts by phosphorylation of the myosin light chain, which decreases vasoconstriction (Gao et al., 2016).

Specific flavanols containing compounds have the antihypertensive effect represented by quercetin and kaempferol. This antihypertensive mechanism is due to the activation of the synthesis enzyme for NO synthetase 3, which eventually leads to vasodilation and eventually decreases blood pressure (Saponara et al., 2006). Furthermore, other flavonoids with an antihypertensive effect are naringenin, a flavone class of flavonoids that show their vasodilation by hyperpolarization and deactivation of the calcium channel. Moreover, in the same class, another representative is hesperetin, which acts by increasing NO's plasma concentration (Yamamoto et al., 2013).

Additionally, an in vivo study suggested the role of epicatechin as a potent antioxidant and used as an antihypertensive agent, and it mainly acts by quenching superoxide, a reactive species in the left ventricles and aorta. It quenches the reactive species and helps in the production of NO, which eventually reduces blood pressure (Igarashi et al., 2007). Not only does epicatechin help to the production of NO and helps inhibit arginase-2, an enzyme responsible for decreasing NO (Schnorr et al., 2008).

Moreover, numerous studies have claimed the role of flavonoids in atherosclerosis; flavonoids prevent lipid oxidation by the interaction of flavonoids with nonpolar molecules in the hydrophobic region of the membrane. In the hydrophobic zone, it prevents the access of oxidants; therefore, protecting the oxidant from entering the cell and eventually protecting oxidative conditions and preventing the genesis of various pathologies (Kerry and Abbey, 1997). Additionally, an in vivo study on hamsters fed with a cholesterol-rich diet and dietary flavonoids reveals a significant effect on apolipoprotein B, triglycerides, and cholesterol levels. In this case, the dietary supplement increases the HDL level and decreases the free triglycerides, apolipoprotein B, and fatty acids (de Gaetano et al., 2002).

Nevertheless, more concert clinical studies are warranted for a deeper understanding of the flavonoids in CVD supplementations.

5.4.6 COENZYME Q10

CoQ10 is one of the most utilized dietary supplements that have a beneficial role in various pathologies. CoQ10 is the benzoquinone ring with 10 isoprene compounds; therefore, the name Q10 is termed; also, it is ubiquitous; therefore, it is also termed as ubiquinone. Furthermore, the coQ10 is not a vitamin but a so-called vitamin because it is structured similar to many vitamins, and vitamins are taken externally, whereas ubiquinone is endogenously produced inside the body. It has involvement in various bodily functions; firstly, it acts as a cofactor in oxidative phosphorylation in ATP production. Secondly, other than ATP production coQ10 in its reduced form, it is a potent antioxidant and helps scavenge various reactive species (Raizner, 2019). Also, it protects the plasma membrane from peroxidation, thereby preventing lipid peroxidation. The research on supplementation with coQ10 in apolipoprotein-E deficient mice shows a decrease in lipid peroxidation in atherosclerotic lesions (Tsai et al., 2012). As a potent hydrogen donor, it is an effective antioxidant compared with other antioxidants; and also helps to regenerate the other antioxidants; for instance, it helps to regenerate vitamin E. Moreover, one of the major mechanisms for initiation of hypertension is through superoxide anions that enter the endothelial cell and react with NO forms $ONOO^-$ that eventually decreases the intracellular NO level and thereby induces vasoconstriction and increases blood pressure (Zozina et al., 2018).

The systolic blood pressure was shown to be reduced to normal levels following 12 weeks of CoQ10 treatment in a randomized, double-blind, placebo-controlled study (Ho et al., 2009). Another systematic review found that CoQ10 can lower systolic blood pressure by 11 mm Hg and diastolic blood pressure by 7 mm Hg. Furthermore, when blood pressure is normal in patients with illnesses such as type 2 diabetes mellitus and ischemic left ventricular systolic dysfunction, injection of CoQ10 did not affect blood pressure (Dai et al., 2011). To put it another way, CoQ10's antihypertensive action is limited to patients with hypertension and does not lower systemic pressure in people who do not have hypertension.

Furthermore, the coQ10 has a protective role in coronary artery disease (CAD), which can cause MI. The study investigated the effect of CoQ10 oral administration at doses of 100 mg on the endothelium-dependent vasodilation activity of extracellular SOD in patients with CAD. The results showed that in the CoQ10-treated group, endothelium-dependent arterial relaxation was higher than in the placebo group (Tiano et al., 2007).

Lastly, discussing the studies and the role of coQ10 in cardiovascular disease, there are still limitations and an in-depth clinical studies, mainly focusing on the antioxidant properties of coQ10 in various CVD, are required which might help get a concrete conclusion. Also, helps to get the specific dose of supplementation required for the intended activity.

5.5 CONCLUSION

Thoroughly discussing all the nutraceuticals and their potential role in CVD. We can firmly conclude that nutraceuticals as an antioxidant have a role in preventing and treating various pathological conditions related to CVD. However, all of the above nutraceuticals lack the specific dose and the exact regimen for the administration. Therefore, the exact need for the specific disease condition is unknown. More extensive clinical trials are needed to overcome this, with a large population and majorly studied for specific disease and antioxidizing capacity. This study would help design the dose regimen and generalize the study further; it would also help develop natural therapeutic supplements in the form of nutraceuticals.

KEYWORDS

- **nutraceutical antioxidant**
- **cardiovascular disease**
- **selenoproteins**
- **lycopene**
- **coenzyme Q10**
- **flavonoids**

REFERENCES

Arab, L.; Steck, S. Lycopene and Cardiovascular Disease. *Am. J. Clin. Nutr.* **2000,** *71* (6), 1691S–1695S. https://doi.org/10.1093/ajcn/71.6.1691S

Arbogast, S; Ferreiro, A. Selenoproteins and Protection Against Oxidative Stress: Selenoprotein N as A Novel Player at the Crossroads of Redox Signaling and Calcium Homeostasis. *Antioxid. Redox Signal.* **2010,** *12* (7), 893–904. https://doi.org/10.1089/ars.2009.2890

Arts, I. C. W.; Sesink, A. L. A.; Faassen-Peters, M.; Hollman, P. C. H. The Type of Sugar Moiety is a Major Determinant of the Small Intestinal Uptake and Subsequent Biliary Excretion of Dietary Quercetin Glycosides. *Br. J. Nutr.* **2004,** *91* (6), 841–847. https://doi.org/10.1079/BJN20041123

Ashor, A. W.; Lara, J.; Mathers, J. C.; Siervo, M. Effect of Vitamin C on Endothelial Function in Health and Disease: A Systematic Review and Meta-Analysis of Randomised Controlled Trials. *Atherosclerosis.* **2014,** *235* (1), 9–20. https://doi.org/10.1016/j.atherosclerosis.2014.04.004

Azad, G. K.; Tomar, R. S.. Ebselen, A Promising Antioxidant Drug: Mechanisms of Action and Targets of Biological Pathways. *Mol. Biol. Rep.* **2014,** *41* (8), 4865–4879. https://doi.org/10.1007/s11033-014-3417-x

Bahoran, T.; Soobrattee, M. A.; Luximon-Ramma, V.; Aruoma, O. I. Free Radicals and Antioxidants in Cardiovascular Health and Disease. *Int. J. Med. Update - EJOURNAL.* **2006,** *1* (2), Article 2. https://doi.org/10.4314/ijmu.v1i2.39839

Benstoem, C.; Goetzenich, A.; Kraemer, S.; Borosch, S.; Manzanares, W.; Hardy, G.; Stoppe, C. Selenium and Its Supplementation in Cardiovascular Disease—What do we Know? *Nutrients* **2015,** *7* (5), 3094–3118. https://doi.org/10.3390/nu7053094

Boaz, M.; Smetana, S.; Weinstein, T.; Matas, Z.; Gafter, U.; Iaina, A.; Knecht, A.; Weissgarten, Y.; Brunner, D.; Fainaru, M.; Green, M. S. Secondary Prevention with Antioxidants of Cardiovascular Disease in Endstage Renal Disease (SPACE): Randomised Placebo-Controlled Trial. *Lancet (London, England).* **2000,** *356* (9237), 1213–1218. https://doi.org/10.1016/s0140-6736(00)02783-5

Briones, A. M.; Touyz, R. M. Oxidative Stress and Hypertension: Current Concepts. *Curr. Hypertens. Rep.* **2010,** *12* (2), 135–142. https://doi.org/10.1007/s11906-010-0100-z

Ciumărnean, L.; Milaciu, M. V.; Runcan, O.; Vesa, Ștefan C.; Răchișan, A. L.; Negrean, V.; Perné, M.-G.; Donca, V. I.; Alexescu, T.-G.; Para, I.; Dogaru, G. The Effects of Flavonoids in Cardiovascular Diseases. *Molecules.* **2020,** *25* (18), 4320. https://doi.org/10.3390/molecules25184320

Croft, L.; Lu, J.; Holmgren, A.; Khanna, K. From Selenium to Selenoproteins: Synthesis, Identity, and Their Role in Human Health. *Antioxid. Redox Signal.* **2007,** *9,* 775–806. https://doi.org/10.1089/ars.2007.1528

Dai, Y.-L.; Luk, T.-H.; Yiu, K.-H.; Wang, M.; Yip, P. M. C.; Lee, S. W. L.; Li, S.-W.; Tam, S.; Fong, B.; Lau, C.-P.; Siu, C.-W.; Tse, H.-F. Reversal of Mitochondrial Dysfunction by Coenzyme Q10 supplement Improves Endothelial Function in Patients with Ischaemic Left Ventricular Systolic Dysfunction: A Randomized Controlled Trial. *Atherosclerosis.* **2011,** *216* (2), 395–401. https://doi.org/10.1016/j.atherosclerosis.2011.02.013

De Gaetano, G.; De Curtis, A.; Di Castelnuovo, A.; Donati, M. B.; Iacoviello, L.; Rotondo, S. Antithrombotic Effect of Polyphenols in Experimental Models: A Mechanism of Reduced

Vascular Risk by Moderate Wine Consumption. *Ann. N Y Acad. Sci.* **2002,** *957,* 174–188. https://doi.org/10.1111/j.1749-6632.2002.tb02915.x

Di Mascio, P.; Kaiser, S.; Sies, H. Lycopene as the Most Efficient Biological Carotenoid Singlet Oxygen Quencher. *Arch. Biochem. Biophys.* **1989,** *274* (2), 532–538. https://doi.org/10.1016/0003-9861(89)90467-0

Di Meo, S.; Reed, T. T.; Venditti, P.; Victor, V. M. Role of ROS and RNS Sources in Physiological and Pathological Conditions. *Oxid. Med. Cell. Longev.* **2016,** 1245049. https://doi.org/10.1155/2016/1245049

Doughan, A. K.; Harrison, D. G.; Dikalov, S. I. Molecular Mechanisms of Angiotensin II-mediated Mitochondrial Dysfunction: Linking Mitochondrial Oxidative Damage and Vascular Endothelial Dysfunction. *Circ. Res.* **2008,** *102* (4), 488–496. https://doi.org/10.1161/CIRCRESAHA.107.162800

Ferré, N.; Camps, J.; Paul, A.; Cabré, M.; Calleja, L.; Osada, J.; Joven, J. Effects of High-Fat, Low-Cholesterol Diets on Hepatic Lipid Peroxidation and Antioxidants in Apolipoprotein E-deficient Mice. *Mol. Cell. Biochem.* **2001,** *218* (1–2), 165–169. https://doi.org/10.1023/a:1007296919243

Flores-Mateo, G.; Navas-Acien, A.; Pastor-Barriuso, R.; Guallar, E. Selenium and Coronary Heart Disease: A Meta-Analysis. *Am. J. Clin. Nutr.* **2006,** *84* (4), 762–773. https://doi.org/10.1093/ajcn/84.4.762

Förstermann, U.; Sessa, W. C. Nitric Oxide Synthases: Regulation and Function. *Eur. Heart J.* **2012,** *33* (7), 829–837, 837a–837d. https://doi.org/10.1093/eurheartj/ehr304

Fuhrman, B.; Elis, A.; Aviram, M. Hypocholesterolemic Effect of Lycopene and Beta-Carotene is Related to Suppression of Cholesterol Synthesis and Augmentation of LDL Receptor Activity in Macrophages. *Biochem. Biophys. Res. Commun.* **1997,** *233* (3), 658–662. https://doi.org/10.1006/bbrc.1997.6520

Gao, Y.; Chen, T.; Raj, J. U. Endothelial and Smooth Muscle Cell Interactions in the Pathobiology of Pulmonary Hypertension. *Am. J. Respir. Cell Mol. Biol.* **2016,** *54* (4), 451–460. https://doi.org/10.1165/rcmb.2015-0323TR

Ghaffari, S.; Roshanravan, N. The Role of Nutraceuticals in Prevention and Treatment of Hypertension: An Updated Review of the Literature. *Food Res. Int.* **2020,** *128,* 108749. https://doi.org/10.1016/j.foodres.2019.108749

Ghani, U.; Naeem, M.; Rafeeq, H.; Imtiaz, U.; Amjad, A.; Ullah, S.; Rehman, A.; Qasim, F. A Novel Approach towards Nutraceuticals and Biomedical Applications. *Sch. Int. J. Biochem.* **2019,** *02* (10), 245–252. https://doi.org/10.36348/SIJB.2019.v02i10.001

Gorecki, G. P.; Elena, R.; Moldovan, H.; Tudorache, I. Reactive Nitrogen Species and Cardiovascular Diseases. *Rom. J. Mil. Med.* **2018,** *CXXI,* No-2.

Guan, Y.; Dai, P.; Wang, H. Effects of vitamin C supplementation on Essential Hypertension: A Systematic Review and Meta-Analysis. *Medicine.* **2020,** *99* (8), e19274. https://doi.org/10.1097/MD.0000000000019274

Hak, A. E.; Stampfer, M. J.; Campos, H.; Sesso, H. D.; Gaziano, J. M.; Willett, W.; Ma, J. Plasma Carotenoids and Tocopherols and Risk of Myocardial Infarction in a Low-Risk Population of US Male Physicians. *Circulation.* **2003,** *108* (7), 802–807. https://doi.org/10.1161/01.CIR.0000084546.82738.89

Heller, R.; Münscher-Paulig, F.; Gräbner, R.; Till, U. L-Ascorbic Acid Potentiates Nitric Oxide Synthesis in Endothelial Cells*. *J. Biol. Chem.* **1999,** *274* (12), 8254–8260. https://doi.org/10.1074/jbc.274.12.8254

Ho, M. J.; Bellusci, A.; Wright, J. M. Blood Pressure Lowering Efficacy of Coenzyme Q10 for Primary Hypertension. *Cochrane Database Syst. Rev.* **2009,** *4,* CD007435. https://doi.org/10.1002/14651858.CD007435.pub2

Igarashi, K.; Honma, K.; Yoshinari, O.; Nanjo, F.; Hara, Y. Effects of Dietary Catechins on Glucose Tolerance, Blood Pressure and Oxidative Status in Goto-Kakizaki Rats. *J. Nutr. Sci. Vitaminol.* **2007,** *53* (6), 496–500. https://doi.org/10.3177/jnsv.53.496

Kerry, N. L.; Abbey, M. Red Wine and Fractionated Phenolic Compounds Prepared from Red Wine Inhibit Low Density Lipoprotein Oxidation In Vitro. *Atherosclerosis.* **1997,** *135* (1), 93–102. https://doi.org/10.1016/s0021-9150(97)00156-1.

Keservani, R. K.; Kesharwani, R. K.; Vyas, N.; Jain, S.; Raghuvanshi, R.; Sharma, A. K. Nutraceutical and Functional Food as Future Food: A Review. *Der Pharm. Lettre* **2010a,** *2* (1), 106–116.

Keservani, R. K.; Kesharwani, R. K.; Sharma, A. K.; Vyas, N.; Chadoker, A. Nutritional Supplements: An Overview. *Int. J. Curr. Pharm. Rev. Res.* **2010b,** *1* (1), 59–75.

Keservani, R. K.; Sharma, A. K.; Kesharwani, R. K. An overview and Therapeutic Applications of Nutraceutical and Functional Foods. In *Recent Advances in Drug Delivery Technology*; 2017; pp 160–201. ISBN:9781522507543.

Keservani, R. K.; Sharma, A. K.; Kesharwani, R. K.; (Eds.). *Nutraceuticals and Dietary Supplements: Applications in Health Improvement and Disease Management*; CRC Press, 2020; pp 1–342.

Keservani, R. K.; Sharma, A. K. Flavonoids: Emerging Trends and Potential Health Benefits. *J. Chin. Pharm. Sci.* **2014,** *23* (12), 815.

Keservani, R. K.; Sharma, A. K.; Kesharwani, R. K. Nutraceutical and Functional Foods for Cardiovascular Health. In *Food Process Engineering (pp. 291–312)*; Apple Academic Press, CRC Press, 2016a; pp 257–278. ISBN: 9781771884020.

Keservani, R. K.; Sharma, A. K.; Kesharwani, R. K. Medicinal Effect of Nutraceutical Fruits for the Cognition and Brain Health. *Scientifica*, 2016b; Article ID 3109254, 10. https://doi.org/10.1155/2016/3109254.

Kim, H.-Y.; Gladyshev, V. N. Methionine Sulfoxide Reduction in Mammals: Characterization of Methionine-R-sulfoxide Reductases. *Mol. Biol. Cell.* **2004,** *15* (3), 1055–1064. https://doi.org/10.1091/mbc.e03-08-0629

Kim, O. Y.; Yoe, H. Y.; Kim, H. J.; Park, J. Y.; Kim, J. Y.; Lee, S.-H.; Lee, J. H.; Lee, K. P.; Jang, Y.; Lee, J. H. Independent Inverse Relationship between Serum Lycopene Concentration and Arterial Stiffness. *Atherosclerosis* **2010,** *208* (2), 581–586. https://doi.org/10.1016/j.atherosclerosis.2009.08.009

Kohlmeier, L.; Kohlmeier, M. Adipose Tissue as a Medium for Epidemiologic Exposure Assessment. *Environ. Health Perspec.* **1995,** *103* (Suppl 3), 99–106. https://doi.org/10.1289/ehp.95103s399

Kurutas, E. B. The Importance of Antioxidants Which Play the role in Cellular Response Against Oxidative/Nitrosative Stress: Current State. *Nutr. J.* **2016,** *15,* 71. https://doi.org/10.1186/s12937-016-0186-5

Lee, B. C.; Péterfi, Z.; Hoffmann, F. W.; Moore, R. E.; Kaya, A.; Avanesov, A.; Tarrago, L.; Zhou, Y.; Weerapana, E.; Fomenko, D. E.; Hoffmann, P. R.; Gladyshev, V. N.' MsrB1 and MICALs Regulate Actin Assembly and Macrophage Function Via Reversible Stereoselective Methionine Oxidation. *Mol. Cell.* **2013,** *51* (3), 397–404. https://doi.org/10.1016/j.molcel.2013.06.019

Libby, P.; Ridker, P. M.; Maseri, A. Inflammation and Atherosclerosis. *Circulation.* **2002,** *105* (9), 1135–1143. https://doi.org/10.1161/hc0902.104353

Lim, C. C.; Bryan, N. S.; Jain, M.; Garcia-Saura, M. F.; Fernandez, B. O.; Sawyer, D. B.; Handy, D. E.; Loscalzo, J.; Feelisch, M.; Liao, R. Glutathione Peroxidase Deficiency Exacerbates Ischemia-Reperfusion Injury in Male but not Female Myocardium: Insights into Antioxidant Compensatory Mechanisms. *Am. J. Physiol. - Heart Circ. Physiol.* **2009,** *297* (6), H2144–H2153. https://doi.org/10.1152/ajpheart.00673.2009

Loscalzo, J. Keshan Disease, Selenium Deficiency, and the Selenoproteome. *N. Engl. J. Med.* **2014,** *370* (18), 1756–1760. https://doi.org/10.1056/NEJMcibr1402199

MacFarquhar, J. K.; Broussard, D. L.; Melstrom, P.; Hutchinson, R.; Wolkin, A.; Martin, C.; Burk, R. F.; Dunn, J. R.; Green, A. L.; Hammond, R.; Schaffner, W.; Jones, T. F. Acute Selenium Toxicity Associated with a Dietary Supplement. *Arch. Intern. Med.* **2010,** *170* (3), 256–261. https://doi.org/10.1001/archinternmed.2009.495

Mangge, H.; Becker, K.; Fuchs, D.; Gostner, J. M. Antioxidants, Inflammation and Cardiovascular Disease. *World J. Cardiol.* **2014,** *6* (6), 462–477. https://doi.org/10.4330/wjc.v6.i6.462

McKenzie, R. C.; Rafferty, T. S.; Beckett, G. J. Selenium: An Essential Element for Immune Function. *Immunology Today.* **1998,** *19* (8), 342–345. https://doi.org/10.1016/s0167-*5699*(98)01294-8

McLaren, J. E.; Michael, D. R.; Ashlin, T. G.; Ramji, D. P. Cytokines, Macrophage Lipid Metabolism and Foam Cells: Implications for Cardiovascular Disease Therapy. *Prog. Lipid Res.* **2011,** *50* (4), 331–347. https://doi.org/10.1016/j.plipres.2011.04.002

Mervaala, E. M.; Cheng, Z. J.; Tikkanen, I.; Lapatto, R.; Nurminen, K.; Vapaatalo, H.; Müller, D. N.; Fiebeler, A.; Ganten, U.; Ganten, D.; Luft, F. C. Endothelial Dysfunction and Xanthine Oxidoreductase Activity in Rats with Human Renin and Angiotensinogen Genes. *Hypertension (Dallas, Tex.: 1979).* **2001,** *37* (2 Pt 2), 414–418. https://doi.org/10.1161/01.hyp.37.2.414

Moss, J. W. E.; Ramji, D. P. Nutraceutical Therapies for Atherosclerosis. *Nat. Rev. Cardiol.* **2016,** *13* (9), 513–532. https://doi.org/10.1038/nrcardio.2016.103

Mügge, A. The Role of Reactive Oxygen Species in Atherosclerosis. *Z. Kardiol.* **1998,** *87* (11), 851–864. https://doi.org/10.1007/s003920050241

Napoli, C.; Paolisso, G.; Casamassimi, A.; Al-Omran, M.; Barbieri, M.; Sommese, L.; Infante, T.; Ignarro, L. J. Effects of Nitric Oxide on Cell Proliferation: Novel Insights. *J. Am. Coll. Cardiol.* **2013,** *62* (2), 89–95. https://doi.org/10.1016/j.jacc.2013.03.070

Napolitano, M.; De Pascale, C.; Wheeler-Jones, C.; Botham, K. M.; Bravo, E. Effects of lycopene on the Induction of Foam Cell Formation by Modified LDL. *Am. J. Physiol. Endocrinol. Metab.* **2007,** *293* (6), E1820–E1827. https://doi.org/10.1152/ajpendo.00315.2007

Noguchi, T.; Ikeda, K.; Sasaki, Y.; Yamamoto, J.; Seki, J.; Yamagata, K.; Nara, Y.; Hara, H.; Kakuta, H.; Yamori, Y. Effects of vitamin E and Sesamin on Hypertension and Cerebral Thrombogenesis in Stroke-Prone Spontaneously Hypertensive Rats. *Hypertens. Res.* **2001,** *24* (6), 735–742. https://doi.org/10.1291/hypres.24.735

Padayatty, S. J.; Katz, A.; Wang, Y.; Eck, P.; Kwon, O.; Lee, J.-H.; Chen, S.; Corpe, C.; Dutta, A.; Dutta, S. K.; Levine, M. Vitamin C as an Antioxidant: Evaluation of Its Role in Disease Prevention. *J. Am. Coll. Nutr.* **2003,** *22* (1), 18–35. https://doi.org/10.1080/07315724.2003.10719272

Piepoli, M. F.; Hoes, A. W.; Agewall, S.; Albus, C.; Brotons, C.; Catapano, A. L.; Cooney, M.-T.; Corrà, U.; Cosyns, B.; Deaton, C.; Graham, I.; Hall, M. S.; Hobbs, F. D. R.; Løchen, M.-L.; Löllgen, H.; Marques-Vidal, P.; Perk, J.; Prescott, E.; Redon, J. 2016 European Guidelines on Cardiovascular Disease Prevention in Clinical Practice. *Eur. Heart J.* **2016,** *37* (29), 2315–2381. https://doi.org/10.1093/eurheartj/ehw106

Plantinga, Y.; Ghiadoni, L.; Magagna, A.; Giannarelli, C.; Franzoni, F.; Taddei, S.; Salvetti, A. Supplementation With Vitamins C and E Improves Arterial Stiffness and Endothelial Function in Essential Hypertensive Patients: *Am. J. Hypertens.* **2007,** *20* (4), 392–397. https://doi.org/10.1016/j.amjhyper.2006.09.021

Raizner, A. E. Coenzyme Q10. *Methodist DeBakey Cardiovasc. J.* **2019,** *15* (3), 185–191. https://doi.org/10.14797/mdcj-15-3-185

Rane, B. R.; Gujarathi, N. A.; Patel, J. K. Biodegradable Anionic Acrylic Resin based Hollow Microspheres of Moderately Water Soluble Drug Rosiglitazone Maleate: Preparation and In Vitro Characterization. *Drug Dev. Ind. Pharm.* **2012,** *38* (12), 1460–1469. https://doi.org/10.3109/03639045.2011.653811

Rees, A.; Dodd, G. F.; Spencer, J. P. E. The Effects of Flavonoids on Cardiovascular Health: A Review of Human Intervention Trials and Implications for Cerebrovascular Function. *Nutrients* **2018,** *10* (12), E1852. https://doi.org/10.3390/nu10121852

Rees, K.; Hartley, L.; Day, C.; Flowers, N.; Clarke, A.; Stranges, S. Selenium Supplementation for the Primary Prevention of Cardiovascular Disease. *Cochrane Database Syst. Rev.* **2013,** *1,* CD009671. https://doi.org/10.1002/14651858.CD009671.pub2

Riemersma, R. A.; Wood, D. A.; Macintyre, C. C.; Elton, R.; Gey, K. F.; Oliver, M. F. Low plasma vitamins E and C. Increased Risk of Angina in Scottish Men. *Ann. N Y Acad. Sci.* **1989,** *570,* 291–295. https://doi.org/10.1111/j.1749-6632.1989.tb14928.x

Rimm, E. B.; Stampfer, M. J.; Ascherio, A.; Giovannucci, E.; Colditz, G. A.; Willett, W. C. Vitamin E Consumption and the Risk of Coronary Heart Disease in Men. *N. Engl. J. Med.* **1993,** *328* (20), 1450–1456. https://doi.org/10.1056/NEJM199305203282004

Rissanen, T. H.; Voutilainen, S.; Nyyssönen, K.; Lakka, T. A.; Sivenius, J.; Salonen, R.; Kaplan, G. A.; Salonen, J. T. Low Serum Lycopene Concentration is Associated with an Excess Incidence of Acute Coronary Events and Stroke: The Kuopio Ischaemic Heart Disease Risk Factor Study. *Br. J. Nutr..* **2001,** *85* (6), 749–754. https://doi.org/10.1079/bjn2001357

Rodrigo, R.; Prat, H.; Passalacqua, W.; Araya, J.; Guichard, C.; Bächler, J. P. Relationship between Oxidative Stress and Essential Hypertension. *Hypertens. Res.* **2007,** *30* (12), 1159–1167. https://doi.org/10.1291/hypres.30.1159

Sánchez, M.; Romero, M.; Gómez-Guzmán, M.; Tamargo, J.; Pérez-Vizcaino, F.; Duarte, J. Cardiovascular Effects of Flavonoids. *Curr. Med. Chem.* **2019,** *26* (39), 6991–7034. https://doi.org/10.2174/0929867326666181220094721

Saponara, S.; Testai, L.; Iozzi, D.; Martinotti, E.; Martelli, A.; Chericoni, S.; Sgaragli, G.; Fusi, F.; Calderone, V. (+/-)-Naringenin as Large Conductance Ca(2+)-activated K+ (BKCa) Channel Opener in Vascular Smooth Muscle Cells. *Br. J. Pharmacol.* **2006,** *149* (8), 1013–1021. https://doi.org/10.1038/sj.bjp.0706951

Saremi, A.; Arora, R. Vitamin E and Cardiovascular Disease. *Am. J. Ther.* **2010,** *17* (3), e56. https://doi.org/10.1097/MJT.0b013e31819cdc9a

Schnorr, O.; Brossette, T.; Momma, T. Y.; Kleinbongard, P.; Keen, C. L.; Schroeter, H.; & Sies, H.' Cocoa Flavanols Lower Vascular Arginase Activity in Human Endothelial Cells In

Vitro and in Erythrocytes In Vivo. *Arch. Biochem. Biophys.* **2008,** *476* (2), 211–215. https://doi.org/10.1016/j.abb.2008.02.040

Sorriento, D.; De Luca, N.; Trimarco, B.; Iaccarino, G. The Antioxidant Therapy: New Insights in the Treatment of Hypertension. *Front. Physiol.* **2018,** *9,* 258. https://doi.org/10.3389/fphys.2018.00258

Stephens, N. G.; Parsons, A.; Brown, M. J.; Schofield, P. M.; Kelly, F.; Cheeseman, K.; Mitchinson, M.' Randomised Controlled Trial of Vitamin E in Patients with Coronary Disease: Cambridge Heart Antioxidant Study (CHAOS). *Lancet.* **1996,** *347* (9004), 781–786. https://doi.org/10.1016/S0140-6736(96)90866-1

Subramani, T.; Yeap, S. K.; Ho, W. Y.; Ho, C. L.; Omar, A. R.; Aziz, S. A.; Rahman, N. M. A. N. A.; Alitheen, N. B. Vitamin C suppresses Cell Death in MCF-7 Human Breast Cancer Cells Induced by Tamoxifen. *J. Cell. Mol. Med.* **2014,** *18* (2), 305–313. https://doi.org/10.1111/jcmm.12188

Tanguy, S.; Toufektsian, M.-C.; Besse, S.; Ducros, V.; De Leiris, J.; Boucher, F. Dietary Selenium Intake Affects Cardiac Susceptibility to Ischaemia/Reperfusion in Male Senescent Rats. *Age and Ageing.* **2003,** *32* (3), 273–278. https://doi.org/10.1093/ageing/32.3.273

Thomas, S. R.; Leichtweis, S. B.; Pettersson, K.; Croft, K. D.; Mori, T. A.; Brown, A. J.; Stocker, R. Dietary Cosupplementation with Vitamin E and Coenzyme Q(10) Inhibits Atherosclerosis in Apolipoprotein E Gene Knockout Mice. *Arterioscler. Thromb. Vasc. Biol.* **2001,** *21* (4), 585–593. https://doi.org/10.1161/01.atv.21.4.585

Tiano, L.; Belardinelli, R.; Carnevali, P.; Principi, F.; Seddaiu, G.; Littarru, G. P. Effect of Coenzyme Q10 Administration on Endothelial Function and Extracellular Superoxide Dismutase in Patients with Ischaemic Heart Disease: A Double-Blind, Randomized Controlled Study. *Eur. Heart J.* **2007,** *28* (18), 2249–2255. https://doi.org/10.1093/eurheartj/ehm267

Tinggi, U. Selenium: Its Role as Antioxidant in Human Health. *Environ. Health Preventive Med.* **2008,** *13* (2), 102–108. https://doi.org/10.1007/s12199-007-0019-4

Touyz, R. M.; Schiffrin, E. L. Reactive Oxygen Species in Vascular Biology: Implications in Hypertension. *Histochem. Cell Biol.* **2004,** *122* (4), 339–352. https://doi.org/10.1007/s00418-004-0696-7

Tsai, K.-L.; Huang, Y.-H.; Kao, C.-L.; Yang, D.-M.; Lee, H.-C.; Chou, H.-Y.; Chen, Y.-C.; Chiou, G.-Y.; Chen, L.-H.; Yang, Y.-P.; Chiu, T.-H.; Tsai, C.-S.; Ou, H.-C.; Chiou, S. H. A Novel Mechanism of Coenzyme Q10 Protects Against Human Endothelial Cells from Oxidative Stress-Induced Injury by Modulating NO-Related Pathways. *J. Nutr. Biochem.* **2012,** *23* (5), 458–468. https://doi.org/10.1016/j.jnutbio.2011.01.011

Venardos, K.; Harrison, G.; Headrick, J.; Perkins, A. Effects of Dietary Selenium on Glutathione Peroxidase and Thioredoxin Reductase Activity and Recovery From Cardiac Ischemia-Reperfusion. *J. Trace Elem. Med. Biol.* **2004,** *18* (1), 81–88. https://doi.org/10.1016/j.jtemb.2004.01.001

Viel, E. C.; Benkirane, K.; Javeshghani, D.; Touyz, R. M.; Schiffrin, E. L. Xanthine Oxidase and Mitochondria Contribute to Vascular Superoxide Anion Generation in DOCA-salt Hypertensive Rats. *Am. J. Physiol. Heart Circ. Physiol.* **2008,** *295* (1), H281–H288. https://doi.org/10.1152/ajpheart.00304.2008

Ward, N. C.; Hodgson, J. M.; Croft, K. D.; Burke, V.; Beilin, L. J.; Puddey, I. B. The Combination of Vitamin C and Grape-Seed Polyphenols Increases Blood Pressure: A Randomized, Double-Blind, Placebo-Controlled Trial. *J. Hypertens.* **2005,** *23* (2), 427–434. https://doi.org/10.1097/00004872-200502000-00026

Yamamoto, M.; Jokura, H.; Hashizume, K.; Ominami, H.; Shibuya, Y.; Suzuki, A.; Hase, T.; Shimotoyodome, A. Hesperidin Metabolite Hesperetin-7-O-glucuronide, but not Hesperetin-3'-O-Glucuronide, Exerts Hypotensive, Vasodilatory, and Anti-Inflammatory Activities. *Food Funct.* **2013,** *4* (9), 1346–1351. https://doi.org/10.1039/c3fo60030k

Yang, G.; Ge, K.; Chen, J.; Chen, X. Selenium-Related Endemic Diseases and the Daily Selenium Requirement of Humans. *Soc. Med. Aspects Nutr.* **1988,** *55,* 98–152. https://doi.org/10.1159/000415560.

Zorov, D. B.; Juhaszova, M.; Sollott, S. J. Mitochondrial Reactive Oxygen Species (ROS) and ROS-Induced ROS Release. *Physiol. Rev.* **2014,** *94* (3), 909–950. https://doi.org/10.1152/physrev.00026.2013.

Zozina, V. I.; Covantev, S.; Goroshko, O. A.; Krasnykh, L. M.; Kukes, V. G. Coenzyme Q10 in Cardiovascular and Metabolic Diseases: Current State of the Problem. *Curr. Cardiol. Rev.* **2018,** *14* (3), 164–174. https://doi.org/10.2174/1573403X14666180416115428.

CHAPTER 6

NOVEL STRATEGIES OF ANTIOXIDANTS IN CHRONIC INFLAMMATORY DISEASES

SUMIT RATHOD[1], UJWAL KATOLKAR[2], VINIT AGNIHOTRI[1], MRUGENDRA POTDAR[1], and YOGEETA GOYAL[1]

[1]*Department of Pharmacy, SVKM's Institute of Pharmacy, Dhule, Maharashtra, India*

[2]*Department of Pharmacology, R. C. Patel Institute of Pharmaceutical Education and Research, Shirpur, Maharashtra, India*

ABSTRACT

The pharmaceutical industry needs to develop effective and economical drug candidates with improved action, and minimal or no side effects for the treatment of chronic inflammatory diseases. Mother Nature has its vast unidentified and unrecognized resources which have a vital scope for beneficial effects, and that could be imparted as an efficient tool for the betterment of mankind. The use of commercially available allopathic drug treatment for chronic illness is limited because of its long-term untoward effects on health. So, there is a need for good alternatives such as nutraceuticals that have significant antioxidant properties that could minimize the problems associated with commercially available treatment options. Through this chapter, we had the goal of improving our scientific knowledge regarding the development of natural products as future anti-inflammatory drugs for various chronic inflammatory disorders and diseases.

Antioxidants as Nutraceuticals. Nayan A. Gujarathi, Raj K. Keservani, Rajesh K. Kesharwani, Bhushan R. Rane, Yogeeta Sameer Goyal (Eds.)

6.1 INTRODUCTION

Since the early 19th century, biomedical researchers have developed a special interest in inflammation. Microcirculation is the main location for analyzing and evaluating the inflammatory cascade (Schmid-Schönbein, 2006). As an immune response, inflammation represents the host's defense against foreign pathogens. An immune system that facilitates tissue repair has been evolved by vertebrates to enable survival. An organism's immune system recognizes and eliminates pathogens through two complementary mechanisms: an innate immune system and an adaptive immune system (Clark and Kupper, 2005). Different tissue regeneration therapies have been developed as a consequence of inflammation to help mend skin injuries, accelerate tissue regeneration after delivery, or repair burns. An inflammatory pathway within a cell or tissue entails a series of processes that include increased blood vessel permeability, blood flow, and leukocyte inclusion into cells and their components (Arulselvan et al., 2016). In recent years, biomedical scientists have concentrated on inflammation as a significant target study field, which encompasses a variety of cellular mechanisms such as (e.g., phagocytic processes, chemotaxis, mitosis, and differentiation of tissue cells) (Schmid-Schönbein, 2006).

6.1.1 CLASSIFICATION OF INFLAMMATION

It is important to understand that inflammation has two stages depending on its duration as well as a variety of immune factors, and it is divided into acute and chronic stages.

6.1.1.1 ACUTE INFLAMMATION

The acute form of inflammation is marked with water and protein infiltration, in addition to the extravasation of leukocytes at the site of inflammation (Arulselvan et al., 2016). Inflammation is triggered by a biological response regulated by various chemicals released by tissues and fluid that produces edema, burning, discomfort, heat, and loss of cellular activity. The characteristic of an inflammatory reaction is vascularized connective tissue reaction. Inflammation can indeed be caused by any injurious stimulus (Arulselvan et al., 2016). The inflammatory process entails three phases greater blood flow to the inflammatory cells, vasodilation, vascular remodeling, and recruitment of phagocytic granulocytes to the deeper structures (Clark and Kupper, 2005; Markiewski and Lambris, 2007; Schmid-Schönbein, 2006) as depicted in Figure 6.1.

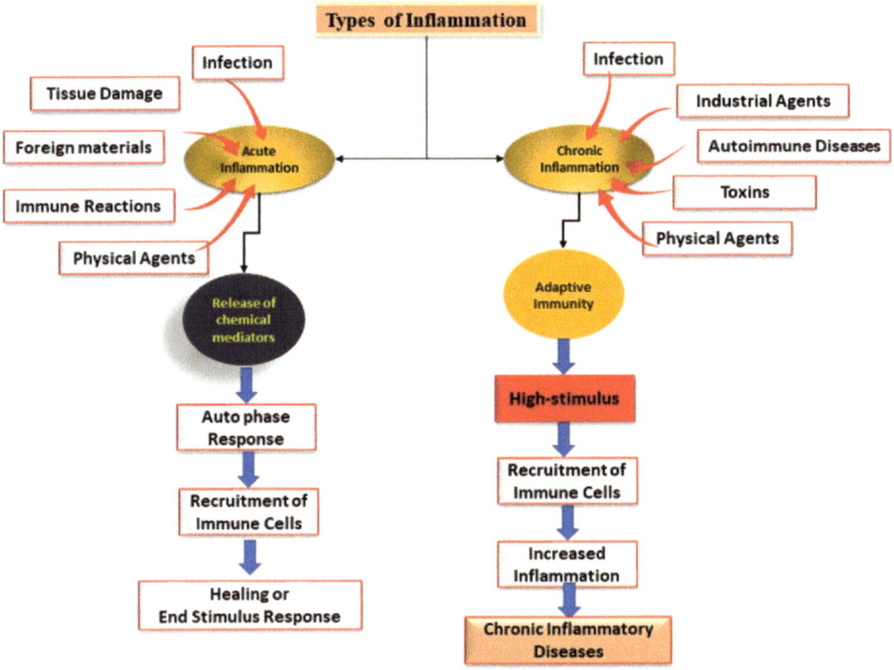

FIGURE 6.1 Types of inflammation.

Source: Adapted from Arulselvan et al., 2016

6.1.1.2 CHRONIC INFLAMMATION

The human immune system vitally responds to chronic inflammation. Despite this, chronic inflammation can have a variety of secondary effects on the body, such as a higher risk of chronic diseases and disorders. Inflammatory responses that are unresponsive to a stimulus usually lead to chronic inflammation. Most often, it results from infections that cannot be resolved by either internal mechanisms of protection or external mechanisms of resistance (Eaves-Pyles et al., 2008). Also, genetic susceptibility can result from agents that are hard to decompose, as well as physical or chemical agents. There are many factors responsible for chronic inflammation, including foreign bodies, ongoing chemicals, recurrent acute inflammation, or specific pathogens (Ferguson, 2010) Figure 6.1. It depends on the type of inflamed cells and organs on how chronic inflammation is mediated at the cellular and molecular level (Weber et al., 2011). In Western countries, the most common causes of chronic liver disease (CLD) include viral hepatitis, metabolic illness, alcoholic consumption, drug-induced liver damage, and autoimmune diseases. As a result, CLD is one of the main causes of morbidity and death around the globe (Czaja and Manns, 2010).

Hepatocellular carcinoma and fibrogenesis are both caused by inflammatory hepatitis, one of the most common liver diseases (Berasain et al., 2009). Studies also evident that chronic inflammatory conditions lead to CLD via abnormal immune responses. Further, the natural immune system is critical to life since it is the body's first line of defense against infections. Earlier studies also postulated the significance of biological mediators in triggering inflammatory responses in the hepatocytes via cytokine production including natural killer T cells, Kupffer cells, neutrophils, and monocytes (Liaskou et al., 2012). Several chronic and acute liver illnesses are directly related to abnormalities in cytokine production after liver injury (Schattenberg et al., 2011). A persistent inflammatory process or an inflammation that fails to resolve will cause a large number of hepatocytes to die and damage the liver parenchyma (Schattenberg et al., 2006). Irreversible decreases in liver function tests can be used to distinguish fibrotic/cirrhotic lesions from any other forms of fibrosis. Because osteoblasts may reproliferate from hepatocellular cell lines and replenish deceased hepatocytes, uncontrolled inflammation can result in fibrotic/cirrhotic plaques (Iwaisako et al., 2012).

6.1.2 HISTORY OF FREE RADICALS

The previous finding suggested that there is a free radical called triphenyl methyl radical (Ph3C•) in biological systems (Gomberg, 1900). Furthermore, researchers also proposed that oxygen may form free radicals as the cause of oxygen toxicity (Gerschman et al., 1954). This result was based on electron spin resonance (ESR) studies of frozen-dried samples conducted by Commoner et al. in the same year (Commoner et al., 1954). A previous line of research proposed the free-radical theory of aging. In line with that, the researcher also revealed the superoxide dismutase in 1969 (McCord and Fridovich, 1969). However, some research groups have discovered that free radicals are also involved in fighting infection as part of the cellular immune response, where reactive oxygen species (ROS) and reactive nitrogen species (RNS) work together to combat invading microorganisms (Babior et al., 1973, 1975; Hassett et al., 1987). Previous studies have discovered that ROS comprises both free radicals and nonradical oxygen derivatives (Halliwell and Gutteridge, 1989).

6.1.3 PRINCIPLES OF FREE-RADICAL BIOLOGY

ROS accumulate in cells and tissues under oxidative stress when the antioxidant (Singh et al., 2017) system fails to counteract them. Unstable protective systems can affect DNA, proteins, and lipids, causing damage to them (Ďuračková, 2010). Signal transduction, gene expression, and receptor activation are all regulated by ROS, which are key chemicals in the process of cell homeostasis. They are generally created in small amounts within the body (Kumar and Pandey, 2015). ROS and organic peroxides are produced by mitochondrial oxidative metabolism during cell respiration (Goossens et al., 1999). Furthermore, taking into consideration the hypoxic environment, nitric oxide (NO) can be produced as well during the respiratory chain reaction (Poyton et al., 2009). By interacting with these RNS, reactive species may result, such as reactive aldehydes, malondialdehydes, and 4-hydroxynonenals (Hussain et al., 2003). In addition to causing cellular damage, ROS/RNS overproduction for long periods can also cause neoplastic changes, preneoplastic changes, and somatic mutations. Cells and tissues that generate excessive ROS may then be harmed if they are left unnoticed (Chang et al., 2011). Cell death may occur through necrosis and apoptosis when ROS/RNS production is excessive (Wang et al., 2004).

Polyphenolic compounds are plant-derived active ingredients with a wide range of biological properties. In response to ROS/RNS, flavonoids (Keservani and Sharma, 2014; Keservani et al., 2016a, 2016b), and phenolic chemicals can stop the chain reaction before it adversely affects the viability of cells (Kumar and Pandey, 2013). Numerous inflammatory stimuli, such as ROS generated during oxidative metabolism as well as a few natural or manufactured substances, are documented to recruit the inflammatory procedure and crop proinflammatory cytokines. Previous data suggested that nuclear factor-kappa B (NF-κB) and the beginning of tumor necrosis factor-alpha (TNF-α) production have been shown to play a key part in the inflammatory progression (Kim et al., 2009).

6.1.4 TYPES OF FREE RADICALS

6.1.4.1 REACTIVE OXYGEN SPECIES (ROS)

A reaction of oxygen-derived radicals, known as ROS, is the primary source of radical species in living systems (Lushchak, 2014; Miller et al., 1990; Phaniendra et al., 2015; Valko et al., 2007). Due to a partial reduction in molecular oxygen, ROS is produced during normal physiological conditions (Nita and Grzybowski, 2016). Previous investigations also identify the important endogenous sources of ROS such as xanthine oxidase, catecholamine oxidation, cyclooxygenase (COX), ischemic reperfusion injury, iron, fatty acid, mitochondrial oxidation, cytochrome oxidase (Bagheri et al., 2016; Bandyopadhyay et al., 1999; Inoue et al., 2003; Lobo et al., 2010; Shinde et al., 2012; Tripathy, 2016). ROS is primarily produced in eukaryotic cells by the electron-transport chain of mitochondria (Dröse and Brandt, 2012). Extracellular sources such as smoking cigarettes, X-ray contact, chemical products, ozone, and air pollutants, in addition to natural or synthetic sources, promote ROS generation (Lobo et al., 2010; Sies, 1997; Slater et al., 1987; Valko et al., 2006). There are two forms of ROS: oxygen-centered, noncentered radicals, and nonradicals (Phaniendra et al., 2015). Radicals-centered oxygen includes superoxide anion ($O_2\bullet^-$), hydroxyl radical (OH), alkoxyl radical (RO), and peroxyl radical (ROO)•, whereas, in addition to NO and nitric dioxide, peroxynitrite (ONOO) is also a RNS. Hydrogen peroxide (H_2O_2) and singlet oxygen ($1O_2$), hypochlorous acid, and ozone are examples of oxygen-centered nonradicals (Halliwell et al., 1995; Is and Woodside, 2001; Simon et al., 2000; Sisein, 2014). ROS can cause cellular damage via several mechanisms such as DNA methylation, peroxidation, peptide breakdown, proteinaceous degradation, inflammatory cytokines release, and NF-κB engagement (Katakwar et al., 2016; Shetti and Patil, 2011).

6.1.4.2 SUPEROXIDE

The most common ROS in biological systems is superoxide ion ($O_2\bullet^-$) (Hayyan et al., 2016). It is produced through a variety of enzymatic (autoxidation reaction) and nonenzymatic processes (an electron is transferred to molecular oxygen) (McCord and FRIDOVICH, 1978). As a dioxygen anion radical, superoxide is the precursor of diamagnetic molecules such as H_2O_2 (and ONOO), as well as paramagnetic reactive free radicals (OH). Radical anion superoxide is a powerful nucleophile as well. Using nucleophilic substitution and free-radical abstraction mechanisms, contributed to DNA methylation, acetylation, and histone methylation (Afanas'ev, 2015). Xanthine oxidase is an enzyme that produces superoxide (Ardan et al., 2004; Muller et al., 2007), lipoxygenase (LOX), COX (Kontos et al., 1985; McIntyre et al., 1999; Muller et al., 2007), and nicotinamide adenine dinucleotide phosphate (NADPH) dependent oxidase (Montezano and Touyz, 2014; Roy et al., 1994). It can occur as an $O_2^{\bullet}$- or hydroperoxyl radical at low pH (HO_2) (Bielski and Cabelli, 1995).

6.1.4.3 PEROXYL RADICAL (ROO.)

In biological systems, peroxyl radicals are formed by oxygen. A peroxyl radical is a protonated form of superoxide, called a per hydroxyl radical (HOO•) (De Grey, 2002). Protonated $O_2^{\bullet-}$ accounts for about 0.3% of total $O_2^{\bullet-}$ in the cytosol of a typical cell. Initiates fatty acid peroxidation, which contributes to tumor development (Cerruti, 1985).

6.1.4.4 HYDROGEN PEROXIDE (H_2O_2)

Data suggested that xanthine oxidase produces hydrogen as its primary oxidant (Kelley et al., 2010). Moreover, a variety of biological catalysts as oxygenase, notably glycollate, and monoamine oxidases, directly create H_2O_2 (Chance et al., 1979; Halliwell et al., 2000). Living cells can be damaged by H_2O_2 even at concentrations as low as 10 M, inactivating enzymes that produce energy within the cell. It is capable of easily penetrating biological membranes. It can cause DNA damage in the presence of transition metal ions by producing OH radicals (Fisher et al., 2004). Several antioxidant enzymes can protect cells from the damaging effects of H_2O_2, including catalase, glutathione peroxidase, and peroxiredoxins (Chae et al., 1999; Matés et al., 1999).

6.2 CELLULAR EVENTS IN OXIDATIVE STRESS

6.2.1 TARGETS FOR OXIDATIVE DAMAGE

Mutagenesis is likely to increase as oxidative stress affects proteins, lipids, and DNA/RNA.

6.2.1.1 LIPIDS

It is principally easy for cellular membranes to oxidize due to their high content of unsaturated fatty acids. Lipid peroxidation, or damage to lipids, occurs in three stages (Halliwell and Gutteridge, 2015). As an initial step, an oxygen metabolite attacks the lipid methylene group to extract a hydrogen atom. Methylene molecules are easily removed due to the occurrence of a double bond adjacent to the methylene group. Upon hydrogenation, a conjugate diene is generated by the biochemical rearranging of the residual lipids radicals. If there is sufficient oxygen in the atmosphere, some fatty acid radicals can combine with oxygen during the dissemination phase to generate ROO• Radicals may extract hydrogen from surrounding fatty acids, resulting in the production of additional radicals that react with oxygen in the same manner they did previously (Henderson et al., 1998). In addition to aldehydes and cyclic endoperoxides, isoprostanes, and hydrocarbons can be formed from lipid hydroperoxides (ROO•). The reaction can continue during the propagation stage. All unsaturated lipids in the membrane can be peroxidized by a single initiation. There is no chain lipid peroxidation process available for oxidizing fatty acids that have no double bonds or one double bond; oleic acid is one such example. The final stage, chain termination, occurs after one ROO• interacts with other radicals or antioxidants (Halliwell and Gutteridge, 2015; Henderson et al., 1998).

6.2.1.2 PROTEINS

Proteins, which are also important components of membranes, could be targets for ROS attacks. It is whispered that the OH radical, RO radical, and nitrogen-reactive radical are the most likely to damage proteins among the various ROS. Proteins with SH groups are more susceptible to oxidation by H_2O_2 and superoxide radicals if they interact with H_2O_2 in physiological concentrations (Dhalla et al., 2000). In addition to damage caused by ROS directly and indirectly, proteins can also be degraded through degradation and fragmentation, including peroxidation. Protein damage reduces enzyme performance, affects energy generation, interferes with membrane potential, and causes alterations in cellular proteins (Grune et al., 1997). Carbonyl, keto, and aldehydes are the most common byproducts of oxidative stress. 3-nitrotyrosine is a usually capable dimer as a signal for proteins' oxidative stress. Whenever ONOO as well as other nitrogen-reactive superoxide combine with the amino acid tyrosine, this compound is generated. Following the OH• attack, a variety of compounds such as hydroxyproline, glutamyl semi-aldehyde, and others can be formed. After protein oxidation, altered protein molecules are susceptible to a wide range of functional changes (Stadtman, 1986).

6.2.1.3 DNA

Previous studies suggested that ROS can cause multiple problems by interacting with DNA such as strand breakage, base modification, loss of purine, breakage to deoxyribose sugars, DNA-protein loss, and interference with DNA repair mechanisms (Ames, 2001). The majority of ROS are OH radicals, which can cause harm. A variety of adducts are created when DNA is exposed to OH radicals, such as those produced by ionizing irradiation. The 8-hydroxydeoxyguanosine (8-OHdG), is obtained as a result of the interaction between OH· and the C-8 position of guanine (Jaffe, 1976). Other positions might be targeted, and new goods could emerge. Other bases can also be attacked by OH radicals, including adenine resulting in 8-hydroxyadenine (or 4-, 5-hydroxyadenine). In addition to pyrimidine peroxide, thymine glycols, 5-(hydroxymethyl) uracyl, and other products are created when pyrimidines react with OH radicals. DNA does not have any direct contact with other less reactive ROS, such as $O_{2\bullet}$ and H_2O_2 when they are present in healthy quantities; however, they may provide sources for other reactive intermediates that are more likely to damage DNA in the future (Halliwell, 1999). H_2O_2 and superoxide, for instance, can cause the synthesis of OH· via the Haber-Weiss reaction, whereas NO and $O\bullet_2^-$ can trigger the development of ONOO, which can easily cause DNA damage akin to that produced by OH radicals (Ames, 2001; Halliwell, 1999). Transition metals with a high affinity for DNA locations, such as iron, can catalyze the synthesis of OH· near the DNA molecule, assuring recurrent assault on the DNA by an outflow of OH radicals (Kasprzak, 2002; Poulsen et al., 2000).

6.2.2 BIOLOGICAL ACTIONS OF REACTIVE OXYGEN SPECIES

ROS affects cell activity at the homeostatic level in some ways, such as activating oxidative transcription factors and protein kinases (Droge, 2002; Halliwell and Gutteridge, 1989). These are described below.

6.2.2.1 STIMULATION OF REDOX-SENSITIVE TRANSCRIPT FACTORS

In addition to regulating cytokine production, redox-sensitive transcription factors such as AP-1 and p53 also influence the differentiation and death of cells (Arrigo and Kretz-Remy, 1998). When its inhibitory subunit I B binds to NF-κB, it becomes inactive. As a consequence, IB becomes phosphorylated and separates from NF-κB, which then translocates to the nucleus and causes cytokine release in response to stress. In mature placental explants treated with hypoxia-reoxygenation in vitro, increased phosphorylation of IκB is found, providing a model for placental malperfusion in vivo (Hung et al., 2001). The proinflammatory enzyme COX-2, interleukin 1β (IL-1β), and the apoptotic cascade are activated by the activation of the pathway (Cindrova-Davies, 2009; Cindrova-Davies et al., 2007). Vitamins C and E, or the inhibitor of NF-κB activation sulfasalazine, can block all of these abnormalities.

6.2.2.2 TRIGGERING OF PROTEIN KINASES

Protein kinase engagement allows the cells to respond to a wide range of external signals and triggers via a number of mitogen-activated protein kinases (MAPK). On the contrary, ROS excitation of ERK1/2 increases cell proliferation and survival whereas p38MAPK (p38) and stress-activated protein kinase c-Jun N-terminal kinase (SAPK-JNK) activation increases death. Apoptosis-regulating signal kinase 1 (ASK1) promotes p38 and SAPK-JNK by phosphorylating proteins. When $O_2^{\bullet}$ oxidizes thiol groups in thioredoxin (TRX), ASK1 releases its conformational shift and becomes active. Compared to control subjects delivered through cesarean section, the term placenta exhibits increased phosphorylation of p38 but not SAPK (Cindrova-Davies et al., 2007). Studies suggested that ASK1 is also triggered in oxygen deprivation or H_2O_2-treated explants, and it is inhibited by vitamins C and E (Cindrova-Davies et al., 2007). Previous data also suggested that preeclampsia pathogenesis has been linked to the upregulation of the sFlt-1 soluble receptor for vascular endothelial growth factor. The addition of vitamins C and E, in addition to p38 pathway inhibitors, can lower sFlt-1 levels. They may also be lowered by adding sulfasalazine, indicating that there are significant connections and joint corroboration between the NF-κB and MAPK signal transduction in the placenta (Cindrova-Davies et al., 2007). The reactions described above might be thought of as physiological adaptations to environmental changes bound for reinstating equilibrium. Further, higher ROS attacks may result in additional widespread and irreversible cell injury, eventually leading to cell loss via necrosis or apoptosis. These lead to serious consequences caused by ion channel opening, lipid peroxidation, protein changes, and DNA damage.

6.2.2.3 OPENING OF ION CHANNELS

ROS alterations cause a breakdown in intracellular Ca^{2+} homeostasis, resulting in the discharge of Ca^{2+} ions from the various reservoirs including the endoplasmic reticulum. A millimolar concentration of calcium exists in the ER lumen, substantially more than in the cytoplasm. This amount is essential for the normal functioning of the protein-folding mechanism and is sustained by exchangers from the cytosolic and endoplasmic reticulum calcium adenosine triphosphatase (ATPase) families. Earlier data revealed that ROS can trigger the release of calcium from the ER membrane, via several receptor modulations including the inositol-1,4,5-triphosphate receptor, and the ryanodine receptor (Hool and Corry, 2007).

The absence of facilitator activity causes a buildup of misfolded proteins inside the lumen, which causes more ROS production. The resulting Ca^{2+} release from the ER activates a variety of Ca^{2+}-sensitive activities within the cell (Berridge et al., 2003; Hool and Corry, 2007), counting several of the signaling pathways with a significant impact on their functions (Hool and Corry, 2007). In addition to the unfolded protein response (UPR), the buildup will also activate a series of signaling pathways aimed at maintaining homeostasis, in case of failure leads to apoptosis (Ron and Walter, 2007; Xu et al., 2005). Furthermore, an increase in cytosolic Ca^{2+} ion concentration will negatively impact mitochondrial function and may cause them to generate more ROS and open the permeability transition pore. The oxidation of thiol groups on mitochondrial proteins and the increase in Ca^{2+} ions cause the transition to open up membrane permeability (Kowaltowski et al., 2001). Consequently, the mitochondrial membrane potential and adenosine triphosphate (ATP) production decline. In case mitochondria are damaged across the cells, concentrations of ATP fall, ionic equilibrium is disrupted, and the cell dies. The engrossment of a smaller quantity of organelles or temporary pore opening may permit ATP to be preserved at levels adequate to allow apoptosis (Leist et al., 1997).

6.2.2.4 LIPID PEROXIDATION

Those organelles with high polyunsaturated fatty acid side chains are susceptible to lipid peroxidation by hydrogen radicals. A fatty acid's hydrocarbon side-chain is hydrogenated to form a carbon-centered radical, $C^{\bullet}$. The creation of peroxyl radicals can be perpetuated by the presence of oxygen in the mix

(–C–O–O•), which can then extract hydrogen from a nearby fatty acid, thus generating more hydrogen. Due to its hydrophobic tail and lipid-soluble nature, vitamin E prefers to collect inside lipid membranes. Moreover, it breaks the chain of lipid peroxyl radicals four times faster than neighboring fatty acid chains because it reacts with them four times quicker (Halliwell and Gutteridge, 2015). Antibodies targeted against one of the main products, 4-hydroxynonenal, can identify evidence of lipid peroxidation. A glutathione S-transferase enzyme group in cells can efficiently detoxify it, however, high levels of glutathione have resulted in a decline in membrane function and apoptosis (Halliwell and Gutteridge, 1989).

6.2.2.5 PROTEIN MODIFICATIONS

Proteins as well as free amino acids can be damaged by oxidation. Studies also show that proline, arginine, lysine, and threonine are particularly vulnerable to the formation of carbonyl groups (aldehydes and ketones) (Dalle-Donne et al., 2003). Western blotting and enzyme-linked immunosorbent assays are commonly used to detect protein oxidation. Similar to how ASK1 is activated, disulfide bonds can be created when hydrogen atoms are removed from the cysteine thiol group. In addition to protein aggregation and cell death, abnormal folding can result in loss of function. Besides endogenous ONOO, 3-nitrotyrosine is produced from ONOO when it reacts with tyrosine residues; so, it can be detected immunohistochemically. Since protein nitration is a selective and reversible activity, it might be as deleterious as phosphorylation at high massive doses. The protein oxidation process in the placenta can thus have a variety of impacts, including both increases and decreases in function (Myatt, 2010).

6.2.2.6 DNA OXIDATION

Deoxyribose sugars and DNA bases react to produce a variety of products. Research indicates that radicals with the OH• charge attack DNA primarily (Halliwell et al., 2000). It is possible to measure biochemically and immunohistochemically 8-hydroxy-2'-deoxyguanosine as a result of OH• adding to guanine. Sugar moiety attacks may lead to strand breaks, while histone protein attacks may result in the cross-linking of DNA, interfering with DNA repair mechanisms including transcription and chromatin folding. As a result, mutations or anomalous gene manifestations may arise. Recent data suggested that in addition to its proximity to the electron transport system that produces $O_2^{\bullet}$, mitochondrial DNA lacks histone shielding and repair mechanisms, making it particularly vulnerable to ROS assault (Halliwell et al., 2000). Consequently, even under ordinary circumstances, mitochondrial DNA is severely damaged, and abnormalities are twice as common in the mitochondrial genome as in the nuclear genome (Richter et al., 1988). Considering that mitochondrial DNA includes numerous proteins, notably electron-transport chain enzymes, a mutation in mitochondrial DNA might impair energy generation or cause further electron leakage, exacerbating the initial stress.

6.3 INFLAMMATION: A MECHANISTIC INSIGHT OF OXIDATIVE STRESS

Inflammation is a usual protective mechanism counter to pathogens and is connected to several pathogens such as microbial and pathogenic organisms, allergen and radioactivity exposure, toxic chemical exposure, autoimmune and prolonged diseases, obesity, alcohol, and tobacco dependence. Numerous prolonged disorders related to increased ROS generation result in oxidative damage and a range of protein oxidations (Entman et al., 1991). Furthermore, protein oxidation leads to the generation of inflammatory cytokine signaling, and peroxiredoxins-2 (PRDX2) has been identified as an inflammatory indication (Salzano et al., 2014). Earlier data revealed connections between inflammation and oxidative stress. According to the evidence, ROS has a harmful function in chronic inflammatory disorders. Neuron death is caused by oxidative stress injury including peroxidation, glycosylated chemicals, and lipid peroxidation, which is most commonly found in neurological diseases (Popa-Wagner et al., 2013). ROS generated in cells can interfere with synaptic and nonsynaptic signaling, culminating in inflammatory conditions, and induce apoptosis, neurodegeneration, and cognitive problems (Popa-Wagner et al., 2013). Increasing ROS intensities caused by low tripeptide glutathione (GSH) increases inflammation, weakens immune function, and increases infection susceptibility (Ghezzi, 2011). Concerning GSH, free-radical scavenging characteristics, experts looked into the functions of GSH and its oxidized state, as well as its framework and epigenetics. Through mixed disulfides, GSH regulates immune function (Ghezzi, 2013), through proteins cysteine and glutathione. This process is also known as glutathionylation, which activates transcription factors and signaling molecules (Fratelli et al., 2002). As a result of inflammation, PRDX2, a ubiquitous redox-active enzyme, is released. Released from macrophages, it turns into an inflammatory mediator that is redox dependent which leads to the release of proinflammatory markers. The regulation of immunity occurs by the oxidative linking of GSH to PRDX2 protein glutathionylation. An earlier proteomics investigation using mass spectrometry discovered PRDX2 as one of the glutathionylated proteins released in vitro by LPS-induced macrophages (Salzano et al., 2014). Furthermore, PRDX2 can also trigger the release of TNF-α as part of the inflammatory cascade. When oxidized and released from macrophages, PRDX2 does not alter mRNA or protein synthesis mediated by liposaccharide (LPS), although it constantly exists in macrophages but at a lower level. A novel therapeutic approach to chronic inflammatory diseases may be found in PRDX2 and TRX from macrophages (Salzano et al., 2014). Data revealed that the overproduction of oxidative stress in diabetes leads to severe cellular damage in the brain (Reagan et al., 1999). Several studies have demonstrated that the brains of diabetic rats had a greater accumulation of lipid peroxidation, nitrites, malondialdehyde, and total enzymes with antioxidant properties (Acar et al., 2012). Diabetes-induced chronic stress raises the levels of proinflammatory factors such as TNF-αand IL-6, as well as biochemical messengers such as vascular cell adhesion molecule-1 (VCAM-1) and NF-κB. In rodents, these chemicals produce neurodegeneration and diabetic encephalopathy, which can lead to brain damage (Prabhakar, 2013). Figure 6.1 portrays some of the disorders induced by chronic inflammation, including type 2 diabetes mellitus, glucose intolerance, and heart diseases. It is important to understand that inflammation is not a disease, but a biological process rather than a disease. Published data explored that in lungs treated with cotreatment, there was a significant reduction in TBARS concentrations and DNA fragmentation (Khan, 2012). Researchers examined whether lemon verbena extract reduced the accumulation of triglycerides in insulin-resistant hypertrophic 3T3-L1 adipocytes. In hypertrophic adipocytes, polyphenols from lemon verbena reduced triglyceride accumulation and ROS production (Herranz-López et al., 2015).

Inflammation caused by ROS toxicity has a substantial impact on the tumor microenvironment (TME). Cancer initiation and progress significantly carry forward through inflammatory responses which are generated via TME and vascularization cascades. Proinflammatory cells that produce a lot of ROS and RNS cause DNA fragmentation and upregulation of signaling pathways, cytokines, and cell survival proteins (Salzano et al., 2014). Previous research looked at the role of G-MDSCs as suppressor cells on clusters of differentiation ($CD8^+$) T-cells, which significantly contributed to ROS production (Popa-Wagner et al., 2013). Additionally, noteworthy initiation of

NF-κB, COX-2, LOX, and inducible nitric oxide synthase (iNOS) in inflammatory tissues, as well as overexpression of oncogenes such as c-Jun and c-Fos, causes ROS and RNS overproduction. In these cells, ROS/RNS are created by activating oxidant-producing enzymes such as NOX, XO, iNOS, and MPO, which enhance nitration, oxidation, and mutation (Ghezzi, 2011). LPS, TNF, TGF, hyperoxia, and hypoxia may all cause a rise in ROS through NOX4. Mitochondrial ROS (MtROS) activates redox-sensitive transcription factors including HIF-1 as well as some other proinflammatory mediators and NLRP3. MtROS stimulates TNF-converting enzymes that degrade the TNF receptor-1 (TNFR1), which would be necessary for the aggregation of inflammatory responses (Reagan et al., 1999). Previous research has revealed the involvement of inflammatory mediators in reducing inflammation by activating suppressors of cytokine signaling (SOCS), which are connected to JAKs and disrupt the JAK-STAT pathway (Acar et al., 2012). ROS-mediated MAPKs circuit activation contributes to the generation of inflammatory mediators such as TNF-α, TGF-β, IL-1β, and IL-6, resulting in transcription factor NFB activation (Prabhakar, 2013). Overexpression of proinflammatory cytokines, chemokines, and antiapoptotic genes is mediated by oxidative stress (OS). Despite this, OS inhibits JNK activity, which lowers TNF-induced ROS buildup. ROS has been demonstrated to behave as immunosuppressive agents in TME, allowing tumor invasion and metastasis to occur (Khan, 2012). A mechanistic insight of oxidative stress leads to chronic inflammatory diseases is depicted in Figure 6.2.

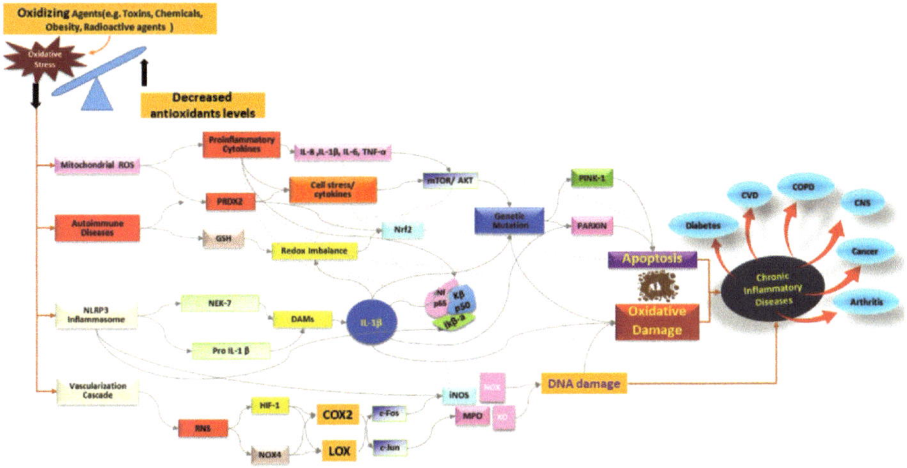

FIGURE 6.2 Molecular mechanism of oxidative stress and chronic inflammatory diseases.

6.4 DISEASES OF CHRONIC INFLAMMATION

Inflammation exists in individuals suffering from infections, and environmental and chronic disorders such as immunological diseases, diabetes, gout, and rheumatoid arthritis (Engler et al., 1983; Schmid-Schönbein and Hugli, 2005; Schmid-Schönbein et al., 2001). Nowadays, it is vibrant that a range of disorders, including venous and chronic artery diseases, Alzheimer's disease, stroke, and cancer, have an inflammatory response (Anselmi et al., 2004; Entman et al., 1991; Suematsu et al., 2002). Since many decades, variety of clinical data postulated the connection of inflammation with osteoarthritis (Benito et al., 2005; Stürmer et al., 2004). Besides, chronic depressive patients have occasional signs of inflammation (Toker et al., 2005). The involvement of molecular mediators of inflammation in pathogenies of a variety of diseases is huge. Previous data suggested the role of inflammatory responses in obesity and physical inactivity (Calabro et al., 2005; Colbert et al., 2004; Nicklas et al., 2004). Inflammation research is becoming increasingly important in the management of human diseases. Anti-inflammatory substances that have shown effectiveness in one condition may turn out to be beneficial in another. This might offer up a wide range of intervention opportunities in the use of anti-inflammatory compounds for dealing with several diseases.

6.4.1 DISEASES ASSOCIATED WITH CHRONIC INFLAMMATION

6.4.1.1 CANCER

Since around 1863, it has been postulated that chronic infection and inflammation are responsible for 20% of all cancer-related fatalities. Autoimmune illnesses including bone, colon malignancy, and microbial infections are both familiar as major sources of chronic inflammation linked with cancer advancement (Tilley et al., 2001). Previous research revealed that TNF-α serves a dual function in carcinogenesis, with high concentrations designed to kill both endothelium and tumor cells. It has been reported to activate fibroblasts or tumor cells and boost tumor cell growth in some different cancers (Mantovani et al., 2008). It is demonstrated that macrophages indorse tumor cell invasiveness in vitro via TNF-dependent matrix metalloproteinase activation (Gaiotti et al., 2000).

Inflammation associated with cancer is questionable with IL-1; low doses promote inflammation, resulting in a protective immune response, but large quantities counteract inflammation-induced cancer (Apte and Voronov, 2002; Pollard, 2004). The transcription factor NF-K is also intricate in the regulation of innate immunity and inflammation. This transcription factor can bridge the gap between inflammation and malignancy (Grivennikov et al., 2009). In preneoplastic and malignant cells, NF-K promotes the production of inflammatory cytokines, adhesion molecules, and enzymes (iNOS and COX-2) (Karin, 2008).

6.4.1.2 CARDIOVASCULAR DISEASE (CVD)

A myocardial infarction (MI) raises circulating C-reactive protein (CRP) levels significantly (Anzai et al., 1997; Courtois and Gilmore, 2006; Kroop and Shackman, 1954). In 1954, a substantial relationship between cardiovascular vulnerability and CRP was identified. Individuals over the age of 65 who have greater levels of IL-6, IL-18, 1-antitrypsin, and ICAM-1 in their blood are at an higher danger of developing cognitive heart disease (Vasan et al., 2003; Willerson and Ridker, 2004). Cardiovascular complications are significantly higher in the population's deals with chronic inflammatory diseases including atherosclerosis (van Eijk et al., 2009). The pravastatin trial in the aged populations postulated the significant contribution of inflammatory markers in CVD-associated mortalities (Sattar et al., 2009).

6.4.1.3 DIABETES

Increased secretion of proinflammatory cytokines along with microphage impeding into adipose tissues of type 2 diabetic is on the higher side as compared to normal people (Pickup et al., 2000). Proinflammatory cytokines revealed to diminish insulin sensitivity (Bastard et al., 2006), and several studies have connected insulin sensitivity with prominent TNF-α, IL-6, macrophages, and decreased adiponectin (Kershaw and Flier, 2004). Augmented plasma levels of CRP and proinflammatory mediators such as IL-1, IL-6, and TNF- in diabetes enhance vascular permeability, alter vasoregulatory reactions, and upsurge leukocyte adherence to the endothelium. Diabetes, through increasing procoagulant activity, can cause thrombus development (Folsom et al., 1999; Grau et al., 1996; Shurtz-Swirski et al., 2001).

6.4.1.4 OBESITY

Among other metabolic disorders, obesity is associated with insulin resistance, diabetes, hypertension, cancer, stroke, osteoarthritis, asthma, and neurodegeneration (Hotamisligil, 2006). Obesity and inflammation are linked by the overexpression of proinflammatory cytokines (Hotamisligil et al., 1993). TNF-α and IL-6 are two major proinflammatory mediators generated by macrophages (Karastergiou and Mohamed-Ali, 2010). TNF-α levels rise with obesity and fall with lowering of weight. TNF-α increases inflammation-induced mediators such as IL-6 and TNF-α while decreasing anti-inflammatory cytokines such as adiponectin (Hotamisligil et al., 1996). It has been found that TNF-α inhibits the insulin receptor substrate-1 (IRS-1) signaling pathway and induces apoptosis and insulin resistance in adipocytes (Hotamisligil et al., 1996; Wang and Trayhurn, 2006). As well as controlling energy and inflammation throughout the body, IL-6 also plays a role in regulating homeostasis and energy (Stenlöf et al., 2003). The utmost vital activity of IL-6 is regulating hepatic CRP synthesis, which is an inflammation indicator strongly associated with obesity and is positively correlated with obesity degree (Pradhan et al., 2001). When CRP is combined with other inflammation-related factors such as VCAM-1, inflammation and atherosclerosis are apparent (Gabay and Kushner, 1999).

6.4.1.5 OSTEOPOROSIS

A strong association has been shown between osteoporosis and inflammatory diseases, including colitis, rheumatoid arthritis, COPD, and autoimmune disorders (Mundy, 2007). It is common in various illnesses and diseases to have cytokines that promote osteoclastic activity, such as TNF- and IL-6 (Ishihara and Hirano, 2002; Moschen et al., 2005). IL-6, IL-1, and TNF-α all enhance hepatic CRP synthesis, which is an appropriate marker of the inflammatory process (Koh et al., 2005; Müller, 2002). Bone mineral density is positively correlated with circulating high-sensitivity C-reactive protein (hs-CRP) levels in inflammatory patients and healthy adults (Ganesan et al., 2005).

6.4.1.6 RHEUMATOID ARTHRITIS (RA)

Persistent autoimmune illness is marked by cytokine production responses that destroy synovial cartilage and bones (Cunnane et al., 1998; Vervoordeldonk and Tak, 2002). In recent years, IL-17 has been recognized as one of the cytokines that may contribute to rheumatoid arthritis. Inflammation, cartilage breakdown, bone erosion, and the production of proinflammatory factors have been reported as side effects of this drug. Although synovial melanocytes are the predominant makers of IL-17, T-cells are also key generators (Suurmond et al., 2011).

6.4.1.7 INFLAMMATORY BOWEL DISEASE (IBD)

Inflammatory bowel diseases are divided into two major types, namely, IBD and IBS. Inflammatory conditions of the intestine, such as Crohn's disease and ulcerative colitis, cause chronic intestinal inflammation. Additionally, the breaching of the intestinal epithelial barrier during the inflammation process, and the resulting abnormality in innate and adaptive immunity is considered to be one of the first etiological factors for IBD (Kaser et al., 2010). Proinflammatory cytokines, including IL-6, IL-1, and TNF-α are associated with chronic IBD that activate hepatic organization to elevate CRP above basal values, that are typically less than 1 mg/L (Darlington et al., 1986). Additional gastric biomarkers currently investigated in IBD include lysozyme, leukocyte esterases, elastase, TNF-α, IL-1β, IL-4, IL-10, β1 antitrypsin, and 2-macroglobulin (Desai et al., 2007; Judd et al., 2011; Lewis, 2011; Mendoza and Abreu, 2009).

6.4.1.8 CHRONIC OBSTRUCTIVE PULMONARY DISEASE (COPD)

Previous data suggested that COPD causes generalized inflammation of the respiratory system, such as the bronchi, alveoli, and pulmonary circulation that is characterized by circulatory free-radical and inflammatory cytokines (Noguera et al., 2001; Saetta et al., 1993). Increased neutrophils, macrophages, and T-lymphocytes are characteristic features of lung inflammation(Saetta et al., 1993), and augmented intensities of proinflammatory mediators such as LTB4, TNF-α, IL-1, and IL-8 (Chung, 2005; Keatings et al., 1996; Profita et al., 2005). Several data suggested that COPD patients had higher systemic CRP levels than healthy controls (de Torres et al., 2006).

6.4.1.9 ASTHMA

Airway mucus metaplasia, eosinophilia, and mucus hypersecretion are some of the pathological changes associated with asthma in the lungs (Boulet et al., 2019). This immune response in the lung is characterized by the production of IL-5, IL-4, and IL-13, and is associated with $CD4^+$ TH2 cells (Kay, 2001).

As compared with healthy participants, asthmatic patients have higher levels of IL-6, a type of cytokine generated by the lung tissues (Kicic et al., 2006; Marini et al., 1992). Earlier data was also evident that IL-6 independently and in combination with IL-1 could selectively convert $CD4^+$ T-cells in TH2 (Acosta-Rodriguez et al., 2007; Dienz and Rincon, 2009).

6.4.1.10 CNS RELATED DISEASES

Neurons and glial cells interact with cytokine receptors to produce cognitive impairment through inflammation in the central nervous system (CNS). A number of cytokines are required to activate the hypothalamus–pituitary–adrenal (HPA) axis, which is involved in the regulation of mood and stress. CNS and peripheral immune systems communicate bidirectionally with cytokines, thus helping facilitate bidirectional communication. Sleep and appetite can be affected by peripheral and central cytokines imbalances (Wilson et al., 2002). TNF-α, IL-1, IL-6, and prostaglandins have all been identified as targets in the treatment of many CNS illnesses such as AD, PD, epilepsy, stroke, schizophrenia, and depression (Lucas et al., 2006).

6.4.1.11 DEPRESSION

Studies have known for more than a decade that there is a relationship between stress, inflammation, and behavioral indicators of depression (Capuron et al., 2008; Dantzer et al., 2011; Raison et al., 2006, 2010). In addition to higher levels of TNF-α and IL-6 in the blood of people with depression and anxiety, such indicators as soluble ICAM-1, CRP, and MCAP-1 are also higher in these individuals (Pace et al., 2006). In addition to persons who show indicators of depression, the function of people who are under stress has been studied. When leukocytes were examined, it was shown that those who experienced loneliness had higher NF-Kβ activity(Cole et al., 2007, 2011).

6.4.1.12 PARKINSON'S DISEASE

A dopamine pathway failure in the substantia nigra pars compacta (SNPC) in the midbrain is the hallmark of Parkinson's disease, a chronic and progressive neurodegenerative condition. PD illness may be associated with a slow but consistent deterioration of nigrostriatal circuitry, contributing to motor, cognitive, and psychological indications (Braak et al., 2003). Nearly 20 years ago, post-mortem studies found that Parkinson's patients' SNPCs contained activated microglia, confirming that inflammation is a factor in Parkinson's development (McGeer et al., 1988). Furthermore, multiple in vivo investigations have revealed overexpression of proinflammatory cytokine values in PD patients while screening their brains, blood, and cerebrospinal fluid (Dobbs et al., 1999; Stypuła et al., 1996).

6.5 ANTIOXIDANTS IN INFLAMMATION

6.5.1 FREE RADICALS

A free radical is a chemical or molecule that may live by itself and comprises one or more lone electron pairs (Poyton et al., 2009). Free radicals, on the contrary, have an uneven number of electrons, which renders them unstable, short-lived, and extremely reactive. As just a consequence, it can respond quickly with other compounds in order to grab the electrons required for persistence. By targeting the nearest stable molecule and "absorbing" its electron, a free radical can become stabilized. Nevertheless, the targeted molecules could be free radical by shedding an electron, triggering a chain reaction cascade that damages the live cell (Reuter et al., 2010). Free radicals include hydroxyl free radical, superoxide free-radical anion, lipid peroxyl, lipid peroxide, and lipid alkoxyl. ROS are oxygen radical intermediates including as protonated H_2O_2 and oxygen (Poyton et al., 2009; Reuter et al., 2010). Radicals are created throughout cell respiration and play crucial roles in signaling pathways engagement in plant and animal cells, affecting intracellular and extracellular physiological functions. The mitochondrial respiratory pathway generates nearly all ROS in organisms (Poyton et al., 2009; Reuter et al., 2010). Aerobic cells create ROS as a normal result of biological molecular oxygen decrease during endogenous metabolic processes. In a hypoxic environment, the mitochondrial respiration chain also produces NO, which can lead to the formation of additional RNS (Poyton et al., 2009). RNS can produce additional superoxide anions such as reactive aldehydes-malondialdehyde and 4-hydroxynonenal by causing massive peroxidation. Lipids and proteins are also key candidates for lipid peroxidation, and altering such components might hasten the mutagenesis pathway (Coussens and Werb, 2002; Hussain and Harris, 2007). In an inflammatory reaction, blood cells and agranulocytes are present in the injured location, causing a "breathing surge" as a consequence of the augmented oxygen endorsement and thereby increasing the generation and production of oxidative stress at the site of damage (Hussain et al., 2003). Cells exhibiting inflammatory responses, produce more soluble inflammatory mediators mainly cytokines, chemokines, and arachidonic acid which significantly causes the release of more ROS nearby to activate inflammatory cells. Mutations in the genes that modify the production of transcriptional regulators such as NF-E2 associated factor-2 and NF-κB, which control critical cellular stress responses, can cause major alterations in the expression of genes. Such crucial indicators can activate signal transduction pathways as well as changes in signaling pathways such as nucleic acid phosphatase (NCP) and protein kinase C (PCR), which are crucial participants in the control of transcriptional as well as cell proliferation and development. Modification in oxidative stress-induced inflammatory processes, including the activation of COX-2, IL-1β, chemokines, and TNF-α, provided to iNOS which lastly leads to inflammation, all have all been linked to the occurrence of disease pathogenesis (Federico et al., 2007; Hussain and Harris, 2007). These systemic inflammatory conditions set off an undesirable cycle that can affect normal stromal cells and adjacent epithelial cells, potentially leading to carcinogenesis over time (Federico et al., 2007; Reuter et al., 2010). Oxidative stress can lead to apoptosis by damaging vital biological elements such as Genetic, protein, and lipid membranes. In a healthy and normal body, there is homeostasis between ROS generation and antioxidative defense systems (Hassan et al., 2018). As a result, it has the potential to cause a variety of diseases such as diabetes, heart disease, inflammatory processes, malignancy, neurological diseases, ischemia events, and vascular diseases (Ravipati et al., 2012).

6.5.2 NATURAL COMPOUNDS AS CONVENIENT ANTIOXIDANT AND ANTI-INFLAMMATORY AGENTS

Based on a WHO assessment, 80% of the worldwide people utilize traditional medicine for basic health care, with the majority of this therapy involving the utilization of medicinal herbs including their bioactive components. WHO in their report revealed that medicinal plant extracts and their active ingredients offer an extensive collection of medicinal as well as pharmacological activities against different forms of diseases and disorders of mankind (Arulselvan et al., 2012, 2014; Huang et al., 2013; Rajasekaran et al., 2007; Sellamuthu et al., 2014; Subramanian et al., 2006; Tan et al.,

2015; Wei et al., 2011; Wen et al., 2011). The influence of oxidative stress as well as its related consequences on human health has recently become a prime area of concern (Gothai et al., 2016). Data also indicate that elevated levels of ROS whenever the body is under stress (Krishnaiah et al., 2011). Intrinsic enzymatic and nonenzymatic scavenger substances are incapable to handle the excess of ROS, resulting in metabolic instabilities and cellular injury, along with several health issues (Krishnaiah et al., 2011). A shortage of antioxidants in nourishment can result in the occurrence of neurodegenerative illnesses (Gothai et al., 2016) such as AD, CVS complications, inflammatory diseases, and cancer (Krishnaiah et al., 2011). This appears to be a negative link between both the consumption of antioxidant-rich foods and the incidence of diseases in humans. Adding antioxidant elements into the daily diet from natural resources may be a valid solution to various diseases and disorders of mankind. Adding antioxidant elements into the daily diet from natural resources may be a valid solution to various diseases and disorders of mankind. Antioxidants from mother nature have the high potential to be utilized as a preventative medication (Krishnaiah et al., 2011).

The previous line of investigations postulated that polyphenolic and flavone-contenting natural substances have the greatest potential as an antioxidants. Furthermore, additional research has found that trace metals including copper (Mu), zinc (Zn), magnesium (Mg), manganese (Mn), etc. show a dynamic role in the cellular antioxidant (Ravipati et al., 2012). Additionally, natural nutritional components such as carotenoids, ascorbic acid, and tocopherols have been studied for their antioxidant potential (Krishnaiah et al., 2011). Various synthetic antioxidant compounds were developed to treat oxidative stress, however, the primary hurdle in dealing with the problem is nonavailability and exorbitant prices. Synthetic antioxidants have become increasingly essential in the battle against oxidative stress, but their usage is still restricted due to a variety of variables such as scarcity, high price, and side effects. Butylated hydroxyanisole (butylated hydroxytoluene), for example, has been extensively employed as a synthetic antioxidant in the nutrition business, but its use is limited because of its potential ability to cause liver toxicity along with several metabolic diseases (Krishnaiah et al., 2011). Antioxidants from natural origin, on the other hand, are widespread in numerous plant materials, have no adverse effects, and are very cost effective. Naturally occurring antioxidants are described to have a shielding effect in contradiction to the formation of ROS, enabling biologically active antioxidants as emerging novel therapeutic agents for the management of oxidative stress disease (Ravipati et al., 2012). Polyphenolic compounds and flavonoids are good anti-inflammatory mediators in conjunction to their pharmacological properties. Natural substances' anti-inflammatory properties have been documented in multiple research and confirmed in several preclinical trials (Ravipati et al., 2012). The previous line of investigations also highlighted that biologically active extracts and their indigenous constituents exhibit deep pharmacological effects by inhibiting important signal transduction pathways including NF-κB, and MAPKs, both of which play a critical role in the synthesis of numerous inflammatory cytokines Table 6.1.

TABLE 6.1 List of Natural Compounds with Different Biological Activities.

Natural compounds	Cellular mediators	Biological actions	Molecular mechanism	References
Flavocoxid	COX-2; LOX	Septic shock	CoX-2 and 5-LOX inhibitions	(Bitto et al., 2012)
Paeonol	miRNA-30a expression	Decrease oxidative stress	ox-LDL-induced autophagy inhibition	(Li et al., 2018)
ω-3: α-linoleic acid (ALA)	Glutamate receptors	Reduce the effects of oxidative stress and cell death	Reducing glutamate-mediated neurodegeneration and neurogenesis	(Komsiiska, 2019)
(-)Epigallo catechin gallate	IL-1β, NF-κB, GST, NQO1, MCP-1, ICAM-1	Melanoma growth inhibition and PCB 126-induced inflammation	Modulation of the AhR/ Nrf2 pathway as well as inhibition of NLRP3	(Ellis et al., 2011; Han et al., 2012)
Quercetin	p53 expression	Reduces the extent of the infarct and the neurological impairments in terms of behavior	Anti-oxidant, anti-inflammatory, anti-blood coagulation	(Wang et al., 2012)
Apigenin	Casp-1, IL-1β	LPS-induced inflammation inhibition	Inhibiting NLRP3 inflammasome activation	(Zhang et al., 2014)
Green tea	SOD1, GSR, NQO1, GST	Reducing PCB 126 induced oxidative damage.	Stimulating AhR/Nrf2 pathway	(Newsome et al., 2014)
Resveratrol	IL-1, TNF-α, IL-6	Reducing hepatic metaflammation	Suppressing NLRP3	(Yang and Lim, 2014)

TABLE 6.1 *(Continued)*

Natural compounds	Cellular mediators	Biological actions	Molecular mechanism	References
Genistein	NF-kB, JNK1, ERK/PI3K/AKT	Antiestrogenic	Both tyrosine kinase and TNF-α, mRNA expression are inhibited	(John et al., 2016)
Ginkgo biloba	Akt-CREB-BDNF	Decrease oxidative stress	Improve the antioxidant status of the mito-chondria, most likely by triggering a GSH antioxidant response	(Wu et al., 2020)
Allicin	TNF-α	Colon cancer	Inhibition of cytokine secretion	(Langa et al., 2004)
Catechin	IL-1β	Against monosodium urate-induced inflammation	Modulating NLRP3 inflammasome	(Jhang et al., 2015)
Polyphenols	MCP-1, IL-10, IL-8, TNF-α, IL-6	Human kerati-nocyte inflam-matory response modulation	EGF induced NFκB via regulating AhR signaling	(Potapovich et al., 2011)
Rutin	Casp-1, IL-1β, ASCNLRP3, IL-18, TNF-α	Reducing inflammation in pancreas	Suppressing NLRP3 inflammasome	(Aruna et al., 2014)
Curcumin	IL-1β, TNF-α	Decrease oxidative stress	Increase GSH cellular levels	(Sharifi-Rad et al., 2020)
Flavonoids	IL-6, IL-1β, TNF-α	Decrease oxidative stress	Reduce ROS inhibiting several enzymes	(Sharifi-Rad et al., 2020)

6.6 CONCLUSION

Antioxidant compounds and anti-inflammatory agents generated from natural substance resources have become the topic of many studies in recent years. In this chapter, we evaluated the anti-inflammatory characteristics of herbs and associated processes, using data from several browsers such as Science Direct, PubMed, Google Scholar, and others. This chapter also looked at the micromolecular foundations of inflammatory pathophysiology, which might lead to new targeted therapies for the management of persistent inflammatory illnesses.

KEYWORDS

- **nutraceuticals**
- **antioxidant**
- **inflammation**
- **chronic inflammatory disorders**
- **free radicals**

REFERENCES

Acar, A.; Akil, E.; Alp, H.; Evliyaoglu, O.; Kibrisli, E.; Inal, A.; Unan, F.; Tasdemir, N. Oxidative Damage is Ameliorated by Curcumin Treatment in Brain and Sciatic Nerve of Diabetic Rats. *Int. J. Neurosci.* **2012,** *122,* 367–372.

Acosta-Rodriguez, E. V.; Napolitani, G.; Lanzavecchia, A. ; Sallusto, F. Interleukins 1beta and 6 but Not Transforming Growth Factor-beta are Essential for the Differentiation of Interleukin 17-Producing Human T Helper Cells. *Nat. Immunol.* **2007,** *8,* 942–949.

Afanas'ev, I. Mechanisms of Superoxide Signaling in Epigenetic Processes: Relation to Aging and Cancer. *Aging Dis.* **2015,** *6,* 216.

Ames, B. N. DNA Damage from Micronutrient Deficiencies is Likely to be a Major Cause of Cancer. *Mutat. Res.* **2001,** *475,* 7–20.

Anselmi, A.; Abbate, A.; Girola, F.; Nasso, G.; Biondi-Zoccai, G. G. L.; Possati, G.; Gaudino, M. Myocardial Ischemia, Stunning, Inflammation, and Apoptosis during Cardiac Surgery: A Review of Evidence. *Eur. J. Cardiothorac. Surg.* **2004,** *25,* 304–311.

Anzai, T.; Yoshikawa, T.; Shiraki, H.; Asakura, Y.; Akaishi, M.; Mitamura, H.; Ogawa, S. C-Reactive Protein as a Predictor of Infarct Expansion and Cardiac Rupture after a First Q-Wave Acute Myocardial Infarction. *Circulation.* **1997,** *96,* 778–784.

Apte, R. N.; Voronov, E. Interleukin-1—A Major Pleiotropic Cytokine in Tumor–Host Interactions. In *Seminars in Cancer Biology*; Elsevier, 2002; pp 277–290.

Ardan, T.; Kovačeva, J.; Čejková, J. Comparative Histochemical and Immunohistochemical Study on Xanthine Oxidoreductase/Xanthine Oxidase in Mammalian Corneal Epithelium. *Acta Histochem.* **2004,** *106,* 69–75.

Arrigo, A. P.; Kretz-Remy, C. Regulation of Mammalian Gene Expression by Free Radicals. In *Molecular Biology of Free Radicals in Human Diseases*; 1998, pp 183–223.

Arulselvan, P.; Fard, M. T.; Tan, W. S.; Gothai, S.; Fakurazi, S.; Norhaizan, M. E.; Kumar, S. S. Role of Antioxidants and Natural Products in Inflammation. *Oxid. Med. Cell. Long.* **2016,** 2016.

Arulselvan, P.; Ghofar, H. A. A.; Karthivashan, G.; Halim, M. F. A.; Ghafar, M. S. A.; Fakurazi, S. Antidiabetic Therapeutics from Natural Source: A Systematic Review. *Biomed. Prevent. Nutr.* **2014,** *4,* 607–617.

Arulselvan, P.; Wen, C.-C.; Lan, C.-W.; Chen, Y.-H.; Wei, W.-C.; Yang, N.-S. Dietary Administration of Scallion Extract Effectively Inhibits Colorectal Tumor Growth: Cellular and Molecular Mechanisms in Mice. **2012**.

Babior, B. M.; Curnutte, J. T.; Kipnes, R. S. Biological Defense Mechanisms. Evidence for the Participation of Superoxide in Bacterial Killing by Xanthine Oxidase. *J. Lab. Clin. Med.* **1975,** *85,* 235–244.

Babior, B. M.; Kipnes, R. S.; Curnutte, J. T. Biological Defense Mechanisms. The Production by Leukocytes of Superoxide, a Potential Bactericidal Agent. *J. Clin. Invest.* **1973,** *52,* 741–744.

Bagheri, F.; Khori, V.; Alizadeh, A. M.; Khalighfard, S.; Khodayari, S.; Khodayari, H. Reactive Oxygen Species-Mediated Cardiac-Reperfusion Injury: Mechanisms and Therapies. *Life Sci.* **2016,** *165,* 43–55.

Bandyopadhyay, U.; Das, D.; Banerjee, R. K. Reactive Oxygen Species: Oxidative Damage and Pathogenesis. *Curr. Sci.* **1999,** 658–666.

Bastard, J.-P.; Maachi, M.; Lagathu, C.; Kim, M. J.; Caron, M.; Vidal, H.; Capeau, J.; Feve, B. Recent Advances in the Relationship between Obesity, Inflammation, and Insulin Resistance. *Eur. Cytokine Netw.* **2006,** *17,* 4–12.

Benito, M. J.; Veale, D. J.; Fitzgerald, O.; Van Den Berg, W. B. ; Bresnihan, B. Synovial Tissue Inflammation in Early and Late Osteoarthritis. *Ann. Rheum. Dis.* **2005,** *64,* 1263–1267.

Berasain, C.; Castillo, J.; Perugorria, M. J.; Latasa, M. U.; Prieto, J.; Avila, M. A. Inflammation and Liver Cancer: New Molecular Links. *Ann. N.Y. Acad. Sci.* **2009,** 1155, 206–221.

Berridge, M. J.; Bootman, M. D.; Roderick, H. L. Calcium Signalling: Dynamics, Homeostasis and Remodelling. *Nat. Rev. Mol. Cell Biol.* **2003,** *4,* 517–529.

Bielski, B. H. J.; Cabelli, D. E. Superoxide and Hydroxyl Radical Chemistry in Aqueous Solution. In *Active Oxygen in Chemistry*; 1995, pp 66–104.

Boulet, L.-P.; Reddel, H. K.; Bateman, E.; Pedersen, S.; Fitzgerald, J. M.; O'Byrne, P. M. The Global Initiative for Asthma (GINA): 25 Years Later. *Eur. Respir. J.* **2019,** 54.

Braak, H.; Del Tredici, K.; Rüb, U.; De Vos, R. A. I.; Jansen Steur, E. N. H.; Braak, E. Staging of Brain Pathology Related to Sporadic Parkinson's Disease. *Neurobiol. Aging.* **2003,** *24,* 197–211.

Calabro, P.; Chang, D. W.; Willerson, J. T.; Yeh, E. T. H. Release of C-Reactive Protein in Response to Inflammatory Cytokines by Human Adipocytes: Linking Obesity to Vascular Inflammation. *J. Am. Coll. Cardiol.* **2005,** *46,* 1112–1113.

Capuron, L.; Su, S.; Miller, A. H.; Bremner, J. D.; Goldberg, J.; Vogt, G. J.; Maisano, C.; Jones, L.; Murrah, N. V; Vaccarino, V. Depressive Symptoms and Metabolic Syndrome: is Inflammation the Underlying Link? *Biol. Psychiatry.* **2008,** *64,* 896–900.

Cerruti, P. A. Prooxidant States and Tumor Promotion. *Science.* **1985,** *227,* 375–381.

Chae, H. Z.; Kang, S. W.; Rhee, S. G. Isoforms of Mammalian Peroxiredoxin That Reduce Peroxides in Presence of Thioredoxin. *Methods Enzymol.* **1999,** *300,* 219–226.

Chance, B.; Sies, H.; Boveris, A. Hydroperoxide Metabolism in Mammalian Organs. *Physiol. Rev.* **1979,** *59,* 527–605.

Chang, C.-H.; Yu, F.-Y.; Wu, T.-S.; Wang, L.-T.; Liu, B.-H. Mycotoxin Citrinin Induced Cell Cycle G2/M Arrest and Numerical Chromosomal Aberration Associated With Disruption of Microtubule Formation in Human Cells. *Toxicol. Sci.* **2011,** *119,* 84–92.

Chung, K. F. Inflammatory Mediators in Chronic Obstructive Pulmonary Disease. *Curr. Drug Targets Inflamm. Allergy* **2005,** *4,* 619–625.

Cindrova-Davies, T. Gabor than Award Lecture 2008: Pre-eclampsia–From Placental Oxidative Stress to Maternal Endothelial Dysfunction. *Placenta* **2009,** *30,* 55–65.
Cindrova-Davies, T.; Spasic-Boskovic, O.; Jauniaux, E.; Charnock-Jones, D. S.; Burton, G. J. Nuclear Factor-κB, p38, and Stress-Activated Protein Kinase Mitogen-Activated Protein Kinase Signaling Pathways Regulate Proinflammatory Cytokines and Apoptosis in Human Placental Explants in Response to Oxidative Stress: Effects of Antioxidant Vitamins. *Am. J. Pathol.* **2007,** *170,* 1511–1520.
Clark, R.; Kupper, T. Old Meets New: The Interaction between Innate and Adaptive Immunity. *J. Invest. Dermatol.* **2005,** *125,* 629–637.
Colbert, L. H.; Visser, M.; Simonsick, E. M.; Tracy, R. P.; Newman, A. B.; Kritchevsky, S. B.; Pahor, M.; Taaffe, D. R.; Brach, J.; Rubin, S. Physical Activity, Exercise, and Inflammatory Markers in Older Adults: Findings from the Health, Aging and Body Composition Study. *J. Am. Geriatr. Soc.* **2004,** *52,* 1098–1104.
Cole, S. W.; Hawkley, L. C.; Arevalo, J. M.; Sung, C. Y.; Rose, R. M.; Cacioppo, J. T. Social Regulation of Gene Expression in Human Leukocytes. *Genome Biol.* **2007,** *8,* R189.
Cole, S. W.; Hawkley, L. C.; Arevalo, J. M. G.; Cacioppo, J. T. Transcript Origin Analysis Identifies Antigen-Presenting Cells as Primary Targets of Socially Regulated Gene Expression in Leukocytes. *Proc. Natl Acad. Sci. U. S. A.* **2011,** *108,* 3080–3085.
Commoner, B.; Townsend, J.; Pake, G. E. Free Radicals in Biological Materials. *Nature.* **1954,** *174,* 689–691.
Courtois, G.; Gilmore, T. D. Mutations in the NF-κ B Signaling Pathway: Implications for Human Disease. *Oncogene* **2006,** *25,* 6831–6843.
Coussens, L. M.; Werb, Z. Inflammation and Cancer. *Nature* **2002,** *420,* 860–867.
Cunnane, G.; Hummel, K. M.; Muller-Ladner, U.; Gay, R. E.; Gay, S. Mechanism of Joint Destruction in Rheumatoid Arthritis. *Arch. Immunol. Ther. Exp. (Warsz.).* **1998,** *46,* 1–7.
Czaja, A. J.; Manns, M. P. Advances in the Diagnosis, Pathogenesis, and Management of Autoimmune Hepatitis. *Gastroenterology* **2010,** *139,* 58–72.
Dalle-Donne, I.; Rossi, R.; Giustarini, D.; Milzani, A.; Colombo, R. Protein Carbonyl Groups as Biomarkers of Oxidative Stress. *Clin. Chim. Acta.* **2003,** *329,* 23–38.
Dantzer, R.; O'Connor, J. C.; Lawson, M. A.; Kelley, K. W. Inflammation-associated Depression: from Serotonin to Kynurenine. *Psychoneuroendocrinology* **2011,** *36,* 426–436.
Darlington, G. J.; Wilson, D. R.; Lachman, L. B. Monocyte-Conditioned Medium, Interleukin-1, and Tumor Necrosis Factor Stimulate the Acute Phase Response in Human Hepatoma Cells In Vitro. *J. Cell Biol.* **1986,** *103,* 787–793.
De Grey, A. D. N. J. HO2•: The Forgotten Radical. *DNA Cell Biol.* **2002,** *21,* 251–257.
de Torres, J. P.; Cordoba-Lanus, E.; López-Aguilar, C.; Muros De Fuentes, M.; Montejo De Garcini, A.; Aguirre-Jaime, A.; Celli, B. R.; Casanova, C. C-Reactive Protein Levels and Clinically Important Predictive Outcomes in Stable COPD Patients. *Eur. Respir. J.* **2006,** *27,* 902–907.Desai, D.; Faubion, W. A.; Sandborn, W. J. Review Article: Biological Activity Markers in Inflammatory Bowel Disease. *Aliment. Pharmacol. Ther.* **2007,** *25,* 247–255.
Dhalla, N. S.; Temsah, R. M.; Netticadan, T. Role of Oxidative Stress in Cardiovascular Diseases. *J. Hypertens.* **2000,** *18,* 655–673.
Dienz, O.; Rincon, M. The Effects of IL-6 on CD4 T Cell Responses. *Clin. Immunol. (Orlando, Fla.).* **2009,** *130,* 27–33.
Dobbs, R. J.; Charlett, A.; Purkiss, A. G.; Dobbs, S. M.; Weller, C.; Peterson, D. W. Association of Circulating TNF-Alpha and IL-6 with Ageing and Parkinsonism. *Acta Neurol. Scand.* **1999,** *100,* 34–41.

Droge, W. Free Radicals in the Physiological Control of Cell Function. *Physiol. Rev.* **2002,** *82,* 47–95.
Dröse, S.; Brandt, U. Molecular Mechanisms of Superoxide Production by the Mitochondrial Respiratory Chain. In *Mitochondrial Oxidative Phosphorylation*; 2012, pp 145–169.
Ďuračková, Z. Some Current Insights into Oxidative Stress. *Physiol. Res.* **2010,** *59.*
Eaves-Pyles, T.; Allen, C. A.; Taormina, J.; Swidsinski, A.; Tutt, C. B.; Jezek, G. E.; Islas-Islas, M.; Torres, A. G. Escherichia Coli Isolated from A Crohn's Disease Patient Adheres, Invades, and Induces Inflammatory Responses in Polarized Intestinal Epithelial Cells. *Int. J. Med. Microbiol.* **2008,** *298,* 397–409.
van Eijk, I. C.; Peters, M. J. L.; Serné, E. H.; van Der Horst-Bruinsma, I. E.; Dijkmans, B. A. C.; Smulders, Y. M.; Nurmohamed, M. T. Microvascular Function is Impaired in Ankylosing Spondylitis and Improves after Tumour Necrosis Factor Alpha Blockade. *Ann. Rheum. Dis.* **2009,** *68,* 362–366.
Engler, R. L.; Schmid-Schönbein, G. W.; Pavelec, R. S. Leukocyte Capillary Plugging in Myocardial Ischemia and Reperfusion in the Dog. *Am. J. Pathol.* **1983,** *111,* 98.
Entman, M. L.; Michael, L.; Rossen, R. D.; Dreyer, W. J.; Anderson, D. C.; Taylor, A. A.; Smith, C. W. Inflammation in the Course of Early Myocardial Ischemia. *FASEB J.* **1991,** *5,* 2529–2537.
Federico, A.; Morgillo, F.; Tuccillo, C.; Ciardiello, F.; Loguercio, C. Chronic Inflammation and Oxidative Stress in Human Carcinogenesis. *Int. J. Cancer.* **2007,** *121,* 2381–2386.
Ferguson, L. R. Chronic Inflammation and Mutagenesis. *Mutat. Res.* **2010,** *690,* 3–11.
Fisher, A. E. O.; Maxwell, S. C.; Naughton, D. P. Superoxide and Hydrogen Peroxide Suppression by Metal Ions and Their EDTA Complexes. *Biochem. Biophys. Res. Commun.* **2004,** *316,* 48–51.
Folsom, A. R.; Rosamond, W. D.; Shahar, E.; Cooper, L. S.; Aleksic, N.; Nieto, F. J.; Rasmussen, M. L.; Wu, K. K. Prospective Study of Markers of Hemostatic Function With Risk of Ischemic Stroke. The Atherosclerosis Risk in Communities (ARIC) Study Investigators. *Circulation* **1999,** *100,* 736–742.
Fratelli, M.; Demol, H.; Puype, M.; Casagrande, S.; Eberini, I.; Salmona, M.; Bonetto, V.; Mengozzi, M.; Duffieux, F.; Miclet, E. Identification by Redox Proteomics of Glutathionylated Proteins in Oxidatively Stressed Human T Lymphocytes. *Proc. Natl. Acad. Sci.* **2002,** *99,* 3505–3510.
Gabay, C.; Kushner, I. Acute-Phase Proteins and Other Systemic Responses to Inflammation. *N. Engl. J. Med.* **1999,** *340,* 448–454.
Gaiotti, D.; Chung, J.; Iglesias, M.; Nees, M.; Baker, P. D.; Evans, C. H.; Woodworth, C. D. Tumor Necrosis Factor-A Promotes Human Papillomavirus (HPV) E6/E7 RNA Expression and Cyclin-Dependent Kinase Activity in HPV-Immortalized Keratinocytes by a Ras-Dependent Pathway. *Mol. Carcinog.* **2000,** *27,* 97–109.
Ganesan, K.; Teklehaimanot, S.; Tran, T.-H.; Asuncion, M.; Norris, K. Relationship of C-reactive Protein and Bone Mineral Density in Community-Dwelling Elderly Females. *J. Natl. Med. Assoc.* **2005,** *97,* 329–333.
Gerschman, R.; Gilbert, D. L.; Nye, S. W.; Dwyer, P.; Fenn, W. O. Oxygen Poisoning and X-Irradiation: A Mechanism in Common. *Science* **1954,** *119,* 623–626.
Ghezzi, P. Protein Glutathionylation in Health and Disease. *Biochim. Biophys. Acta* **2013,** *1830,* 3165–3172.
Ghezzi, P. Role of Glutathione in Immunity and Inflammation in the Lung. *Int. J. Gen. Med.* **2011,** *4,* 105.

Gomberg, M. An Incidence of Trivalent Carbon Trimethylphenyl. *J. Am. Chem. Soc.* **1900,** *22,* 757–771.

Goossens, V.; Vos, K. De; Vercammen, D.; Steemans, M.; Vancompernolle, K.; Fiers, W.; Vandenabeele, P. ; Grooten, J. Redox Regulation of TNF Signaling. *Biofactors* **1999,** *10,* 145–156.

Gothai, S.; Arulselvan, P.; Tan, W. S.; Fakurazi, S. Wound Healing Properties of Ethyl Acetate Fraction of Moringa Oleifera in Normal Human Dermal Fibroblasts. *J. Intercult. Ethnopharmacol.* **2016,** *5,* 1.

Grau, A. J.; Buggle, F.; Becher, H.; Werle, E.; Hacke, W. The Association of Leukocyte Count, Fibrinogen and C-Reactive Protein with Vascular Risk Factors and Ischemic Vascular Diseases. *Thromb. Res.* **1996,** *82,* 245–255.

Grivennikov, S.; Karin, E.; Terzic, J.; Mucida, D.; Yu, G.-Y.; Vallabhapurapu, S.; Scheller, J.; Rose-John, S.; Cheroutre, H.; Eckmann, L. IL-6 and Stat3 are Required for Survival of Intestinal Epithelial Cells and Development of Colitis-Associated Cancer. *Cancer Cell.* **2009,** *15,* 103–113.

Grune, T.; Reinheckel, T.; Davies, K. J.A. Degradation of Oxidized Proteins in Mammalian Cells. *FASEB J.* **1997,** *11,* 526–534.

Halliwell, B. Oxygen and Nitrogen are Pro-Carcinogens. Damage to DNA by Reactive Oxygen, Chlorine and Nitrogen Species: Measurement, Mechanism and the Effects of Nutrition. *Mutat. Res.* **1999,** *443,* 37–52.

Halliwell, B.; Clement, M. V.; Long, L. H. Hydrogen Peroxide in the Human Body. *FEBS Lett.* **2000,** *486,* 10–13.

Halliwell, B.; Gutteridge, J. M. C. *Free Radicals in Biology and Medicine*, 2nd ed.; Clarendon, 1989.

Halliwell, B.; Gutteridge, J. M. C. *Free Radicals in Biology and Medicine*; 2015; Oxford University Press: USA.

Halliwell, B.; Murcia, M. A.; Chirico, S.; Aruoma, O. I. Free Radicals and Antioxidants in Food and In Vivo: What They do and How They Work. *Crit. Rev. Food Sci. Nutr.* **1995,** *35,* 7–20.

Hassan, S.; Sajjad, N.; Ali, R.; Ganie, S. A.; Hamid, R. In Vitro Antioxidant Potential of Various Extracts of Meconopsis Aculeata. *Int. J. Adv. Res. Sci. Eng.* **2018,** *7,* 1984–1995.

Hassett, D. J.; Britigan, B. E.; Svendsen, T.; Rosen, G. M.; Cohen, M. S. Bacteria Form Intracellular Free Radicals in Response to Paraquat and Streptonigrin. Demonstration of the Potency of Hydroxyl Radical. *J. Biol. Chem.* **1987,** *262,* 13404–13408.

Hayyan, M.; Hashim, M. A.; Alnashef, I. M. Superoxide Ion: Generation and Chemical Implications. *Chem. Rev.* **2016,** *116,* 3029–3085.

Henderson, C. J.; Mclaren, A. W.; Moffat, G. J.; Bacon, E. J.; Wolf, C. R. Pi-Class Glutathione S-Transferase: Regulation and Function. *Chem. Biol. Interact.* **1998,** *111,* 69–82.

Herranz-López, M.; Barrajón-Catalán, E.; Segura-Carretero, A.; Menéndez, J. A.; Joven, J.; Micol, V. Lemon Verbena (Lippia Citriodora) Polyphenols Alleviate Obesity-Related Disturbances in Hypertrophic Adipocytes Through AMPK-Dependent Mechanisms. *Phytomedicine* **2015,** *22,* 605–614.

Hool, L. C.; Corry, B. Redox Control of Calcium Channels: From Mechanisms to Therapeutic Opportunities. *Antioxid. Redox Signal.* **2007,** *9,* 409–435.

Hotamisligil, G. S. Inflammation and Metabolic Disorders. *Nature* **2006,** *444,* 860–867.

Hotamisligil, G. S.; Peraldi, P.; Budavari, A.; Ellis, R.; White, M. F.; Spiegelman, B. M. IRS-1-Mediated Inhibition of Insulin Receptor Tyrosine Kinase Activity in TNF-Alpha- and Obesity-Induced Insulin Resistance. *Science (New York, N.Y.)* **1996,** *271,* 665–668.

Hotamisligil, G. S.; Shargill, N. S.; Spiegelman, B. M. Adipose Expression of Tumor Necrosis Factor-Alpha: Direct Role in Obesity-Linked Insulin Resistance. *Science (New York, N.Y.).* **1993,** *259,* 87–91.

Huang, Y.-T.; Wen, C.-C.; Chen, Y.-H.; Huang, W.-C.; Huang, L.-T.; Lin, W.-C.; Arulselvan, P.; Liao, J.-W.; Lin, S.-H.; Hsiao, P.-W. Dietary Uptake of Wedelia Chinensis Extract Attenuates Dextran Sulfate Sodium-Induced Colitis in Mice. *PLoS One.* **2013,** *8,* E64152.

Hung, T.-H.; Skepper, J. N.; Burton, G. J. In Vitro Ischemia-Reperfusion Injury in Term Human Placenta as a Model for Oxidative Stress in Pathological Pregnancies. *Am. J. Pathol.* **2001,** *159,* 1031–1043.

Hussain, S. P.; Harris, C. C. Inflammation and Cancer: An Ancient Link with Novel Potentials. *Int. J. Cancer.* **2007,** *121,* 2373–2380.

Hussain, S. P.; Hofseth, L. J.; Harris, C. C. Radical Causes of Cancer. *Nat. Rev. Cancer.* **2003,** *3,* 276–285.

Inoue, M.; Sato, E. F.; Nishikawa, M.; Park, A.-M.; Kira, Y.; Imada, I.; Utsumi, K. Mitochondrial Generation of Reactive Oxygen Species and Its Role in Aerobic Life. *Curr. Med. Chem.* **2003,** *10,* 2495–2505.

Is, Y. ; Woodside, J. V Antioxidant in Health and Disease. *J. Clin. Pathol.* **2001,** *54,* 176–186.

Ishihara, K.; Hirano, T. IL-6 in Autoimmune Disease and Chronic Inflammatory Proliferative Disease. *Cytokine Growth Factor Rev.* **2002,** *13,* 357–368.

Iwaisako, K.; Brenner, D. A.; Kisseleva, T. What's New in Liver Fibrosis? The Origin of Myofibroblasts in Liver Fibrosis. *J. Gastroenterol. Hepatol.* **2012,** *27,* 65–68.

Jaffe, B. *Crucibles: The Story of Chemistry from Ancient Alchemy to Nuclear Fission*; Courier Corporation, 1976.

Judd, T. A.; Day, A. S.; Lemberg, D. A.; Turner, D.; Leach, S. T. Update of Fecal Markers of Inflammation in Inflammatory Bowel Disease. *J. Gastroenterol. Hepatol.* **2011,** *26,* 1493–1499.

Karastergiou, K.; Mohamed-Ali, V. The Autocrine and Paracrine Roles of Adipokines. *Mol. Cell. Endocrinol.* **2010,** *318,* 69–78.

Karin, M. The Iκb Kinase—A Bridge between Inflammation and Cancer. *Cell Res.* **2008,** *18,* 334–342.

Kaser, A.; Zeissig, S.; Blumberg, R. S. Inflammatory Bowel Disease. *Annu. Rev. Immunol.* **2010,** *28,* 573–621.

Kasprzak, K. S. Oxidative DNA and Protein Damage in Metal-Induced Toxicity and Carcinogenesis. *Free Radical Biol. Med.* **2002,** *32,* 958–967.

Katakwar, P.; Metgud, R.; Naik, S.; Mittal, R. Oxidative Stress Marker in Oral Cancer: A Review. *J. Cancer Res. Therapeut.* **2016,** *12,* 438.

Kay, A. B. Allergy and Allergic Diseases. First of Two Parts. *N. Engl. J. Med.* **2001,** *344,* 30–37.

Keatings, V. M.; Collins, P. D.; Scott, D. M.; Barnes, P. J. Differences in Interleukin-8 and Tumor Necrosis Factor-Alpha in Induced Sputum from Patients with Chronic Obstructive Pulmonary Disease or Asthma. *Am. J. Respir. Crit. Care Med.* **1996,** *153,* 530–534.

Kelley, E. E.; Khoo, N. K. H.; Hundley, N. J.; Malik, U. Z.; Freeman, B. A.; Tarpey, M. M. Hydrogen Peroxide is the Major Oxidant Product of Xanthine Oxidase. *Free Radical Biol. Med.* **2010,** *48,* 493–498.

Keservani, R. K; Sharma, A. K. Flavonoids: Emerging Trends and Potential Health Benefits. *J. Chin. Pharmaceut. Sci.* **2014,** *23* (12), 815.
Keservani, R. K.; Sharma, A. K.; Kesharwani, R. K. Nutraceutical and Functional Foods for Cardiovascular Health. In *Food Process Engineering*; Apple Academic Press, CRC Press, 2016a; pp 291–312, pp 257–278).
Keservani, R. K.; Sharma, A. K.; Kesharwani, R. K. Medicinal Effect of Nutraceutical Fruits for the Cognition and Brain Health. *Scientifica* **2016b,** *3109254,* 10. DOI: 10.1155/2016/3109254.
Kershaw, E. E.; Flier, J. S. Adipose Tissue as an Endocrine Organ. *J. Clin. Endocrinol. Metab.* **2004,** *89,* 2548–2556.
Khan, R. A. Protective Effect of Launaea Procumbens (L.) on Lungs Against CCl 4-Induced Pulmonary Damages in Rat. *BMC Complement. Altern. Med.* **2012,** *12,* 1–7.
Kicic, A.; Sutanto, E. N.; Stevens, P. T.; Knight, D. A.; Stick, S. M. Intrinsic Biochemical and Functional Differences in Bronchial Epithelial Cells of Children with Asthma. *Am. J. Respir. Crit. Care Med.* **2006,** *174,* 1110–1118.
Kim, Y. S.; Young, M. R.; Bobe, G.; Colburn, N. H.; Milner, J. A. Bioactive Food Components, Inflammatory Targets, and Cancer Prevention. *Cancer Prev. Res.* **2009,** *2,* 200–208.
Koh, J.-M.; Khang, Y.-H.; Jung, C.-H.; Bae, S.; Kim, D. J.; Chung, Y.-E.; Kim, G. S. Higher Circulating Hscrp Levels are Associated with Lower Bone Mineral Density in Healthy Pre- and Postmenopausal Women: Evidence for a Link between Systemic Inflammation and Osteoporosis. *Osteoporos. Int.* **2005,** *16,* 1263–1271.
Kontos, H. A.; Wei, E. P.; Ellis, E. F.; Jenkins, L. W.; Povlishock, J. T.; Rowe, G. T.; Hess, M. L. Appearance of Superoxide Anion Radical in Cerebral Extracellular Space during Increased Prostaglandin Synthesis in Cats. *Circ. Res.* **1985,** *57,* 142–151.
Kowaltowski, A. J.; Castilho, R. F.; Vercesi, A. E. Mitochondrial Permeability Transition and Oxidative Stress. *FEBS Lett.* **2001,** *495,* 12–15.
Krishnaiah, D.; Sarbatly, R.; Nithyanandam, R. A Review of the Antioxidant Potential of Medicinal Plant Species. *Food Bioprod. Process.* **2011,** *89,* 217–233.
Kroop, I. G.; Shackman, N. H. Level of C-Reactive Protein as a Measure of Acute Myocardial Infarction. *Proc. Soc. Exp. Biol. Med.* **1954,** *86,* 95–97.
Kumar, S.; Pandey, A. K. Chemistry and Biological Activities of Flavonoids: An Overview. *Sci. World J.* **2013,** 2013.
Kumar, S.; Pandey, A. K. Free Radicals: Health Implications and Their Mitigation by Herbals. *J. Adv. Med. Med. Res.* **2015,** 438–457.
Leist, M.; Single, B.; Castoldi, A. F.; Kühnle, S.; Nicotera, P. Intracellular Adenosine Triphosphate (ATP) Concentration: A Switch in the Decision between Apoptosis and Necrosis. *J. Exp. Med.* **1997,** *185,* 1481–1486.
Lewis, J. D. The Utility of Biomarkers in the Diagnosis and Therapy of Inflammatory Bowel Disease. *Gastroenterology* **2011,** *140,* 1817–1826.e2.
Liaskou, E.; Wilson, D. V; Oo, Y. H. Innate Immune Cells in Liver Inflammation. *Mediators Inflamm.* **2012,** *2012.*
Lobo, V.; Patil, A.; Phatak, A.; Chandra, N. Free Radicals, Antioxidants and Functional Foods: Impact on Human Health. *Pharmacogn. Rev.* **2010,** *4,* 118.
Lucas, S.-M.; Rothwell, N. J.; Gibson, R. M. The Role of Inflammation in CNS Injury and Disease. *Br. J. Pharmacol.* **2006,** *147* (Suppl), S232-S240.
Lushchak, V. I. Classification of Oxidative Stress Based on Its Intensity. *Excli. J.* **2014,** *13,* 922.

Mantovani, A.; Allavena, P.; Sica, A.; Balkwill, F. Cancer-Related Inflammation. *Nature* **2008,** *454,* 436–444.
Marini, M.; Vittori, E.; Hollemborg, J.; Mattoli, S. Expression of the Potent Inflammatory Cytokines, Granulocyte-Macrophage-Colony-Stimulating Factor and Interleukin-6 and Interleukin-8, in Bronchial Epithelial Cells of Patients with Asthma. *J. Allergy Clin. Immunol.* **1992,** *89,* 1001–1009.
Markiewski, M. M.; Lambris, J. D. The Role of Complement in Inflammatory Diseases from Behind the Scenes Into the Spotlight. *Am. J. Pathol.* **2007,** *171,* 715–727.
Matés, J. M.; Pérez-Gómez, C.; De Castro, I. N. Antioxidant Enzymes and Human Diseases. *Clin. Biochem.* **1999,** *32,* 595–603.
Mccord, J. M.; Fridovich, I. Superoxide Dismutase. An Enzymic Function for Erythrocuprein (Hemocuprein). *J. Biol. Chem.* **1969,** *244,* 6049–6055.
Mccord, J. M.; Fridovich, I. The Biology and Pathology of Oxygen Radicals. *Ann. Intern. Med.* **1978,** *89,* 122–127.
Mcgeer, P. L.; Itagaki, S.; Boyes, B. E.; Mcgeer, E. G. Reactive Microglia are Positive for HLA-DR in the Substantia Nigra of Parkinson's and Alzheimer's Disease Brains. *Neurology* **1988,** *38,* 1285–1291.
Mcintyre, M.; Bohr, D. F.; Dominiczak, A. F. Endothelial Function in Hypertension: The Role of Superoxide Anion. *Hypertension* **1999,** *34,* 539–545.
Mendoza, J. L.; Abreu, M. T. Biological Markers in Inflammatory Bowel Disease: Practical Consideration for Clinicians. *Gastroenterol. Clin. Biol.* **2009,** *33* (Suppl 3), S158–S173.
Miller, D. M.; Buettner, G. R.; Aust, S. D. Transition Metals as Catalysts of "Autoxidation" Reactions. *Free Radical Biol. Med.* **1990,** *8,* 95–108.
Montezano, A. C.; Touyz, R. M. Reactive Oxygen Species, Vascular Noxs, and Hypertension: Focus on Translational and Clinical Research. *Antioxid. Redox Signal* **2014,** *20,* 164–182.
Moschen, A. R.; Kaser, A.; Enrich, B.; Ludwiczek, O.; Gabriel, M.; Obrist, P.; Wolf, A. M.; Tilg, H. the RANKL/OPG System is Activated in Inflammatory Bowel Disease and Relates to the State of Bone Loss. *Gut.* **2005,** *54,* 479–487.
Müller, B. Cytokine Imbalance in Non-immunological Chronic Disease. *Cytokine* **2002,** *18,* 334–339.
Muller, F. L.; Lustgarten, M. S.; Jang, Y.; Richardson, A.; Van Remmen, H. Trends in Oxidative Aging Theories. *Free Radic. Biol. Med.* **2007,** *43,* 477–503.
Mundy, G. R. Osteoporosis and Inflammation. *Nutr. Rev.* **2007,** *65,* S147–S151.
Myatt, L. Review: Reactive Oxygen and Nitrogen Species and Functional Adaptation of the Placenta. *Placenta* **2010,** *31* (Suppl), S66–S69.
Nicklas, B. J.; Ambrosius, W.; Messier, S. P.; Miller, G. D.; Penninx, B. W. J. H.; Loeser, R. F.; Palla, S.; Bleecker, E.; Pahor, M. Diet-Induced Weight Loss, Exercise, and Chronic Inflammation in Older, Obese Adults: A Randomized Controlled Clinical Trial. *Am. J. Clin. Nutr.* **2004,** *79,* 544–551.
Nita, M.; Grzybowski, A. The Role of the Reactive Oxygen Species and Oxidative Stress in the Pathomechanism of the Age-Related Ocular Diseases and Other Pathologies of the Anterior and Posterior Eye Segments in Adults. *Oxid. Med. Cell. Long.* **2016,** 2016.
Noguera, A.; Batle, S.; Miralles, C.; Iglesias, J.; Busquets, X.; Macnee, W.; Agustí, A. G. Enhanced Neutrophil Response in Chronic Obstructive Pulmonary Disease. *Thorax* **2001,** *56,* 432–437.

Pace, T. W. W.; Mletzko, T. C.; Alagbe, O.; Musselman, D. L.; Nemeroff, C. B.; Miller, A. H.; Heim, C.M. Increased Stress-Induced Inflammatory Responses in Male Patients with Major Depression and Increased Early Life Stress. *Am. J. Psychiatry*. **2006,** *163,* 1630–1633.

Phaniendra, A.; Jestadi, D. B.; Periyasamy, L. Free Radicals: Properties, Sources, Targets, and Their Implication in Various Diseases. *Indian J. Clin. Biochem.* **2015,** *30,* 11–26.

Pickup, J. C.; Chusney, G. D.; Thomas, S. M. ; Burt, D. Plasma Interleukin-6, Tumour Necrosis Factor Alpha and Blood Cytokine Production in Type 2 Diabetes. *Life Sci.* **2000,** *67,* 291–300.

Pollard, J. W. Tumour-Educated Macrophages Promote Tumour Progression and Metastasis. *Nat. Rev. Cancer*. **2004,** *4,* 71–78.

Popa-Wagner, A.; Mitran, S.; Sivanesan, S.; Chang, E.; Buga, A.-M. ROS and Brain Diseases: The Good, the Bad, and the Ugly. *Oxid. Med. Cell. Long.* **2013,** 2013.

Poulsen, H. E.; Jensen, B. R.; Weimann, A.; Jensen, S. A.; Sorensen, M. ; Loft, S. A, DNA Damage and Gene Expression. *Free Radical Res.* **2000,** *33,* S33–S40.

Poyton, R. O.; Ball, K. A.; Castello, P. R. Mitochondrial Generation of Free Radicals and Hypoxic Signaling. *Trends Endocrinol. Metab.* **2009,** *20,* 332–340.

Prabhakar, O. Cerebroprotective Effect of Resveratrol Through Antioxidant and Anti-inflammatory Effects in Diabetic Rats. *Naunyn Schmiedebergs Arch. Pharmacol.* **2013,** *386,* 705–710.

Pradhan, A. D.; Manson, J. E.; Rifai, N.; Buring, J. E.; Ridker, P. M. C-Reactive Protein, Interleukin 6, and Risk of Developing Type 2 Diabetes Mellitus. *JAMA* **2001,** *286,* 327–334.

Profita, M.; Giorgi, R. Di; Sala, A.; Bonanno, A.; Riccobono, L.; Mirabella, F.; Gjomarkaj, M.; Bonsignore, G.; Bousquet, J. ; Vignola, A. M. Muscarinic Receptors, Leukotriene B4 Production and Neutrophilic Inflammation in COPD Patients. *Allergy* **2005,** *60,* 1361–1369.

Raison, C. L.; Capuron, L.; Miller, A. H. Cytokines Sing the Blues: Inflammation and the Pathogenesis of Depression. *Trends Immunol.* **2006,** *27,* 24–31.

Raison, C. L.; Lowry, C. A.; Rook, G. A. W. Inflammation, Sanitation, and Consternation: Loss of Contact with Coevolved, Tolerogenic Microorganisms and the Pathophysiology and Treatment of Major Depression. *Arch. Gen. Psychiatry* **2010,** *67,* 1211–1224.

Rajasekaran, S.; Sriram, N.; Arulselvan, P.; Subramanian, S. Effect of Aloe Vera Leaf Gel Extract on Membrane Bound Phosphatases and Lysosomal Hydrolases in Rats With Streptozotocin Diabetes. *Pharmazie* **2007,** *62,* 221–225.

Ravipati, A. S.; Zhang, L.; Koyyalamudi, S. R.; Jeong, S. C.; Reddy, N.; Bartlett, J.; Smith, P. T.; Shanmugam, K.; Münch, G.; Wu, M. J. Antioxidant and Anti-inflammatory Activities of Selected Chinese Medicinal Plants and Their Relation With Antioxidant Content. *BMC Complement. Altern. Med.* **2012,** *12,* 1–14.

Reagan, L. P.; Magariños, A. M.; Mcewen, B. S. Neurological Changes Induced by Stress in Streptozotocin Diabetic Rats. *Ann. N.Y. Acad. Sci.* **1999,** *893,* 126–137.

Reuter, S.; Gupta, S. C.; Chaturvedi, M. M.; Aggarwal, B. B. Oxidative Stress, Inflammation, and Cancer: How are they Linked? *Free Radical Biol. Med.* **2010,** *49,* 1603–1616.

Richter, C.; Park, J.-W.; Ames, B. N. Normal Oxidative Damage to Mitochondrial and Nuclear DNA is Extensive. *Proc. Natl. Acad. Sci.* **1988,** *85,* 6465–6467.

Ron, D.; Walter, P. Signal Integration in the Endoplasmic Reticulum Unfolded Protein Response. *Nat. Rev. Mol. Cell Biol.* **2007,** *8,* 519–529.

Roy, P.; Roy, S. K.; Mitra, A.; Kulkarni, A. P. Superoxide Generation by Lipoxygenase in the Presence of NADH and NADPH. *Biochim. Biophys. Acta* **1994,** *1214,* 171–179.

Saetta, M.; Di Stefano, A.; Maestrelli, P.; Ferraresso, A.; Drigo, R.; Potena, A.; Ciaccia, A.; Fabbri, L. M. Activated T-Lymphocytes and Macrophages in Bronchial Mucosa of Subjects with Chronic Bronchitis. *Am. Rev. Respirat. Dis.* **1993,** *147*, 301–306.

Salzano, S.; Checconi, P.; Hanschmann, E.-M.; Lillig, C. H.; Bowler, L. D.; Chan, P.; Vaudry, D.; Mengozzi, M.; Coppo, L.; Sacre, S. Linkage of Inflammation and Oxidative Stress via Release of Glutathionylated Peroxiredoxin-2, which Acts as a Danger Signal. *Proc. Natl. Acad. Sci.* **2014,** *111,* 12157–12162.

Sattar, N.; Murray, H. M.; Welsh, P.; Blauw, G. J.; Buckley, B. M.; Cobbe, S.; de Craen, A. J. M.; Lowe, G. D.; Jukema, J. W.; Macfarlane, P. W.; et al. Are Markers of Inflammation More Strongly Associated with Risk for Fatal Than for Nonfatal Vascular Events? *PLoS Med.* **2009,** *6,* e1000099.

Schattenberg, J. M.; Galle, P. R.; Schuchmann, M. Apoptosis in Liver Disease. *Liver Int.* **2006,** *26,* 904–911.

Schattenberg, J. M.; Schuchmann, M.; Galle, P. R. Cell Death and Hepatocarcinogenesis: Dysregulation of Apoptosis Signaling Pathways. *J. Gastroenterol. Hepatol.* **2011,** *26,* 213–219.

Schmid-Schönbein, G. W. Analysis of Inflammation. *Annu. Rev. Biomed. Eng.* **2006,** *8,* 93–151.

Schmid-Schönbein, G. W.; Hugli, T. E. A New Hypothesis for Microvascular Inflammation in Shock and Multiorgan Failure: Self-Digestion by Pancreatic Enzymes. *Microcirculation (New York, N.Y. : 1994).* **2005,** *12,* 71–82.

Schmid-Schönbein, G. W.; Takase, S.; Bergan, J. J. New Advances in the Understanding of the Pathophysiology of Chronic Venous Insufficiency. *Angiology* **2001,** *52* (Suppl 1), S27–S34.

Sellamuthu, P. S.; Arulselvan, P.; Fakurazi, S.; Kandasamy, M. Beneficial Effects of Mangiferin Isolated from Salacia Chinensis on Biochemical and Hematological Parameters in Rats with Streptozotocin-Induced Diabetes. *Pak. J. Pharm. Sci.* **2014,** *27,* 161–167.

Shetti, N.; Patil, R. Antioxidants: Its Beneficial Role against Health Damaging Free Radical. *World J. Sci. Technol.* **2011,** *1,* 46–51.

Shinde, A.; Ganu, J.; Naik, P. Effect of Free Radicals & Antioxidants on Oxidative Stress: A Review. *J. Dent. Allied Sci.* **2012,** *1,* 63.

Shurtz-Swirski, R.; Sela, S.; Herskovits, A. T.; Shasha, S. M.; Shapiro, G.; Nasser, L.; Kristal, B. Involvement of Peripheral Polymorphonuclear Leukocytes in Oxidative Stress and Inflammation in Type 2 Diabetic Patients. *Diabetes Care* **2001,** *24,* 104–110.

Sies, H. Oxidative Stress: Oxidants and Antioxidants. *Exp. Physiol.* **1997,** *82,* 291–295.

Simon, H.-U.; Haj-Yehia, A.; Levi-Schaffer, F. Role of Reactive Oxygen Species (ROS) in Apoptosis Induction. *Apoptosis.* **2000,** *5,* 415–418.

Singh, P.; Kesharwani, R. K.; Keservani, R. K. Antioxidants and Vitamins: Roles in Cellular Function and Metabolism. In *Sustained Energy for Enhanced Human Functions and Activity*; Academic Press, pp 385–407; 2017.

Sisein, E. A. Biochemistry of Free Radicals and Antioxidants. *Sch. Acad. J. Biosci.* **2014,** *2,* 110–118.

Slater, T. F.; Cheeseman, K. H.; Davies, M. J.; Proudfoot, K.; Xin, W. Free Radical Mechanisms in Relation to Tissue Injury. *Proc. Nutr. Soc.* **1987,** *46,* 1–12.

Stadtman, E. R. Oxidation of Proteins by Mixed-Function Oxidation Systems: Implication in Protein Turnover, Ageing and Neutrophil Function. *Trends Biochem. Sci.* **1986,** *11,* 11–12.

Stenlöf, K.; Wernstedt, I.; Fjällman, T.; Wallenius, V.; Wallenius, K.; Jansson, J.-O. Interleukin-6 Levels in the Central Nervous System are Negatively Correlated with Fat Mass in Overweight/Obese Subjects. *J. Clin. Endocrinol. Metab.* **2003,** *88,* 4379–4383.

Stürmer, T.; Brenner, H.; Koenig, W.; Günther, K. P. Severity and Extent of Osteoarthritis and Low Grade Systemic Inflammation as Assessed by High Sensitivity C Reactive Protein. *Ann. Rheum. Dis.* **2004,** *63,* 200–205.

Stypuła, G.; Kunert-Radek, J.; Stepień, H.; Zylińska, K.; Pawlikowski, M. Evaluation of Interleukins, ACTH, Cortisol and Prolactin Concentrations in the Blood of Patients with Parkinson's Disease. *Neuroimmunomodulation* **1996,** *3,* 131–134.

Subramanian, S.; Sathishkumar, D.; Arulseelvan, P.; Senthilkumar, G. P. Invitro Antibacterial and Antifungal Activities of Ethanolic Extracts of Aloe Vera Leaf Gel. *J. Plant Sci.* **2006,** *1,* 348–355.

Suematsu, M.; Suzuki, H.; Delano, F. A.; Schmid-Schönbein, G. W. The Inflammatory Aspect of the Microcirculation in Hypertension: Oxidative Stress, Leukocytes/Endothelial Interaction, Apoptosis. *Microcirculation* **2002,** *9,* 259–276.

Suurmond, J.; Dorjée, A. L.; Boon, M. R.; Knol, E. F.; Huizinga, T. W. J.; Toes, R. E. M.; Schuerwegh, A. J. M. Mast Cells are the Main Interleukin 17-Positive Cells in Anticitrullinated Protein Antibody-Positive and -Negative Rheumatoid Arthritis and Osteoarthritis Synovium. *Arthritis Res. Ther.* **2011,** *13,* R150.

Tan, W. S.; Arulselvan, P.; Karthivashan, G.; Fakurazi, S. Moringa Oleifera Flower Extract Suppresses the Activation of Inflammatory Mediators in Lipopolysaccharide-Stimulated RAW 264.7 Macrophages Via NF-Kb Pathway. *Mediators Inflamm.* **2015,** 2015.

Tilley, S. L.; Coffman, T. M.; Koller, B. H. Mixed Messages: Modulation of Inflammation and Immune Responses by Prostaglandins and Thromboxanes. *J. Clin. Invest.* **2001,** *108,* 15–23.

Toker, S.; Shirom, A.; Shapira, I.; Berliner, S.; Melamed, S. The Association between Burnout, Depression, Anxiety, and Inflammation Biomarkers: C-Reactive Protein and Fibrinogen in Men and Women. *J. Occup. Health Psychol.* **2005,** *10,* 344.

Tripathy, A. O. S. Reactive Oxygen Species (ROS) and Antioxidative Defense System, with Special Reference to Fish. *Int. J. Curr. Res. Biosci. Plant Biol.* **2016,** *3,* 79–89.

Valko, M.; Leibfritz, D.; Moncol, J.; Cronin, M. T. D.; Mazur, M.; Telser, J. Free Radicals and Antioxidants in Normal Physiological Functions and Human Disease. *Int. J. Biochem. Cell Biol.* **2007,** *39,* 44–84.

Valko, M.; Rhodes, C. J. B.; Moncol, J.; Izakovic, M. M.; Mazur, M. Free Radicals, Metals and Antioxidants in Oxidative Stress-Induced Cancer. *Chem. Biol. Interact.* **2006,** *160,* 1–40.

Vasan, R. S.; Sullivan, L. M.; Roubenoff, R.; Dinarello, C. A.; Harris, T.; Benjamin, E. J.; Sawyer, D. B.; Levy, D.; Wilson, P. W. F.; D'Agostino, R. B. Inflammatory Markers and Risk of Heart Failure in Elderly Subjects Without Prior Myocardial Infarction: The Framingham Heart Study. *Circulation* **2003,** *107,* 1486–1491.

Vervoordeldonk, M. J. B. M.; Tak, P. P. Cytokines in Rheumatoid Arthritis. *Curr. Rheumatol. Rep.* **2002,** *4,* 208–217.

Wang, B.; Trayhurn, P. Acute and Prolonged Effects of TNF-Alpha on the Expression and Secretion of Inflammation-Related Adipokines by Human Adipocytes Differentiated in Culture. *Pflugers Arch.* **2006,** *452,* 418–427.

Wang, C.; Levis, G. B. S.; Lee, E. B.; Levis, W. R.; Lee, D. W.; Kim, B. S.; Park, S. Y.; Park, E. Platycodin D and D3 Isolated from the Root of Platycodon Grandiflorum Modulate the

Production of Nitric Oxide and Secretion of TNF-A in Activated RAW 264.7 Cells. *Int. Immunopharmacol.* **2004,** *4,* 1039–1049.

Weber, A.; Boege, Y.; Reisinger, F.; Heikenwalder, M. Chronic Liver Inflammation and Hepatocellular Carcinoma: Persistence Matters. *Swiss Med. Wkly.* **2011,** *141,* W13197.

Wei, W.-C.; Lin, S.-Y.; Chen, Y.-J.; Wen, C.-C.; Huang, C.-Y.; Palanisamy, A.; Yang, N.-S.; Sheu, J.-H. Topical Application of Marine Briarane-Type Diterpenes Effectively Inhibits 12-O-Tetradecanoylphorbol-13-Acetate-Induced Inflammation and Dermatitis in Murine Skin. *J. Biomed. Sci.* **2011,** *18,* 1–13.

Wen, C.-C.; Shyur, L.-F.; Jan, J.-T.; Liang, P.-H.; Kuo, C.-J.; Arulselvan, P.; Wu, J.-B.; Kuo, S.-C.; Yang, N.-S. Traditional Chinese Medicine Herbal Extracts of Cibotium Barometz, Gentiana Scabra, Dioscorea Batatas, Cassia Tora, and Taxillus Chinensis Inhibit SARS-Cov Replication. *J. Tradit. Complement. Med.* **2011,** *1,* 41–50.

Willerson, J. T.; Ridker, P. M. Inflammation as a Cardiovascular Risk Factor. *Circulation* **2004,** *109,* II2–II10.

Wilson, C. J.; Finch, C. E.; Cohen, H. J. Cytokines and Cognition—The Case for a Head-to-Toe Inflammatory Paradigm. *J. Am. Geriatr. Soc.* **2002,** *50,* 2041–2056.

Xu, C.; Bailly-Maitre, B.; Reed, J. C. Endoplasmic Reticulum Stress: Cell Life and Death Decisions. *J. Clin. Invest.* **2005,** *115,* 2656–2664.

CHAPTER 7

PLANT-DERIVED ANTIOXIDANT NUTRACEUTICALS FOR THE TREATMENT OF NEURODEGENERATIVE DISORDERS

PRASHANT AMALE[1], KUSHAGRA NAGORI[2], HEMANT BADWAIK[3], MADHURI BAGHEL[3], and KARTIK NAKHATE[4]

[1]*Priyadarshini J. L. College of Pharmacy, Electronic Zone Building, MIDC, Hingna Road, Nagpur, Maharashtra, India*

[2]*Rungta College of Pharmaceutical Sciences and Research, Kohka–Kurud Road, Bhilai, Chhattisgarh, India*

[3]*Shri Shankaracharya Institute of Pharmaceutical Sciences and Research, Junwani, Bhilai, Chhattisgarh, India*

[4]*Shri Vile Parle Kelavani Mandal's Institute of Pharmacy, Mumbai–Agra Highway, Behind Gurudwara, Dhule, Maharashtra, India*

ABSTRACT

Treatment of neurodegenerative disorders (NDs) such as Alzheimer's disease (AD) and Parkinson's disease (PD) has become one of the most challenging issues for clinicians as their progression can only be slowed up by the currently marketed drugs, but cannot be stopped completely. Therefore, the need for better treatment approaches, particularly herbal-based medicines, to fight with NDs seems necessary. The development of oxidative stress is considered one of the hallmark signs of neurodegenerative diseases. Several plant-based nutraceuticals possess antioxidant potential; therefore, they can

Antioxidants as Nutraceuticals. Nayan A. Gujarathi, Raj K. Keservani, Rajesh K. Kesharwani, Bhushan R. Rane, Yogeeta Sameer Goyal (Eds.)

be used for the effective management of NDs. In the present chapter, several findings and recent trends in antioxidant nutraceuticals with reference to their potential in the treatment of NDs have been elaborated.

7.1 INTRODUCTION

Neurodegenerative disorders (NDs), including Alzheimer's disease (AD), Parkinson's disease (PD), Huntington's disease (HD), spinal muscular atrophy (SMA), amyotrophic lateral sclerosis (ALS), and spinocerebellar ataxia (SCA) are characterized by progressive destruction of neurons in the central nervous system (CNS). Neurodegeneration can occur due to injury to the nervous system, neuroinflammation, ischemia, oxidative stress, abnormal protein deposition in neural tissue, endoplasmic reticulum stress, autoimmune-mediated neuronal loss, viral or prion infections, and family history (Muddapu et al., 2020; Sharifi-Rad et al., 2020). The neurodegenerative abnormalities generally start in the subcortical regions, and as the condition progresses, it spreads to the cortical regions. In each ND, the part of the brain varies, for example, hippocampal and cortical areas in AD, striatal areas in PD, striatal and cortical areas in HD, and spinal motor neurons and cortical areas in ALS (Muddapu et al., 2020). In addition to this, neuronal selectivity has also been observed; for example, in Alzheimer's, the destruction of cholinergic neurons takes place due to amyloid-β (Aβ) plaques accumulation, while Parkinsonian is associated with loss of dopaminergic neurons due to the accumulation of Lewy bodies (Nakhate et al., 2020).

Worldwide millions of people suffer from NDs, and the incidences of the most common diseases such as AD and PD are predicted to increase significantly with the rising population. NDs pose a serious health challenge as the progressive neurodegeneration can only be slow-up by the currently marketed drugs, but cannot be stopped completely (Nakhate et al., 2020, 2018). Therefore, the therapy of NDs has become one of the most challenging issues for clinicians and researchers. Therefore, the need for better therapeutic approaches, particularly herbal-based medicines, to fight with NDs seems necessary. Indeed, the effectiveness of phytoconstituents has been suggested for the prevention and treatment of various illnesses (Arora et al., 2021; Badwaik et al., 2019; Kamdi et al., 2021b, 2021c; Lu and Lu, 2019; Sharma et al., 2021). Several studies support the efficiency of phytochemicals in the treatment of NDs. The majority of the medicinal plant compounds including polyphenols, flavonoids, alkaloids, and terpenes possess therapeutic properties and can be utilized as an alternative for the treatment of NDs (Pérez-Hernández et al., 2016; Ratheesh et al., 2017). The main challenge for the delivery of drugs including phytoconstituents into the CNS is to overcome their poor blood–brain barrier penetration ability and possible side effects when reaching nontarget peripheral tissues (Badwaik et al., 2013, 2018; Tonda-Turo et al., 2018). To address these issues, attempts have been made by the researchers to develop the nanocarrier based delivery for the phytochemicals.

In recent times, plant-based nutraceuticals have drawn the attention of several researchers. A nutraceutical (Keservani et al., 2010a, 2010b, 2017, 2020) is any compound other than pharmaceutical; it may be a food or part of food that is used in the prevention and treatment of disease. It includes isolated nutrients, dietary supplements, genetically engineered "designer" foods, herbal products, and processed foods (cereals, soups, and beverages). Moreover, antioxidants such as carotenoids, flavonoids, glucosinolates, vitamins, minerals etc. also considered as nutraceuticals (DeFelice, 2002; Dudeja and Gupta, 2017). In terms of safety, they are publicly accepted (but not approved) products as compared to pharmaceuticals; and hence, the frequency of their use is around 50–70% or more in developed countries. Globally nutraceuticals market has become a multibillion-dollar industry. Taking nutraceuticals with the pharmaceuticals may cause interactions (beneficial/harmful) in vulnerable populations. Nowadays, nutraceuticals are used for the prevention and treatment of conditions such as pain, spasms, arthritis, inflammation, allergy, polycystic ovary disorders, AD, PD, depression, cardiovascular disorders, cancer, diabetes, hyperlipidemia, and obesity. Curcumin, lutein, lycopene, turmerin, vitamin C, vitamin E, phloridzin, berberine, resveratrol (RSV), omega-3-fatty acid, and β-carotene are the nutraceuticals that exhibit antioxidant potential; hence, used in the management of diseases that are caused due to oxidative stress (Advani et al., 2020; Glenville, 2006; Kamdi et al., 2021a, 2021c, 2021b; Rajasekaran, 2017). They can also been used in the pharmaceutical formulations to enhance the pharmacokinetics profile and therapeutic potential of the drugs (Khan et al., 2019). The list of some plant-based nutraceuticals and their probable modes of action of nutraceuticals on neurodegenerative illnesses are outlined in Table 7.1 and Figure 7.1.

4-HNE, 4-hydroxy-2-nonenal; 8-OHdG, 8-hydroxy-2′-deoxyguanosine; AD, Alzheimer's disease; APP, amyloid precursor protein; APPswe/PS1dE9, a mutant AD mouse model with increased A plaque caused by Swedish

TABLE 7.1 Plant-derived antioxidant nutraceuticals for the treatment of NDs. 4-HNE, 4-hydroxy-2-nonenal; 8-OHdG, 8-hydroxy-2′-deoxyguanosine; AD, Alzheimer disease; APP, amyloid precursor protein; APPswe/PS1dE9, a mutant AD mouse model with increased A plaque caused by Swedish mutation in APP and exon 9 deletion of presenilin-1; $A\beta_1$, Aβ; IsoPs, isoprostanes; ICV-STZ, intracerebroventricular streptozotocin; LPO, lipid peroxides; MDA, malondialdehyde; MPTP, 1-methyl-4-phenyl-1,2,3,6-tetrahydropyridine; PC, protein carbonyls; ROS, Reactive oxygen species; TBARC, 2-ThioBarbituric Acid Reactive components.

S. No.	Phytonutraceutical	Antioxidant Effects	Experimental Models	References
1.	RSV	Decreased superoxide levels in the nucleus tractus solitarius and hippocampus.	Angiotensin II-induced early AD rats	(Lin et al., 2018)
2.	Lycopene	Elevated GSH level and reduced levels of TBARC and some proapoptotic proteins	MPTP-induced PD in mice	(D. Chen et al, 2019)
3.	Curcumin	Decreased IsoPs levels in rat brains.	Aβ-induced cognitive deficits in rat	(Frautschy et al., 2001)
		Decreased LPO in the spinal cord.	APP transgenic mouse	(Seo et al., 2010)
4.	*Ginkgo biloba* flavonols (kaempferol, quercetin and isorhamnetin), 6% terpene lactones (ginkgolide-A, -B, -C-M, and -J and bilobalide B)	Decreased intracellular ROS levels	Aβ-secreting mutant cells	(Singh et al., 2019)
5.	Vitamin C	Decreased soluble and insoluble $A\beta_{1\text{-}42}$ and a higher $A\beta_{1\text{-}42/1\text{-}40}$ ratio	$APP_{SWE}/PSEN1_{deltaE9}$ mouse model	(Dixit et al., 2015b)
6.	Magnolol	Decreased lipid peroxidation in the striatum	MPTP-induced PD in mice	(Muroyama et al., 2012)
		Decreased PC, HNE, and superoxide levels	Acrolein-induced oxidative damage in neuroblastoma cells	(Dong et al., 2013)
7.	Grape seed extract; Proanthocyanidins	Decreased 8-OHdG and DNA protein cross-links levels in the rat brains and spinal cords	Aged rats	(Balu et al., 2006)
		Decreased ROS and PC levels in the rat brains and spinal cords	Aged rats	(Balu et al., 2005)

TABLE 7.1 *(Continued)*

S. No.	Phytonutraceutical	Antioxidant Effects	Experimental Models	References
8.	Green tea Polyphenols	Levels of MDA, 8-OHdG, and PC decreased significantly as compared to baseline values and increased value in FRAP assay	Severe AD patients	(Arab et al., 2016)
9.	Pycnogenol®; Procyanidins, phenolic acids, and polyphenols (catechin, epicatechin, and taxifolin)	Decreased ROS, superoxide, PC, and 4-HNE levels	Acrolein-induced oxidative damage in neuroblastoma cells	(Arab et al., 2016)
		Decreased PC and LPO in the hippocampus and cerebral cortex	ICV-STZ induced AD in rats	(Ishrat et al., 2009)
		Increased antioxidant capacity of plasma compared to baseline	Healthy subjects	(Devaraj et al., 2002)
		Decreased plasma reactive oxygen metabolites and increased antioxidant potential compared to smokers taking placebo.	Human subjects; smokers	(Belcaro et al., 2013)
10.	Xanthorrhizol	Decreased LPO in the rat brains	H_2O_2-induced lipid peroxidation in rat brain homogenate	(Lim et al., 2005)
		Decreased intracellular ROS generation in the hippocampal neurons	Glutamate-induced cytotoxicity in hippocampal neurons	(Lim et al., 2005)
11.	Vitamin E; α, β, γ tocopherol and α, β, γ tocotrienol	Decreased plasma MDA and DNA damage.	Older adults aged 50–55 years old	(Goon et al., 2017)
		Decreased DNA strand breaks in the blood.	APPswe/PS1dE9 transgenic mouse model of AD	(Damanhuri et al., 2016)
12.	Guarana seed extract polyphenols (catechins and epicatechins)	Decreased intracellular ROS production	*Caenorhabditis elegans* models of AD	(Boasquívis et al., 2018)
		Decreased intracellular ROS production	Acrolein-induced cytotoxicity on neuronal cells	(Beyaz Coşkun and Şanlıer, 2020)

mutation in APP and exon 9 deletion of presenilin-1; $A\beta_1$, $A\beta$; IsoPs, isoprostanes; ICV-STZ, intracerebroventricular streptozotocin; LPO, lipid peroxides; MDA, malondialdehyde; MPTP, 1-methyl-4-phenyl-1,2,3,6-tetrahydropyridine; PC, protein carbonyls; ROS, Reactive oxygen species; TBARC, 2-Thiobarbituric acid reactive components.

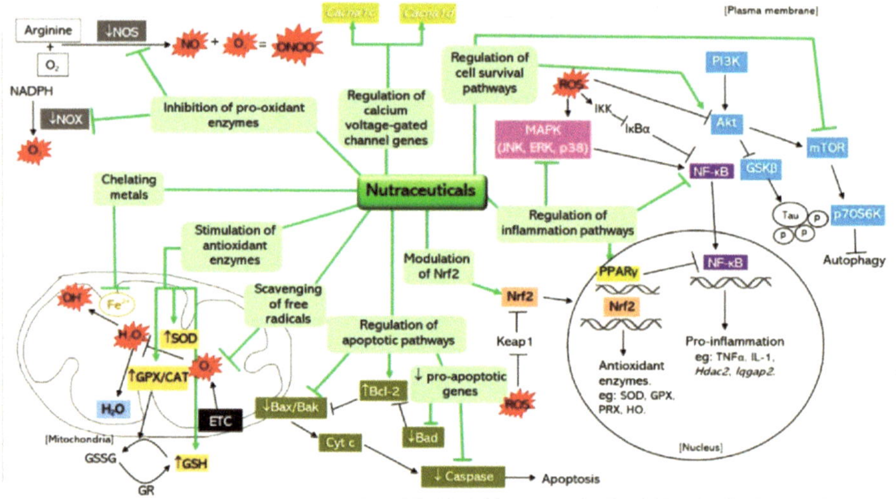

FIGURE 7.1 The suggested mode of nutraceutical action in the treatment of NDs. Akt, protein kinase B; Bad, BCL-2 related agonist of cell death; Bak, BCL2 Antagonist; Bax, Bcl-2-linked X protein; Bcl 2, B-cell lymphoma 2; caspase, cysteine aspartic proteases; Cacna1c, calcium-voltage-gated channel subunit of alpha-1C genes; Cyt c, cytochrome C; Cacna1d, calcium-voltage-gated channel subunit alpha-1D genes; CAT, catalase; ERK, extracellular signal regulated kinase; ETC, electron transport chain; Fe^{2+}, ferrous ion; GSH, glutathione; GPX, glutathione peroxidase; GSSG, oxidized glutathione; GSK3, glycogen synthase kinase 3; GR, glutathione reductase; HO, heme oxygenase; Hdac2, histone deacetylase 2 encoding genes; H_2O_2, hydrogen peroxide; IκBα, nuclear factor kappa light chain enhancer of activated B cells inhibitor-alpha; IKK, IkappaB kinase; Iqgap2, ras GTPase activating such as protein encoding genes; IL-1, interleukin-1; JNK, c-Jun N-terminal kinases; Keap-1, Kelch-like ECH associated protein-1; MAPK, mitogen activated protein kinase; mTOR, rapamycin's mammalian target; NADPH, reduced nicotinamide adenine dinucleotide phosphate; NF-κB, nuclear factor kappa-light-chain-enhancer of activated B cells; NOS, nitric oxide synthases; Nrf2, nuclear factor erythroid 2 related factor-2; NOX, NADPH oxidase; ONOO, peroxynitrite; NO, nitric oxide; $O2^{\bullet-}$, superoxide anion; O_2, oxygen; $OH^{\cdot}$, hydroxyl radical; PPARγ, peroxisome-proliferator activated receptor gamma; PRX, peroxiredoxin; PI3K, phosphoinositide-3 kinase; ROS, reactive oxygen species; p70S6K, S6 kinase ribosomal protein; TNFα, tumor necrosis factor alpha; SOD, superoxide dismutase; ↑, increased; ↓, decreased. The depicted mechanisms are adapted from earlier publications.

Source: Reprinted with permission from Ramli et al., 2020. Copyright © 2020 by the authors. Licensee MDPI, Basel, Switzerland. http://creativecommons.org/licenses/by/4.0/

The development of oxidative stress is considered one of the hallmark signs of neurodegenerative diseases (Kamdi et al., 2021d; Nakhate et al., 2020, 2018). Several plant-based nutraceuticals possess antioxidant potential; therefore, they can be used for the effective management of the NDs. To assess the potential applications of antioxidant nutraceuticals, a detailed review of the literature is essential. In the present chapter, several findings and recent trends in plant-derived antioxidant nutraceuticals with reference to their potential in the treatment of NDs have been elaborated.

7.2 POTENTIAL OF PHYTOCHEMICALS FOR NEURODEGENERATIVE DISORDERS

Although several drugs are available for the symptomatic treatment of NDs, there are several issues to administrate the progressive and serious symptoms (Chen and Pan, 2014). Currently, several natural agents have been suggested for the management of NDs. In this section, we highlighted some phytochemicals and their role in NDs.

7.2.1 ALZHEIMER'S DISEASE (AD)

Several phytoconstituents can act on multiple targets against AD. Phytomedicines mitigate the oxidative stress, generation or aggregation of Aβ, cholinesterase activity, and inflammation (Hosseinkhani et al., 2017; Kamdi et al., 2021d, 2021a; Ratheesh et al., 2017). In the Ayurveda, several herbs are used to treat AD-related abnormalities including Guduchi (*Tinospora cordifolia*), Yashtimadhu (*Glycyrrhiza glabra*), Padma (*Nelumbo nucifera*), Vacha (*Acorus calamus*), Shankhpushpi (*Convolvulus pluricaulis*), Amalaki (*Phyllanthus emblica*), Arjun (*Terminalia arjuna)*, and Ashwagandha (*Withania somnifera*) (Singhal et al., 2012). Additionally, several medicinal plants are utilized in AD treatment which includes *A. calamus* L. (Araceae), *Angelica archangelica* L. (Umbelliferae), *Bacopa monniera* Wettst. (Scrophulariaceae), *Biota orientalis* L. (Coniferae) Cupressaceae, *Celastrus paniculatus* Willd. (Celastraceae), *Centella asiatica* L. (Umbelliferae), *Clitoria ternatea* L. (Leguminosae), *Codonopsis pilosula* Franch. (Campanulaceae), *C. pluricaulis* Chois. (Convolvulaceae), *Coptis chinensis* Franch. (Ranunculaceae), *Crocus sativus* L. (Iridaceae), *Curcuma longa* L. (Zingeberaceae), *Evodia rutaecarpa* (Juss.) Benth. (Rutaceae), *G. biloba* L. (Ginkgoaceae), *Hypericum perforatum* L. (Clusiaceae) (Hypericaceae).

Magnolia officinalis Rehd. and Wils. (Magnoliaceae), *Melissa officinalis* L. (Lamiaceae), *Piper methysticum* Frost. (Piperaceae), *Polygala tenuifolia* Wild. (Polygalaceae), *Rheum* spp. L. (Polygonaceae), *Salvia lavandulaefolia* Vahl. (Lamiaceae), *Salvia miltiorrhizia* Bung. (Lamiaceae), *Salvia officinalis* L. (Lamiaceae), *Terminalia chebula* L. (Combretaceae), *W. somnifera* L. (Solonaceae) (Hosseinkhani et al., 2017; Ratheesh et al., 2017; Roy, 2018; Singhal et al., 2012).

7.2.2 PARKINSON'S DISEASE (PD)

Phytochemicals have the ability to treat PD, and some of them proved to be effective and more reliable than the current synthetic drugs. These herbs and nutraceuticals include *Erythrina velutin* (Fabaceae), *Peganum harmal* (Nitrariaceae), *C. longa* (Zingiberaceae), *Carthamus tinctorius* L. (Asteraceae), *Pueraria lobate* (Fabaceae), *Juglandis Semen* (Juglandaceae), *Lycium barbarum* L. fruit (Solanaceae), *Mucuna pruriens* (Fabaceae), *Bacopa monnieri* (*Schrophulariaceae*), *Camellia sinensis* (Theaceae), *Coffea arabica* (Rubiaceae), *G. biloba* (Ginkgoaceae), *Fructus alpiniaoxyphylla* (Zingiberaceae), *Delphinium denudatum* (Ranunculaceae), *Panax ginseng* (Araliaceae), Chunghyuldan, Paeoniae Alba Radix, Tianma Gouteng Yin, Baicalei, and RSV (Amro et al., 2018; Sofia et al., 2021).

7.2.3 HUNTINGTON DISEASE (HD)

Natural compounds and herbs have antioxidant, anti-inflammatory, antiapoptotic, and neurofunctional properties that exhibit preventive or therapeutic effects in NDs including HD. Various plants such as *B. monnieri*, *G. biloba*, *C. longa*, *W. somnifera*, *P. ginseng*, *C. asiatica,* and phytochemicals such as flavonoids, lycopene, celastrol, sesamol, and trehalose have shown to be effective against experimental HD. Ginsenosides, obtain from *P. ginseng* (Araliaceae) have shown to have beneficial effects in CNS disorders, including NDs. They show antioxidant, anti-inflammatory, and antiapoptotic activity. Moreover, they have exhibited neuroprotective effects against the experimental HD model (Huang et al., 2019). Flavonoids (Keservani and Sharma, 2014; Keservani et al., 2016a, 2016b), are a group of polyphenolic compounds, that exhibit antioxidant, anti-inflammatory and neuroprotective activity that may be helpful in several NDs, including HDs (Choudhary et al., 2013). Celastrol is a triterpenoid isolated from *Tripterygium wilfordi*

(Thunder of God vine), and *Celastrus regelii* belonging to the Celastraceae family shows potent antioxidant and anti-inflammatory actions. Celastrol is known to prevent the production of proinflammatory cytokines, inducible nitric oxide synthase, and lipid peroxidation and also shows neuroprotection against the neurotoxic HD experimental model (Cleren et al., 2005). Trehalose is a nonreducing disaccharide found in many organism-like bacteria, yeast, fungi, insects, invertebrates, and plants. It protects the integrity of cells by preventing protein denaturation from environmental stresses. A plethora of research has shown that it inhibits the amyloid formation and aggregation, polyglutamine (polyQ)-mediated protein aggregation, decreased Huntington aggregates-induced toxicity, and increases the autophagy activity against several protein aggregates, including Huntington. Thus, it can be useful in the HD (Choudhary et al., 2013; Sarkar et al., 2007). Lycopene, a carotenoid found in tomato (*Solanum lycopersicum*, family Solanaceae) has shown potent antioxidant, anti-inflammatory, antiproliferative, and neuroprotective activities and also mitigates the various behavioral and biochemical changes induced by experimental HD model (Kumar et al., 2009).

7.2.4 AMYOTROPHIC LATERAL SCLEROSIS (ALS)

Complementary and alternative medicine including, acupuncture, natural compounds, phytomedicine, and natural therapy such as yoga has been popular in the treatment of several diseases including ALS. A plethora of research indicated that various phytomedicines and natural compounds such as ginseng (*Panax ginseng*), *C. asiatica*, Epigallocatechin gallate, garlic (*Allium sativum*), curcumin, RSV, obovatol, wogonin, and paeonol have been suggested as nutraceuticals for the prevention of symptoms of ALS by their antioxidant, anti-inflammatory, and neuroprotective action (Khan et al., 2021). Ginseng is composed of a variety of biomolecules such as carbohydrates, proteins, amino acids, vitamins, fatty acids, and ginsenosides. It has been shown to have protective effects against ALS by attenuating neuroinflammation and improving motor neurons (Cai and Yang, 2016). *C. asiatica* increases the protection and survival time in mice against motor neurodegeneration (Khan et al., 2021). Epigallocatechin gallate, an active constituent of green tea and allicin, an active constituent of garlic are antioxidants and show neuroprotection against ALS (Guo et al., 2011; Koh et al., 2006).

7.2.5 SPINAL MUSCULAR ATROPHY (SMA)

A traditional Chinese herbal medicine *Liuwei dihuang* has a variety of therapeutic benefits. Its extract elevates the SMN protein level and protects motor neuron against SMN deficiency-induced neurodegeneration, and improve muscle strength (Tseng et al., 2017). *Brucea javanica* extract and its constituent Bruceine D have the ability to correct the SMN2 spicing defect and improve the symptoms of SMA in mice (Baek et al., 2019). Besides these, oxidative stress is also a prime pathophysiological factor for SMA. It is well established that phytochemicals such as flavonoids (rutin, quercetin, and isoquercetin) have great antioxidant potential, which may also be helpful in the treatment of muscular atrophy.

7.2.6 SPINOCEREBELLAR ATAXIA (SCA)

There is no specific drug and symptomatic treatment is recommended for the SCAs; however, FDA accepted an investigational new drug application for one molecule CAD-1883 for its human testing in SCAs (Keaney et al., 2019). Recent studies suggested that lots of herbs have been shown beneficial effects on SCAs. Examples include *Rehmannia glutinose*, *P. lobate*, *Gastrodia elata*, *Gardenia jasminoides*, *Glycyrrhiza inflata*, *Paeonia lactifora*, *Brassica napus*, and *G. biloba* (Chang et al., 2014, 2013; Chen et al., 2014, 2019a, 2019b; Chou et al., 2015; Huang et al., 2016; Pohl et al., 2019). They reduce oxidative stress, promote proteasome activity, suppress polyQ aggregation, improve motor function, and prevent cell death, which is dysregulated in SCAs (Phang et al., 2021).

7.3 ANTIOXIDANT NUTRACEUTICALS FOR NEURODEGENERATIVE DISORDERS: A NEUROPHARMACOLOGICAL PERSPECTIVE

Antioxidants act by scavenging the species that initiate the peroxidation, breaking the auto-oxidative chain reaction, quenching singlet oxygen, and preventing the formation of peroxides. They also possess the ability to scavenge free radicals and prevent the generation of reactive oxygen species (ROS), and are hence, reported to be used as protective and curative agents for several diseases including neurological disorders (Neves Carvalho et al., 2017). There are two types of antioxidants, that is enzymatic superoxide dismutase, catalase (CAT), glutaredoxins, glutathione peroxidase, and glutathione reductase] and nonenzymatic (vitamin C, vitamin E, selenium, zinc, carotenes, taurine, hypotaurine, and glutathione). Out of these, superoxide dismutase, CAT, and glutathione peroxidase are the primary intracellular antioxidant enzymes in mammalian cells. Generally, the cells possess some antioxidants as protectants, but advancements in age, nutritional deficiency, stress, and other mechanisms may cause a reduction in the levels of antioxidants, or imbalance between prooxidant and antioxidants, or an increase in the generation of ROS, which leads to a development of disease state (Mulgund et al., 2015; Weydert and Cullen, 2010). A plethora of research has demonstrated that plant-derived antioxidant nutraceuticals can reduce the progression of the most common NDs such as AD and PD as discussed in the following.

7.3.1 RESVERATROL

RSV is a plant polyphenol or phytoalexin found richly in red wine and the skin of grapes, berries, and peanuts. A plethora of literature is evident for its antioxidant, antinociceptive, anti-inflammatory, anxiolytic, antidiabetic, antioncogenic, anti-PD, anti-AD, antidepressant, and lipid-lowering effects. These pharmacological activities are mediated through the modulation of some enzymes, neurotransmitters, biogenic amines, cytokines, proteins, receptors, and signaling molecules underlying the specific mechanism (Amale et al., 2021).

PD is a neurodegenerative disease that is associated with dopaminergic neuronal loss caused due to mitochondrial dysfunction, oxidative stress, free radicals, ROS generation, etc. The neuroprotective effects of RSV in a model of PD are exerted via the reduction of oxidative stress, scavenging of the ROS, and suppression of ROS-generating enzymes, followed by the activation of the antioxidant protein (Kung et al., 2021). Research data showed that 20 mg/kg RSV once daily for 15 days showed an antioxidant effect in chronic 6-hydroxydopamine (6-OHDA) infused rats via modulation of the antioxidant enzymes, lipid peroxidation, and glutathione level followed by suppression of the dopaminergic neuronal loss (Khan et al., 2010). RSV restored the malonaldehyde and glutathione levels altered due to neurodegeneration caused by streptozotocin (Sharma and Gupta, 2002). RSV treatment reduces 6-OHDA-increased expression of TNF-α mRNA, COX-2 protein, and COX-2 enzyme level and corrected the behavioral impairment, and damage of the dopaminergic system of substantia nigra by promoting the PI3K/Akt signaling in the rat model of PD (Chen et al., 2017; Huang et al., 2019). In addition, oxidative stress, free radical formation, and mitochondrial dysfunction result in the loss of dopaminergic neurons and cause PD. RSV acts via AKT/GSK-3β pathway and attenuates MPP^+ induced mitochondrial dysfunction and cell apoptosis (Khan et al., 2010; Peng et al., 2016; Zeng et al., 2017).

The accumulation of β-amyloid (Aβ) peptide aggregates in the hippocampus exerts oxidative stress and inflammation that causes neurodegeneration which is a confirmatory parameter of AD. Suppression of the Aβ peptide aggregation has been considered the primary therapeutic strategy for AD treatment. RSV attenuated neuroinflammation, and oxidative stress, suppresses elevated macrophage-derived chemokine (MDC), cytokines (IL-4), Aβ1–42-induced cell death and protect neuronal loss, thus evident as an anti-AD drug (Moussa et al., 2017; Santana and Magalhães, 2020; Wang et al., 2018). In a clinical study, RSV intake may reduce glycated hemoglobin A1c, preserves hippocampus volume, and improve hippocampus RSFC in at-risk patients for dementia (Köbe et al., 2017). RSV and Curcumin are effective against aluminum chloride-induced neuroinflammation in rats (Zaky et al., 2017). RSV at 10 μM concentration exhibited the antioxidant effect by alleviating the membrane lipid peroxidation and enhancing the level of enzymes (CAT, SOD, and glutathione reductase-GR) as well as nonenzymes (glutathione; Vitamins C and E) in hippocampal cell lines (D Rege et al., 2015; Santana and Magalhães, 2020). Moreover, RSV enhanced the expression of CAT, copper chaperone for SOD 1, GST zeta 1, sirtuin 1 and 3, and modulated antioxidant and antiaging factors contributing to AD (Cosín-Tomàs et al., 2019). RSV or Losartan at 10 mg/kg dose increased hippocampal BDNF level while decreasing blood pressure and nucleus tractus solitarius ROS production in the Ang-II. RSV causes the deletion of NADPH oxidase 2 (NOX2) and the elevation of SOD2 results in restoration of hippocampal-dependent contextual memory (Lin et al., 2018). In a study, RSV facilitates clearance of neurotoxic Aβ peptides, breakdown of the amyloid precursor protein (APP), and promotes SIRT1 expression which reduces amyloidogenic plaque formation in AD (Braidy et al., 2016; Sathya et al., 2017). RSV and oxy-RSV cause activation of α-secretase and MMP-9 to lower Aβ levels without causing cell death (Choi et al., 2016). RSV, metalloporphyrins, and nicotinamide riboside synergistically reduced amyloid β protein leading to improvement of mitochondrial and cognitive function in AD (Dragicevic et al., 2017).

7.3.2 LYCOPENE

Lycopene is a naturally occurring nonvitamin A carotenoid compound imparting red color to vegetables and fruits; lycopene is predominantly found in tomatoes, watermelon, papaya, apricots, pink grapefruit, and guava). It is also synthesized by microorganisms (Chen et al., 2016). Lycopene can be used as prophylactic and/or therapeutic in the management of various neurological problems including, AD, PD, HD, cerebral ischemia, spinal cord injury, neuropathy, epilepsy, and depression (Chen et al., 2019). It is a potent antioxidant and also provides neuroprotection by preventing proteinopathies, neuroinflammation, apoptosis, cerebral edema, and restoration of mitochondrial/synaptic dysfunction (Paul et al., 2020). In addition, it causes inhibition of nuclear factor-κB (NF-κB) and c-Jun N-terminal kinase (JNK), activation of the nuclear factor erythroid 2-related factor (Nrf2) and brain-derived neurotrophic factor (BDNF) signaling, and restoration of intracellular Ca^{2+} homeostasis which is equally important in its therapeutic effects (Chen et al., 2019). Lycopene 5 mg/kg and sodium valproate (100 mg/kg) for 29 days reduced kindling score, restored mitochondrial enzyme function and oxidative damage in pentylenetetrazol (PTZ)-induced kindling epilepsy (Bhardwaj and Kumar, 2016).

Consumption of tomato/Lycopene (20 mg/kg) supplement was found to normalize the motor incoordination in 1-methyl-4-phenyl-1,2,3,6-tetrahydropyridine (MPTP) induced PD (Prema et al., 2015). MPTP, being a potential toxicant depletes the striatal dopamine and leads to PD, whereas lycopene by elevating the GSH level and reducing the levels of 2-thiobarbituric acid reactive substances (TBARS) and some proapoptotic proteins, such as Bax, caspases-3, 8 and 9. The neuroprotective effect of lycopene involves oxidative stress inhibition, activation of the adenosine 5′monophosphate-activated protein kinase (AMPK), peroxisome proliferator-activated receptor γ (PPARγ), and phosphatidylinositol-4,5-bisphosphate 3-kinase (PI3K)/protein kinase B (Akt) signaling and activation of microglia (Chen et al., 2019).

Chronic treatment with lycopene is found to be effective in inhibiting oxidative stress. Treatment of lycopene inhibited apoptosis by reducing ROS, and by inhibiting mitochondrial dysfunction and NF-κB-target gene Nucling expression in neuronal cells (Hwang et al., 2017). Lycopene at 1-4mg/kg dose for 14 days inhibiting the neuroinflammation and prevent neuronal damage (Liu et al., 2018; Sachdeva and Chopra, 2015). Treatment with lycopene reversed lipopolysaccharide (LPS)-induced Aβ accumulation and APP/amyloid precursor protein lyase 1 (BACE1) accumulation (Wang et al., 2018). Lycopene prevented malondialdehyde (MDA) and a decrease in glutathione peroxidase (GSH-Px), inhibition of tau protein phosphorylation anti-AD effect (Yu et al., 2017). Regulation of oxidative stress and neuroinflammation by lycopene may be interconnected because the preventive effect of lycopene pre-treatment (0.2 or 0.5 μM) on proinflammatory cytokine production and oxidative stress-triggered Nucling expression in SH-SY5Y cells are both mediated by NF-κB (Hwang et al., 2017).

Research data revealed the ameliorative effect of lycopene on some toxicant-induced cognition and memory impairment. Experimentally induced diabetes mellitus increases the level of NO, tumor necrosis factor-α (TNF-α), interleukin-1β (IL-1β), NF-κB, and Bax, acetylcholinesterase (AchE), blood glucose levels, insulin resistance and thiobarbituric acid-reactive substances, while a decrease in SOD, CAT, GSH-Px, acetylcholine (Ach), and peroxisome proliferator-activated receptor γ (PPARγ) levels, Bcl-2/Bcl-xL ratio which intern causes memory disturbance. Lycopene 4 mg/kg for 4 weeks was found to modulate all the aforementioned-altered parameters that cause diabetes-induced cognitive impairment. Colchicine treatment causes memory impairment by increasing the MDA/NO levels, decrease in SOD, CAT, caspase-3, and AchE activity, proinflammatory cytokines, and GSH levels, decrease in cell viability lycopene 2.5–5 mg/kg treatment alleviated the colchicine induced effects. D galactose exerts oxidative stress and contributes to the aging process in the brain. It also causes neurodegeneration, nucleus shrinkage, increase MDA and proinflammatory mediator levels, and reduction in BDNF expression, GSH, SOD, GSH-Px, HO-1, and quinone oxidoreductase 1 (NQO-1) levels. Lycopene supplementation for 2 months significantly reversed the cognitive and memory impairment caused due to the D-galactose. High-fat diet feeding results in an increase in the in blood or brain levels of total cholesterol (TC), low-density lipoprotein cholesterol (LDL-C), triglyceride (TG), oxidized low-density lipoprotein (ox-LDL), a proinflammatory cytokine, glutamate, N-methyl-D-aspartic acid (NMDA), and dopamine while a reduction in dendritic spine density, gamma-aminobutyric acid (GABA) and serotonin (5-HT) levels. Lycopene treatment for 3 weeks was found to decrease the elevated blood/brain parameter and restore the GABA and 5-HT levels. Thus, lycopene per se ameliorated the HFD-induced cognitive decline and memory impairment (Yin et al., 2014).

3-Nitropropionic acid-induced mitochondrial swelling, cytochrome c release, and caspase-3 expression involved in brain hemorrhage rats. The mechanisms of action of lycopene in these processes include increasing mitochondrial complexes activity and respiration, reducing mitochondrial lipid peroxidation, ROS, and nitric oxide (NO) production, and increasing thiol content and superoxide dismutase (SOD) activity. Experimentally induced bilateral common carotid artery occlusion (BCCAO) decreased neurological score, and GSH contents and increased neuronal degeneration, oxidative stress, lipid peroxidation, ROS levels, and neuronal apoptosis. Continuous administration of lycopene for 7 days reversed these effects by activating the Nrf2, heme oxygenase-1 (HO-1) signaling, free radicals scavenging and inhibiting lipid peroxidation, mitogen-activated protein kinase (MAPK)-c-Jun N-terminal kinase (JNK) activation, caspase-3 activity, and cellular apoptosis (Chen et al., 2019).

7.3.3 CURCUMIN

Curcumin reduces the progression of neuronal damage, inflammation, and aggregation of Aβ along with a destabilization of a formed neurofibrillary tangle (Ambegaokar et al., 2003; Jabir et al., 2018; Tai et al., 2018; Yamazaki et al., 2019). Curcumin exerts strong antioxidant properties via ROS, free radical scavenging, and lipid peroxidation which in turn reduces amyloid accumulation and oxidative stress-mediated neurotoxicity (Nimse and Pal, 2015; Ono et al., 2004; Reddy et al., 2016). Curcumin was found to reduce the oxidative stress elevated (>1 mM) concentration of copper, zinc, or iron in the brain which intern inhibition of peptide aggregation in AD (Bhat et al., 2019).

Curcumin inhibits the neurodegeneration-associated elevation of oxidative stress, free radical level, ROS, iNOS, NF-κB translocation, lipid peroxidation, mitochondrial dysfunction, glial fibrillary acidic protein (GFAP), loss of the dopaminergic neurons while increased in the level of dopamine, Cu-Zn superoxide dismutase, and tyrosine hydroxylase (Fu et al., 2015; Jagatha et al., 2008; Sharma and Nehru, 2018). Deposition of α-synuclein aggregate protein at substantia nigra, thalamus, and cortex results in dopaminergic neuronal loss and takes a part in the pathogenesis of PD. Curcumin at a therapeutic dose prevents α-synuclein aggregation by inhibiting oxidative stress and, generation of ROS and thus provides symptomatic relief in PD (Lee et al., 2013).

Exertion of oxidative stress, microglia, and proinflammatory cytokine activation majorly contributes to pathological epilepsy. Oral administration of curcumin 100 mg/kg was found to restore glutathione, cognitive deficits, and mitochondrial complex activity while the reduction in oxidative stress, ROS generation, NO synthase, lipid peroxidation, and protein carbonyls. It also acts as a modulator of brain monoamine and AchE in an experimental-induced model of epilepsy (Kaur et al., 2014).

Formation of blood clots leads to inadequate blood supply which results in oxidative stress, generation of ROS, free radicals that cause reversible or irreversible cellular damage and malfunction, that is, stroke. People under the influence of the risk factors such as advanced age, atherosclerosis, and metabolic abnormality are highly susceptible to stroke. There are two types of strokes, ischemic (85%) and hemorrhagic (15%). Administration of curcumin after 30 min of ischemic injury inhibits iNOS expression, lipid peroxidation, glial cell activation, and cellular apoptosis, while the increase in phase II enzymatic activity (NADPH: quinone oxidoreductase1-NQO1, glutathione S-transferase-GST, Aldo-keto-reductase-AR, and heme oxygenase-1 HO-1), ultimately results in a decrease in infarct volume and restoration of neuronal function in stroke-associated injury (Jiang et al., 2007).

7.3.4 GINKGO BILOBA

G. Biloba extracts contain flavonoids as major (24%) constituents such as ginkgolides and bilobalide are well known for their antioxidant activity. GB possesses an antioxidant property as it can modulate oxidative stress, free radicals (superoxide), lipoperoxide, hydrogen peroxide, peroxynitrite, nitrogen species, mitochondrial function, proinflammatory cytokines, enzymes (caspases, GSH, and SOD). The continuous 12–26 weeks treatment of *G. Biloba* is useful in the treatment of dementia associated with AD (Montes et al., 2015). Moreover, the efficacy of *G. biloba* extracts in the treatment of AD via its multidimensional mechanisms including reduction of the Aβ-induced fibrogenesis, toxicity, oxidative stress, caspase 3 and 12 activity, apoptosis along with restoration of mitochondrial function (Singh et al., 2019).

7.3.5 VITAMIN C (ASCORBIC ACID)

AD have lower cerebrospinal fluid (CSF)/brain availability of docosahexaenoic acid, choline, vitamin B_{12}, folate, vitamin C, and vitamin E. Directionally, brain nutrient status appears to parallel the lower circulatory nutrient status (de Wilde et al., 2017). About 5% of the population above 65 years of age suffer from AD worldwide. Ascorbic acid deficiency may lead to memory impairment, amyloid accumulation, and enhancement of oxidative stress in mice (Dixit et al., 2015). The oral AlCl3, 100 mg/kg daily for 15 days in rats showed neurodegeneration, significant weight loss, memory impairment, cognitive decline, motor deficits, and anxiety. These effects may be seen due to oxidative impairment depleted SOD and lipid peroxidation, increased neural AChE expression, and lactate dehydrogenase. On the contrary, ascorbic acid administration of 100 mg/kg daily for 15 days was found to reverse these alterations (Olajide et al., 2017).

7.3.6 MAGNOLOL

A bioactive polyphenolic, 5,50-diallyl-2,20-dihydroxy biphenyl (Magnolol), obtained from the stem bark of *M. officinalis*, has been used in traditional Chinese and Japanese medicine to treat a number of ailments, including respiratory and gastrointestinal disorders. Magnolol bark extract is also present in chewing gum as a dental and plaque caries preventative. Magnolol has previously been shown to be beneficial in the treatment of neurodegenerative illnesses. Mice given a single dose of 30 mg/kg BW magnolol after inducing parkinsonism with MPTP (1-methyl-4-phenyl-1,2,3,6-tetrahydropyridine) showed a significant reduction in thiobarbituric acid reactive compounds (TBARC), a marker of lipid peroxidation when compared to rats given a vehicle solution (110 vs 168% of control) (Muroyama et al., 2012). In another investigation, extracts of Magnolia cortex at 1 mg/mL concentration were found to have the largest inhibitory effects on lipid peroxidation as determined by the TBARC assay (73.15% vs 0.00–62.55%) compared to other Kampo medicines (traditional Japanese/Chinese crude medications). Magnolol was identified as one of the principal phenolic compounds in this extract by HPLC. In acrolein-induced oxidative damage in neuroblastoma cells, pretreatment with magnolol (16 and 32 M) significantly reduced superoxide anions, lipid peroxides (LPO), and PC levels in comparison with the control acrolein-exposed cells (Dong et al., 2013).

7.3.7 GRAPE SEED EXTRACT

Because of its proanthocyanidin composition, the grape seed has health benefits in addition to the RSV present in grapes. Proanthocyanidins have been shown to offer efficacy as a nutritional supplement for neurodegenerative disease management. It has been demonstrated that it acts as a radical scavenger in vivo, reducing oxidative DNA and protein degradation. The phenolic component in grape seed extract is responsible for its antioxidant potential since it functions as an in vivo radical scavenger, lowering oxidative DNA and protein damage (El-Beshbishy et al., 2009). In comparison to controls, oral administration of 100 mg/kg BW/day of grape seed extract for 30 days lowered DNA protein cross-links and 8-hydroxy-20-deoxyguanosine levels in the striatum, spinal cord, hippocampus, and cerebral cortex in elderly rats. Similarly, grape seed extract administration could reduce oxidative-mediated protein degradation in elderly rats (Singh et al., 2016).

7.3.8 GREEN TEA POLYPHENOLS

Green tea polyphenols may also have a beneficial impact on radical scavenging. EC (epicatechin), EGC (epigallocatechin), ECG (epicatechin-3-gallate), and, EGCG (Epigallocatechin-3-gallate), which are flavonols, are examples of green tea polyphenols. An ortho-trihydroxyl, ortho-30,40-dihydroxy moiety in their structures confers a varied degree of lipid and hydroxyl radical scavenging ability to each of them (Balu et al., 2006). In an earlier study (Arab et al., 2016), it was proved that green tea has neuroprotective properties. In this 2-month interventional trial, 30 individuals with severe AD were given four capsules containing 2 g of green tea each day in two divided dosages. Each pill included total polyphenols (50 mg), comprising EC, ECG, and EGCG. The total antioxidant capacity of plasma evaluated by a FRAP assay at the end of the trial was significantly higher than the baseline values. Similarly, there was a significant decrease in the levels of 8-OHdG, MDA (malondialdehyde), and PC (protein carbonyls) (Arab et al., 2016).

7.3.9 PYCNOGENOL®

Pycnogenol is a registered term for a standardized extract derived solely from the bark of a French maritime pine tree. It contains a blend of bioflavonoids such as procyanidins, catechin, phenolic acids, epicatechin, and taxifolin (Coates et al., 2004). Pine bark was once used to cure wounds and scurvy, but it has now evolved into a useful nutritional supplement for a variety of chronic conditions. Pycnogenol has a strong scavenging effect on both oxygen-free radicals and stable radicals. The capacity of pycnogenol to quench DPPH radicals is proportional to Trolox. When acrolein-induced cytotoxicity in neuroblastoma cells was pretreated with 100 g/mL pycnogenol, the generation of ROS, superoxide anions, PC, and 4-HNE bound proteins was significantly reduced compared to untreated acrolein-exposed cells (Ansari et al., 2008). In the hippocampus and cerebral cortex of ICV-STZ induce AD rats, pycnogenol pre-treatment at a dose of 10 mg/kg BW for 3 weeks significantly reduced PC content (PC-hippocampus and PC-cerebral cortex) and TBARC levels (TBARC-hippocampus and TBARS-cerebral cortex), ultimately improving cognitive performance (Khana et al., 2013). Pycnogenol's antioxidant ability has also been established in a clinical investigation. In this study, 25 healthy adults treated with 150 mg of pycnogenol each day for 6 weeks saw a 40% rise in plasma ORAC compared to baseline values. Furthermore, smokers who were given 50 mg of pycnogenol had 25.3% fewer plasma ROS metabolites after 2 weeks as compared to those who were given a placebo (Belcaro et al., 2013).

7.3.10 XANTHORRHIZOL

Curcuma xanthorrhiza Roxb., often known as Javanese turmeric, is a kind of turmeric from the Zingiberaceae family which is normally found on the Indonesian island of Java and nearby Southeast Asian countries. Xanthorrhizol, a sesquiterpenoid isolated from the tuber of *C. xanthorrhiza* Roxb., is one of its bioactive components. In rat brain homogenate, xanthorrhizol in various concentrations significantly inhibited H_2O_2-induced lipid peroxidation in a dose-dependent manner, with the maximum dose reducing lipid peroxidation by 101.87 ± 1.62% of control. Furthermore, 2 M of Xanthorrhizol significantly inhibited glutamate-induced ROS production in mouse hippocampus neuronal HT22 cells (130 vs 210% of control) in a manner akin to curcumin (Lim et al., 2005).

7.3.11 VITAMIN E

A lipid-soluble vitamin; vitamin E, can be found in a variety of vegetable oils, including wheat germ oil, palm, sunflower, coconut, and soybean. Tocopherols and tocotrienols are the two classes of vitamin E. There are four isoforms in each class: α, β, and γ tocopherols, and tocotrienols. They had strong antioxidative capabilities, which had health-promoting effects such as reducing cardiovascular disease, neurological illnesses, and osteoporosis (Sekikawa et al., 2020). Vitamin E's direct antioxidative capabilities include the capacity of its chromanol ring to donate hydrogen atoms, which neutralizes free radicals. Tocopherol and tocotrienol are oxidized in this process, resulting in stable tocopheroxyl- and tocotrienoxyl- radicals. Vitamin E is mostly disseminated in the lipid membrane owing to its lipid solubility, which is critical for arresting lipid peroxidation chain processes. To sustain the scavenging action, these substances can be transformed back to their reduced levels by combining with the other endogenous antioxidant mechanisms. Supplementing healthy older people with tocotrienol-rich fraction (TRF) (150 mg/day) for 6 months reduced MDA (0.14 vs 0.22 nmol/mL) and DNA damage levels (95 vs 125 arbitrary unit, AU) compared to baseline values (Goon et al., 2017). Furthermore, giving TRF (200 mg/kg BW) to healthy Wistar rats for 8 months reduced DNA damage compared to the control group (2.87 0.48 vs 5.96 0.43%), which was linked to enhanced cognitive function (Taridi et al., 2011). APPswe/PS1dE9 mice, a transgenic AD mouse model with increased A plaque due to Swedish mutations in APP and deleted presenilin-1 in exon 9, showed similar results. When mice were given TRF at 200 mg/kg BW daily for 6 months, there was a significant reduction in DNA damage (3.47 0.35 vs 14.04 1.475%) compared to unsupplemented control mice (Nasri et al., 2019).

7.3.12 GUARANA SEED EXTRACT

Guarana seeds are native to South America, particularly the Amazon region, and are predominantly taken as a dietary supplement and energy drink by Brazilians. It has a lot of caffeine in it, as well as polyphenols such as catechins and epicatechins. Guarana seed's antioxidant and antiaging properties, as well as its protective effect against neurological illnesses, have been thoroughly proven (Boasquívis et al., 2018; Sereia et al., 2019). Guarana seed extract has antioxidant properties due to the synergistic action of polyphenol components and its high caffeine level (Peixoto et al., 2017). A TRAP assay that has been comparable to 40 g/mL of caffeine revealed that guarana seed extract (100 and 1000 g/mL) has significant antioxidant potential. Furthermore, in acrolein-induced cytotoxicity on human neuronal-like cells, intracellular ROS generation was significantly reduced compared to control cells. Similarly, in previous study (Boasquívis et al., 2018), it was found that guarana hydroalcoholic extract (5, 10, and 50 mg/mL), which includes 2.49 g/mL of theobromine, 34.59 g/mL of catechin, 36.35 g/mL of EC, and 166.07 g/mL of caffeine has a similar DPPH radical scavenging property to 500 M of Trolox. Furthermore, as compared to untreated controls, a dose of 10 or 50 mg/mL of GHE significantly lowered intracellular ROS levels in C. elegans AD models and eventually extended the worm's lifespan (Boasquívis et al., 2018).

7.4 CONCLUSION

NDs such as AD and PD are the most common health issues associated with cognitive and motor abnormalities in the aging population. Since the pathophysiological mechanisms underlying NDs are very complex, the therapeutic efficacy of currently prescribed drugs used in NDs is very limited. Therefore, the need for effective therapeutic strategies, particularly plant-based medicines, to fight with NDs seems essential. Development of oxidative stress associated complications are considered as the hallmark sign of NDs. Interestingly, several preclinical studies show therapeutic potential of various herbal-based antioxidant nutraceuticals in the management of NDs. Nevertheless, poor penetration of phytonutraceuticals through the BBB is the most challenging issue for the clinical development of NDs. In recent times, enormous advanced technologies have been developed to improve pharmacokinetic profile and therapeutic effects of the nutraceuticals. Several nanocarriers-based delivery systems have been developed to enhance the penetration of nutraceuticals through the BBB in NDs. Nanocarriers-based delivery system of nutraceuticals significantly improves the biocompatibility, biodegradability, pharmacokinetic and therapeutic efficacy, and reduces their peripheral side effects in NDs. Anticipating the recent progress, we hope that the antioxidant potential of herbal nutraceuticals will be helpful in the development of highly effective therapeutic approaches for the treatment of NDs in the near future.

KEYWORDS

- **nutraceuticals**
- **antioxidants**
- **Alzheimer's disease**
- **Parkinson's disease**
- **phytoconstituents**

REFERENCES

Advani, K.; Batra, M.; Tajpuriya, S.; Gupta, R.; Saraswat, A.; Nagar, H. D.; Makwana, L.; Kshirsagar, S.; Kaul, P.; Ghosh, A. K.; Pradhan, S.; Mehta, A.; Jaiswal, A.; Nakhate, K. T.; Kamdi, S. Efficacy of Combination Therapy of Inositols, Antioxidants and Vitamins in Obese and Non-obese Women with Polycystic Ovary Syndrome: An Observational Study. *J. Obstet. Gynaecol.* **2020,** *40* (1), 96–101.

Ambegaokar, S. S.; Wu, L.; Alamshahi, K.; Lau, J.; Jazayeri, L.; Chan, S.; Khanna, P.; Hsieh, E.; Timiras, P. S. Curcumin Inhibits Dose-Dependently and Time-Dependently Neuroglial Cell Proliferation and Growth. *Neuroendocrinol. Lett.* **2003,** *24* (6), 469.

Amale, P. N.; Deshmukh, M.; Budrani, A.; Deshpande, S. A. Resveratrol: A Pleiotropic Phytoconstitunet. *Int. J. Res. Pharmaceut. Sci.* **2021,** *12* (2), 1–7.

Amro, M. S.; Teoh, S. L.; Norzana, A. G.; Srijit, D. The Potential Role of Herbal Products in the Treatment of Parkinson's Disease. *Clin. Therapeut.* **2018,** *169* (1), E23–E33.

Ansari, M. A.; Keller, J. N.; Scheff, S. W. Protective Effect of Pycnogenol in Human Neuroblastoma sh-sy5y Cells Following Acrolein-Induced Cytotoxicity. *Free Radic. Biol. Med.* **2008,** *45* (11), 1510–1519.

Arab, H.; Mahjoub, S.; Hajian-Tilaki, K.; Moghadasi, M. The Effect of Green Tea Consumption on Oxidative Stress Markers and Cognitive Function in Patients with Alzheimer's Disease: A Prospective Intervention Study. *Caspian J. Intern. Med.* **2016,** *7* (3), 188–194.

Arora, S. K.; Verma, P. R.; Itankar, P. R.; Prasad, S. K.; Nakhate, K. T. Evaluation of Pancreatic Regeneration Activity of *Tephrosia purpurea* Leaves in Rats with Streptozotocin-Induced Diabetes. *J. Tradit. Complement. Med.* **2021,** 11 (5), 435–445.

Badwaik, H.; Giri, T.; Nakhate, K.; Kashyap, P.; Tripathi, D. Xanthan Gum and Its Derivatives as a Potential Bio-polymeric Carrier for Drug Delivery System. *Curr. Drug Deliv.* **2013,** *10* (5), 587–600.

Badwaik, H. R.; Kumari, L.; Nakhate, K.; Verma, V. S.; Sakure, K. Phytoconstituent Plumbagin: Chemical, Biotechnological and Pharmaceutical Aspects. In *Studies in Natural Products Chemistry*; 2019; Vol. 63. pp 415–460.

Badwaik, H. R.; Nakhate, K.; Kumari, L.; Sakure, K. Oral Delivery of Proteins and Polypeptides through Polysaccharide Nanocarriers. In *Polysaccharide-Based Nano-Biocarrier in Drug Delivery*; CRC Press, 2018; pp 1–24.

Baek, J.; Jeong, H.; Ham, Y.; Jo, Y. H.; Choi, M.; Kang, M.; Son, B.; Choi, S.; Ryu, H. W.; Kim, J.; Shen, H.; Sydara, K.; Lee, S. W.; Kim, S. Y.; Han, S. B.; Oh, S. R.; Cho, S. Improvement of Spinal Muscular Atrophy via Correction of the SMN2 Splicing Defect by *Brucea javanica* (L.) Merr. Extract and Bruceine D. *Phytomedicine* **2019,** *65,* 153089.

Balu, M.; Sangeetha, P.; Murali, G.; Panneerselvam, C. Modulatory Role of Grape Seed Extract on Age-related Oxidative DNA Damage in Central Nervous System of Rats. *Brain Res. Bull.* **2006,** *68* (6), 469–473.

Belcaro, G.; Hu, S.; Cesarone, M. R.; Dugall, M. A Controlled Study Shows Daily Intake of 50 mg of French Pine Bark Extract (Pycnogenol®) Lowers Plasma Reactive Oxygen Metabolites in Healthy Smokers. *Minerva Medica.* **2013,** *104* (4), 439–446.

Bhardwaj, M.; Kumar, A. Neuroprotective Effect of Lycopene Against PTZ-Induced Kindling Seizures in Mice: Possible Behavioural, Biochemical and Mitochondrial Dysfunction. *Pharmacol. Res.* **2016,** *30* (2), 306–313.

Bhat, A.; Mahalakshmi, A. M.; Ray, B.; Tuladhar, S.; Hediyal, T. A.; Manthiannem, E.; Padamati, J.; Chandra, R.; Chidambaram, S. B.; Sakharkar, M. K. Benefits of Curcumin in Brain Disorders. *Biofactors* **2019,** *45* (5), 666–689.

Boasquívis, P. F.; Silva, G. M. M.; Paiva, F. A.; Cavalcanti, R. M.; Nunez, C. V.; De Paula Oliveira, R. G (Paullinia Cupana) Extract Protects *Caenorhabditis elegans* Models for Alzheimer Disease and Huntington Disease Through Activation of Antioxidant and Protein Degradation Pathways. *Oxid. Med. Cell. Longev.* **2018,** *2018.*

Braidy, N.; Jugder, B. E.; Poljak, A.; Jayasena, T.; Mansour, H.; Mohammad Nabavi, S.; Sachdev, P.; Grant, R. Resveratrol as a Potential Therapeutic Candidate for the Treatment and Management of Alzheimer's Disease. *Curr. Top. Med. Chem.* **2016,** *16* (17), 1951–1960.

Cai, M.; Yang, E. J. Ginsenoside Re-Attenuates Neuroinflammation in a Symptomatic ALS Animal Model. *Am. J. Chin. Med.* **2016,** *44* (2), 401–413.

Chang, K. H.; Chen, W. L.; Lee, L. C.; Lin, C. H.; Kung, P. J.; Lin, T. H.; Wu, Y. C.; Wu, Y. R.; Chen, Y. C.; Lee-Chen, G. J.; Chen, C. M. Aqueous Extract of Paeonia Lactiflora and Paeoniflorin as Aggregation Reducers Targeting Chaperones in Cell Models of Spinocerebellar Ataxia 3. *Evid. Based Complement. Alternat. Med.* **2013,** *2013,* 471659.

Chang, K. H.; Chen, W. L.; Wu, Y. R.; Lin, T. H.; Wu, Y. C.; Chao, C. Y.; Lin, J. Y.; Lee, L. C.; Chen, Y. C.; Lee-Chen, G. J.; Chen, C. M. Aqueous Extract of Gardenia Jasminoides Targeting Oxidative Stress to Reduce polyQ Aggregation in Cell Models of Spinocerebellar Ataxia 3. *Neuropharmacology* **2014,** *81,* 166–175.

Chen, C. M.; Weng, Y. T.; Chen, W. L.; Lin, T. H.; Chao, C. Y.; Lin, C. H.; Chen, I. C.; Lee, L. C.; Lin, H. Y.; Wu, Y. R.; Chen, Y. C.; Chang, K. H.; Tang, H. Y.; Cheng, M. L.; Lee-Chen, G. J.; Lin, J. Y. Aqueous Extract of *Glycyrrhiza inflata* Inhibits Aggregation by Upregulating PPARGC1A and NFE2L2-ARE Pathways in Cell Models of Spinocerebellar Ataxia 3. *Free Radic. Biol. Med.* **2014,** *71,* 339–350.

Chen, D.; Huang, C.; Chen, Z. A Review for the Pharmacological Effect of Lycopene in Central Nervous System Disorders. *Biomed. Pharmacother.* **2019,** *111,* 791–801.

Chen, I. C.; Chang, C. N.; Chen, W. L.; Lin, T. H.; Chao, C. Y.; Lin, C. H.; Lin, H. Y.; Cheng, M. L.; Chiang, M. C.; Lin, J. Y.; Wu, Y. R.; Lee-Chen, G. J.; Chen, C. M. Targeting Ubiquitin Proteasome Pathway with Traditional Chinese Medicine for Treatment of Spinocerebellar Ataxia Type 3. *Am. J. Chin. Med.* **2019,** *47* (1), 63–95.

Chen, I. C.; Chang, K. H.; Chen, Y. J.; Chen, Y. C.; Lee-Chen, G. J.; Chen, C. M. Pueraria Lobata and Daidzein Reduce Cytotoxicity by Enhancing Ubiquitin-Proteasome System Function in SCA3-IPSC-Derived Neurons. In *Oxidative Medicine and Cellular Longevity*; 2019; pp 2019.

Chen, W. J.; Du, J. K.; Hu, X.; Yu, Q.; Li, D. X.; Wang, C. N.; Zhu, X. Y.; Liu, Y. J. Protective Effects of Resveratrol on Mitochondrial Function in the Hippocampus Improves Inflammation-Induced Depressive-Like Behavior. *Physiol. Behav.* **2017,** *182,* 54–61.

Chen, X.; Pan, W. The Treatment Strategies for Neurodegenerative Diseases by Integrative Medicine. *Integr. Med. Int.* **2014,** *1* (4), 223–225.

Chen, Y.; Xiao, W.; Wang, Y.; Liu, H.; Li, X.; Yuan, Y. Lycopene Overproduction in Saccharomyces Cerevisiae Through Combining Pathway Engineering with Host Engineering. *Microb. Cell Factories.* **2016,** *15* (1), 113.

Choi, B.; Kim, S.; Jang, B. G.; Kim, M. J. Piceatannol, a Natural Analogue of Resveratrol, Effectively Reduces Beta-amyloid Levels via Activation of Alpha-Secretase and Matrix Metalloproteinase-9. *J. Func. Foods* **2016,** *23,* 124–134.

Chou, A. H.; Chen, Y. L.; Chiu, C. C.; Yuan, S. J.; Weng, Y. H.; Yeh, T. H.; Lin, Y. L.; Fang, J. M.; Wang, H. L. T1-11 and JMF1907 Ameliorate Polyglutamine-Expanded Ataxin-3-Induced Neurodegeneration, Transcriptional Dysregulation and Ataxic Symptom in the SCA3 Transgenic Mouse. *Neuropharmacology* **2015,** *99,* 308–317.

Choudhary, S.; Kumar, P.; Malik, J. Plants and Phytochemicals for Huntington's Disease. *Pharmacogn. Rev.* **2013,** *7* (14), 81–91.

Cleren, C.; Calingasan, N. Y.; Chen, J.; Beal, M. F. Celastrol Protects Against MPTP- and 3-Nitropropionic Acid-Induced Neurotoxicity. *J. Neurochem.* **2005,** *94* (4), 995–1004.

Coates, P. M.; Blackman, M. R.; Cragg, G. M.; Levine, M.; Moss, J.; White, J. D. Encyclopedia of Dietary Supplements. In *Encyclopedia of Dietary Supplements*; 2004; pp 1–821.

Cosín-Tomàs, M.; Senserrich, J.; Arumí-Planas, M.; Alquézar, C.; Pallàs, M.; Martín-Requero, Á.; Suñol, C.; Kaliman, P.; Sanfeliu, C. Role of Resveratrol and Selenium on Oxidative Stress and Expression of Antioxidant and Anti-aging Genes in Immortalized Lymphocytes from Alzheimer's Disease Patients. *Nutrients* **2019,** *11* (8), 1764.

Rege, S. D.; Geetha, T.; L Broderick, T.; Ramesh Babu, J. Resveratrol Protects β Amyloid-Induced Oxidative Damage and Memory Associated Proteins in h19-7 Hippocampal Neuronal Cells. *Curr. Alzheimer Res.* **2015,** *12* (2), 147–156.

De Wilde, M. C.; Vellas, B.; Girault, E.; Yavuz, A. C.; Sijben, J. W. Lower Brain and Blood Nutrient Status in Alzheimer's Disease: Results from Meta-Analyses. *Alzheimers Dement (N Y).* **2017,** *3* (3), 416–431.

Defelice, S. L. Foundation for Innovation in Medicine Rationale and Proposed Guidelines for the Nutraceutical Research & Education Act. *J. Nutraceut., Funct. Med. Foods* **2002,** *2,* 43–52.

Dixit, S.; Bernardo, A.; Walker, J. M.; Kennard, J. A.; Kim, G. Y.; Kessler, E. S.; Harrison, F. E. Vitamin C Deficiency in the Brain Impairs Cognition, Increases Amyloid Accumulation and Deposition, and Oxidative Stress in APP/PSEN1 and Normally Aging Mice. *ACS Chem. Neurosci.* **2015,** *6* (4), 570–581.

Dong, L.; Zhou, S.; Yang, X.; Chen, Q.; He, Y.; Huang, W. Magnolol Protects against Oxidative Stress-Mediated Neural Cell Damage by Modulating Mitochondrial Dysfunction and PI3K/Akt Signaling. *J. Mol. Neurosci.* **2013,** *50* (3), 469–481.

Dragicevic, N.; Zhang, P.; Bradshaw, P. Synthetic Metalloporphyrins and Resveratrol Act Synergistically as Enhancers of Cognitive Performance through Reduction of Deposited Amyloid Beta and Improvement of Mitochondrial Function in Alzheimer's Mice. *Am. Acad. Neurol.* **2017,** *88* (16), P5.087.

Dudeja, P.; Gupta, R. K. Chapter 40 - Nutraceuticals. In *Food Safety in The 21stcentury*; Gupta, R. K., Dudeja, S. M., Eds.; Academic Press: San Diego, 2017; pp 491–496.

El-Beshbishy, H. A.; Mohamadin, A. M.; Abdel-Naim, A. B. In Vitro Evaluation of the Antioxidant Activities of Grape Seed (Vitis Vinifera) Extract, Blackseed (Nigella Sativa) Extract and Curcumin. *J. Taibah Univ. Med. Sci.* **2009,** *4* (1), 23–35.

Fu, W.; Zhuang, W.; Zhou, S.; Wang, X. Plant-Derived Neuroprotective agents in Parkinson's Disease. *Am. J. Transl. Res.* **2015,** *7* (7), 1189.

Glenville, M. Nutritional Supplements in Pregnancy: Commercial Push or Evidence Based? *Curr. Opin. Obstet. Gynecol.* **2006,** *18* (6), 642–647.

Goon, J. A.; Nor Azman, N. H. E.; Abdul Ghani, S. M.; Hamid, Z.; Wan Ngah, W. Z. Comparing Palm Oil Tocotrienol Rich Fraction with α-Tocopherol Supplementation on Oxidative Stress in Healthy Older Adults. *Clin.Nutr. ESPEN.* **2017,** *21,* 1–12.

Guo, Y.; Zhang, K.; Wang, Q.; Li, Z.; Yin, Y.; Xu, Q.; Duan, W.; Li, C. Neuroprotective Effects of Diallyl Trisulfide in SOD1-G93A Transgenic Mouse Model of Amyotrophic Lateral Sclerosis. *Brain Res.* **2011,** *1374,* 110–115.

Hosseinkhani, A.; Sahragard, A.; Namdari, A.; Zarshenas, M. M. Botanical Sources for Alzheimer's: A Review on Reports from Traditional Persian Medicine. *Am. J. Alzheimers Dis. Other Demen.* **2017,** *32* (7), 429–437.

Huang, D. S.; Lin, H. Y.; Lee-Chen, G. J.; Hsieh-Li, H. M.; Wu, C. H.; Lin, J. Y. Treatment with a *Ginkgo biloba* Extract, EGb 761, Inhibits Excitotoxicity in an Animal Model of Spinocerebellar Ataxia Type 17. *Drug Des. Devel. Ther.* **2016,** *10,* 723–731.

Huang, N.; Zhang, Y.; Chen, M.; Jin, H.; Nie, J.; Luo, Y.; Zhou, S.; Shi, J.; Jin, F. Resveratrol Delays 6-Hydroxydopamine-Induced Apoptosis by Activating Thc PI3K/Akt Signaling Pathway. *Exp. Gerontol.* **2019,** *124,* 110653.

Huang, X.; Li, N.; Pu, Y.; Zhang, T.; Wang, B. Neuroprotective Effects of Ginseng Phytochemicals: Recent Perspectives. *Molecules* **2019,** *24* (16).

Hwang, S.; Lim, J. W.; Kim, H. Inhibitory Effect of Lycopene on Amyloid-β-Induced Apoptosis in Neuronal Cells. *Nutrients* **2017,** *9* (8), 883.

Jabir, N. R.; Khan, F. R.; Tabrez, S. Cholinesterase Targeting by Polyphenols: A Therapeutic Approach for the Treatment of Alzheimer's Disease. *CNS Neurosci. Therapeut.* **2018,** *24* (9), 753–762.

Jagatha, B.; Mythri, R. B.; Vali, S.; Bharath, M. M. S. Curcumin Treatment Alleviates the Effects of Glutathione Depletion In Vitro and In Vivo: Therapeutic Implications for Parkinson's Disease Explained via in Silico Studies. *Free Radic. Biol. Med.* **2008,** *44* (5), 907–917.

Jiang, J.; Wang, W.; Sun, Y. J.; Hu, M.; Li, F.; Zhu, D. Y. Neuroprotective Effect of Curcumin on Focal Cerebral Ischemic Rats by Preventing Blood-Brain Barrier Damage. *Eur. J. Pharmacol.* **2007,** *561* (1–3), 54–62.

Kamdi, S. P.; Badwaik, H. R.; Raval, A.; Ajazuddin; Nakhate, K. T. Ameliorative Potential of Phloridzin in Type 2 Diabetes-Induced Memory Deficits in Rats. *Eur. J. Pharmacol.* **2021,** *913,* 174645.

Kamdi, S. P.; Raval, A.; Nakhate, K. T. Effect of Apple Peel Extract on Diabetes-Induced Peripheral Neuropathy and Wound Injury. *J. Diabetes Metab. Disord.* **2021,** *20* (1), 119–130.

Kamdi, S. P.; Raval, A.; Nakhate, K. T. Phloridzin Ameliorates Type 2 Diabetes-Induced Depression in Mice by Mitigating Oxidative Stress and Modulating Brain-Derived Neurotrophic Factor. *J. Diabetes Metab. Disord.* **2021,** *20* (1), 341–348.

Kamdi, S. P.; Raval, A.; Nakhate, K. T. Phloridzin Attenuates Lipopolysaccharide-Induced Cognitive Impairment via Antioxidant, Anti-Inflammatory and Neuromodulatory Activities. *Cytokine.* **2021,** *139,* 155408.

Kaur, H.; Bal, A.; Sandhir, R. Curcumin Supplementation Improves Mitochondrial and Behavioral Deficits in Experimental Model of Chronic Epilepsy. *Pharmacol. Biochem. Behav.* **2014,** *125,* 55–64.

Keaney, G.; Amrutkar, D.; Christophersen, P.; Curtis, M.; Dagher, B.; Foster, K.; Grayzel, D.; Jacobsen, T.; Jefson, M.; Larsen, J. Discovery of CAD-1883: Clinical-Stage Positive Allosteric Modulator of the SK Channel for the Treatment of Essential Tremor and Spinocerebellar Ataxia. In *Abstracts of Papers of the American Chemical Society*; Amer Chemical Soc 1155 16th St: NW, Washington, DC 20036 USA, **2019**; Vol. 258.

Keservani, R. K.; Kesharwani, R. K.; Vyas, N.; Jain, S.; Raghuvanshi, R.; Sharma, A. K. Nutraceutical and Functional Food as Future Food: A Review. *Der. Pharm. Lett.* **2010a,** *2* (1), 106–116.

Keservani, R. K.; Kesharwani, R. K.; Sharma, A. K.; Vyas, N.; Chadoker, A. Nutritional Supplements: An Overview. *Int. J. Curr. Pharmaceut. Rev. Res.* **2010b,** *1* (1), 59–75.

Keservani, R. K.; Sharma, A. K.; Kesharwani, R. K. An Overview and Therapeutic Applications of Nutraceutical and Functional Foods. In *Recent Advances in Drug Delivery Technology;* 2017; pp 160–201.

Keservani, R. K.; Sharma, A. K.; Kesharwani, R. K.; Eds. *Nutraceuticals and Dietary Supplements: Applications in Health Improvement and Disease Management*; CRC Press, 2020; pp 1–342.

Keservani, R. K.; Sharma, A. K. Flavonoids: Emerging Trends and Potential Health Benefits. *J. Chin. Pharm. Sci.* **2014,** *23* (12), 815.

Keservani, R. K.; Sharma, A. K.; Kesharwani, R. K. Nutraceutical and Functional Foods for Cardiovascular Health. In *Food Process Engineering* (pp 291–312); Apple Academic Press: CRC Press, 2016a; pp 257–278.

Keservani, R. K.; Sharma, A. K.; Kesharwani, R. K. Medicinal Effect of Nutraceutical Fruits for the Cognition and Brain Health. Scientifica, **2016b,** *3109254,* 10. DOI: 10.1155/2016/3109254.

Khan, A.; Jahan, S.; Alshahrani, S.; Alshehri, B. M.; Sameer, A. S.; Arafah, A.; Ahmad, A.; Rehman, M. U. *Chapter 21-Phytotherapeutic Agents For Neurodegenerative Disorders: A Neuropharmacological Review*; Bhat, R. A., Hakeem, K. R., Dervash, M. A. B. T. P., Eds.; Academic Press, 2021; pp 581–620.

Khan, I.; Joshi, G.; Nakhate, K. T.; Ajazuddin; Kumar, R.; Gupta, U. Nano-Co-Delivery of Berberine and Anticancer Drug Using PLGA Nanoparticles: Exploration of Better Anticancer Activity and In Vivo Kinetics. *Pharm. Res.* **2019,** *36* (10).

Khan, M. M.; Ahmad, A.; Ishrat, T.; Khan, M. B.; Hoda, M. N.; Khuwaja, G.; Raza, S. S.; Khan, A.; Javed, H.; Vaibhav, K. Resveratrol Attenuates 6-Hydroxydopamine-Induced Oxidative Damage and Dopamine Depletion in Rat Model of Parkinson's Disease. *Brain Res.* **2010,** *1328,* 139–151.

Khana, M. D.; Kempuraja, D.; Thangavela, R.; Zaheer, A. Protection of MPTP-Induced Neuroinflammation and Neurodegeneration by Pycnogenol. *Neurochem. Int.* **2013,** *62* (4), 379–388.

Köbe, T.; Witte, A. V.; Schnelle, A.; Tesky, V. A.; Pantel, J.; Schuchardt, J. P.; Hahn, A.; Bohlken, J.; Grittner, U.; Flöel, A. Impact of Resveratrol on Glucose Control, Hippocampal Structure and Connectivity, and Memory Performance in Patients with Mild Cognitive Impairment. *Front. Neurosci.* **2017,** *11,* 105.

Koh, S. H.; Lee, S. M.; Kim, H. Y.; Lee, K. Y.; Lee, Y. J.; Kim, H. T.; Kim, J.; Kim, M. H.; Hwang, M. S.; Song, C.; Yang, K. W.; Lee, K. W.; Kim, S. H.; Kim, O. H. The Effect of Epigallocatechin Gallate on Suppressing Disease Progression of ALS Model Mice. *Neurosci. Lett.* **2006,** *395* (2), 103–107.

Kumar, P.; Kalonia, H.; Kumar, A. Lycopene Modulates Nitric Oxide Pathways against 3-Nitropropionic Acid-induced Neurotoxicity. *Life Sci.* **2009,** *85* (19–20), 711–718.

Kung, H. C.; Lin, K. J.; Kung, C. T.; Lin, T. K. Oxidative Stress, Mitochondrial Dysfunction, and Neuroprotection of Polyphenols with Respect to Resveratrol in Parkinson's Disease. *Biomedicines* **2021,** *9* (8), 918.

Lee, W. H.; Loo, C. Y.; Bebawy, M.; Luk, F.; Mason, R. S.; Rohanizadeh, R. Curcumin and Its Derivatives: Their Application in Neuropharmacology and Neuroscience in The 21st Century. *Curr. Neuropharmacol.* **2013,** *11* (4), 338–378.

Lim, C. S.; Jin, D. Q.; Mok, H. Antioxidant and Antiinflammatory Activities of Xanthorrhizol in Hippocampal Neurons and Primary Cultured Microglia. *J. Neurosci. Res.* **2005,** *82,* 831–838.

Lin, Y. T.; Wu, Y. C.; Sun, G. C.; Ho, C. Y.; Wong, T. Y.; Lin, C. H.; Chen, H. H.; Yeh, T. C.; Li, C. J.; Tseng, C. J. Effect of Resveratrol on Reactive Oxygen Species-Induced Cognitive Impairment in Rats with Angiotensin ii-Induced Early Alzheimer's Disease. *J. Clin. Med.* **2018,** *7* (10), 329.

Liu, C. B.; Wang, R.; Yi, Y. F.; Gao, Z.; Chen, Y. Z. Lycopene Mitigates β-Amyloid Induced Inflammatory Response and Inhibits NF-κB Signaling at The Choroid Plexus in Early Stages of Alzheimer's Disease Rats. *J. Nutr. Biochem.* **2018,** *53,* 66–71.

Lu, D. Y.; Lu, T. R. Herbal Medicine in New Era. *Hosp. Palliat. Med. Int. J.* **2019,** *3* (4), 125–130.

Montes, P.; Ruiz-Sanchez, E.; Rojas, C.; Rojas, P. *Ginkgo biloba* Extract 761: A Review of Basic Studies and Potential Clinical Use in Psychiatric Disorders. CNS *Neurol. Disord. Drug Targets* **2015,** *14* (1), 132–149.

Moussa, C.; Hebron, M.; Huang, X.; Ahn, J.; Rissman, R. A.; Aisen, P. S.; Turner, R. S. Resveratrol Regulates Neuro-Inflammation and Induces Adaptive Immunity in Alzheimer's Disease. *J. Neuroinflammation.* **2017,** *14* (1), 1–10.

Muddapu, V. R.; Dharshini, S. A. P.; Chakravarthy, V. S.; Gromiha, M. M. Neurodegenerative Diseases—Is Metabolic Deficiency The Root Cause? *Front. Neurosci.* **2020,** *14,* 213.

Mulgund, A.; Doshi, S.; Agarwal, A. The Role of Oxidative Stress in Endometriosis. In *Handbook of Fertility*; Elsevier, 2015; pp 273–281.

Muroyama, A.; Fujita, A.; Lv, C.; Kobayashi, S.; Fukuyama, Y.; Mitsumoto, Y. Magnolol Protects Against mptp/mpp + -Induced Toxicity via Inhibition of Oxidative Stress in In Vivo and in Vitro Models of Parkinson's Disease. *Parkinson's Dis.* **2012,** 2012.

Nakhate, K.; Borkar, C.; Bharne, A. Functional Neuroanatomy and Disorders of Cognition. In *Cognitive Informatics, Computer Modelling, and Cognitive Science*; Sinha, G. R., Suri, J. S., Eds.; Academic Press, 2020; pp 21–47.

Nakhate, K. T.; Bharne, A. P.; Verma, V. S.; Aru, D. N.; Kokare, D. M. Plumbagin Ameliorates Memory Dysfunction in Streptozotocin Induced Alzheimer's Disease via Activation of Nrf2/ARE Pathway and Inhibition of β-Secretase. *Biomed. Pharmacother.* **2018,** *101,* 379–390.

Nasri, W. N. W.; Makpol, S.; Mazlan, M.; Tooyama, I.; Ngah, W. Z. W.; Damanhuri, H. A. Tocotrienol Rich Fraction Supplementation Modulate Brain Hippocampal Gene Expression in APPswe/PS1dE9 Alzheimer's Disease Mouse Model. *J. Alzheimers Dis.* **2019,** *70* (S1), S239–S254.

Neves Carvalho, A.; Firuzi, O.; Joao Gama, M.; van Horssen, J.; Saso, L. Oxidative Stress and Antioxidants in Neurological Diseases: Is There Still Hope? *Curr. Drug Targets* **2017,** *18* (6), 705–718.

Nimse, S. B.; Pal, D. Free Radicals, Natural Antioxidants, and Their Reaction Mechanisms. *RSC Adv.* **2015,** *5* (35), 27986–28006.

Olajide, O. J.; Yawson, E. O.; Gbadamosi, I. T.; Arogundade, T. T.; Lambe, E.; Obasi, K.; Lawal, I. T.; Ibrahim, A.; Ogunrinola, K. Y. Ascorbic Acid Ameliorates Behavioural Deficits and Neuropathological Alterations in Rat Model of Alzheimer's Disease. *Environ. Toxicol. Pharmacol.* **2017,** *50,* 200–211.

Ono, K.; Hasegawa, K.; Naiki, H.; Yamada, M. Curcumin Has Potent Anti-amyloidogenic Effects for Alzheimer's β-Amyloid Fibrils In Vitro. *J. Neurosci. Res.* **2004,** *75* (6), 742–750.

Paul, R.; Mazumder, M. K.; Nath, J.; Deb, S.; Paul, S.; Bhattacharya, P.; Borah, A. Lycopene-A. Pleiotropic Neuroprotective Nutraceutical: Deciphering Its Therapeutic Potentials in Broad Spectrum Neurological Disorders. *Neurochem. Int.* **2020,** *140,* 104823.

Peixoto, H.; Roxo, M.; Röhrig, T.; Richling, E.; Wang, X.; Wink, M. Anti-Aging and Antioxidant Potential of Paullinia Cupana var. Sorbilis: Findings in *Caenorhabditis elegans* Indicate a New Utilization for Roasted Seeds of Guarana. *Medicines* **2017,** *4* (4), 61.

Peng, K.; Tao, Y.; Zhang, J.; Wang, J.; Ye, F.; Dan, G.; Zhao, Y.; Cai, Y.; Zhao, J.; Wu, Q. Resveratrol Regulates Mitochondrial Biogenesis and Fission/Fusion to Attenuate Rotenone-Induced Neurotoxicity. *Oxid. Med. Cell. Longev.* **2016,** 2016.

Pérez-Hernández, J.; Zaldívar-Machorro, V. J.; Villanueva-Porras, D.; Vega-Ávila, E.; Chavarría, A. A Potential Alternative against Neurodegenerative Diseases: Phytodrugs. *Oxid. Med. Cell. Long.* **2016,** *2016,* 8378613.

Phang, M. W. L.; Lew, S. Y.; Chung, I.; Lim, W. K. S.; Lim, L. W.; Wong, K. H. Therapeutic Roles of Atnural Remedies in Combating Hereditary Ataxia: A Systematic Review. *Chin. Med.* **2021,** *16* (1), 15.

Pohl, F.; Teixeira-Castro, A.; Costa, M. D.; Lindsay, V.; Fiúza-Fernandes, J.; Goua, M.; Bermano, G.; Russell, W.; Maciel, P.; Kong Thoo Lin, P. GST-4-Dependent Suppression of Neurodegeneration in *C. elegans* Models of Parkinson's and Machado-Joseph Disease by Rapeseed Romace Extract Supplementation. *Front. Neurosci.* **2019,** *13,* 1091.

Prema, A.; Janakiraman, U.; Manivasagam, T.; Thenmozhi, A. J. Neuroprotective Effect of Lycopene against mptp Induced Experimental Parkinson's Disease in Mice. *Neurosci. Lett.* **2015,** *599,* 12–19.

Rajasekaran, A. 1.05—Nutraceuticals. in *Comprehensive Medicinal Chemistry III*; Chackalamannil, S.; Rotella, D.; Ward, S. E.; Eds.; Elsevier: Oxford, 2017; pp 107–134.

Ramli, N. Z.; Yahaya, M. F.; Tooyama, I.; Damanhuri, H. A. A Mechanistic Evaluation of Antioxidant Nutraceuticals on Their Potential Against Age-associated Neurodegenerative Diseases. *Antioxidants* **2020,** *9* (10), 1–39.

Ratheesh, G.; Tian, L.; Venugopal, J. R.; Ezhilarasu, H.; Sadiq, A.; Fan, T. P.; Ramakrishna, S. Role of Medicinal Plants in Neurodegenerative Diseases. *Biomanufac. Rev.* **2017,** *2* (1), 2.

Reddy, P. H.; Manczak, M.; Yin, X.; Grady, M. C.; Mitchell, A.; Kandimalla, R.; Kuruva, C. S. Protective Effects of a Natural Product, Curcumin, against Amyloid β Induced Mitochondrial and Synaptic Toxicities in Alzheimer's Disease. *J. Investig. Med.* **2016,** *64* (8), 1220–1234.

Roy, A. Role of Medicinal Plants against Alzheimer's Disease. *Int. J. Complement. Altern. Med.* **2018,** *11* (4), 205–208.

Sachdeva, A. K.; Chopra, K. Lycopene Abrogates aβ(1-42)-Mediated Neuroinflammatory Cascade in an Experimental Model of Alzheimer's Disease. *J. Nutr. Biochem.* **2015,** *26* (7), 736–744.

Santana, A. C. F.; Magalhães, G. J. P. Resveratrol in Alzheimer's Disease: A Review of Pathophysiology and Therapeutic Potential. *Arq. Neuropsiquiatr.* **2020,** *78,* 501–511.

Sarkar, S.; Davies, J. E.; Huang, Z.; Tunnacliffe, A.; Rubinsztein, D. C. Trehalose, A Novel MTOR-Independent Autophagy Enhancer, Accelerates the Clearance of Mutant Huntingtin and Alpha-Synuclein. *J. Biol. Chem.* **2007,** *282* (8), 5641–5652.

Sathya, M.; Moorthi, P.; Premkumar, P.; Kandasamy, M.; Jayachandran, K. S.; Anusuyadevi, M. Resveratrol Intervenes Cholesterol-and Isoprenoid-Mediated Amyloidogenic Processing of aβpp in Familial Alzheimer's Disease. *J. Alzheimers Dis.* **2017,** *60* (S1), S3–S23.

Sekikawa, T.; Kizawa, Y.; Li, Y.; Takara, T. Cognitive Function Improvement with Astaxanthin and Tocotrienol Intake: A Randomized, Double-Blind, Placebo-Controlled Study. *J. Clin. Biochem. Nutr.* **2020,** *67* (3), 307–316.

Sereia, A. L.; de Oliveira, M. T.; Baranoski, A.; Medeiros Marques, L. L.; Ribeiro, F. M.; Isolani, R. G.; De Medeiros, D. C.; Chierrito, D.; Lazarin-Bidóia, D.; Ferreira Zielinski, A. A.; Novello, C. R.; Nakamura, C. V.; Mantovani, M. S.; De Mello, J. C. P. In Vitro Evaluation of the Protective Effects of Plant Extracts Against Amyloid-Beta Peptide-Induced Toxicity in Human Neuroblastoma SH-SY5Y Cells. *PLoS One.* **2019,** *14* (2), 1–24.

Sharifi-Rad, M.; Lankatillake, C.; Dias, D. A.; Docea, A. O.; Mahomoodally, M. F.; Lobine, D.; Chazot, P. L.; Kurt, B.; Boyunegmez Tumer, T.; Catarina Moreira, A.; Sharopov, F.; Martorell, M.; Martins, N.; Cho, W. C.; Calina, D.; Sharifi-Rad, J. Impact of Natural Compounds on Neurodegenerative Disorders: From Preclinical to Pharmacotherapeutics. *J. Clin. Med.* **2020,** *9* (4).

Sharma, M.; Alexander, A.; Saraf, S.; Saraf, S.; Vishwakarma, U. K.; Nakhate, K. T.; Ajazuddin. Mosquito Repellent and Larvicidal Perspectives of Weeds Lantana Camara L. and Ocimum Gratissimum L. Found in Central India. *Biocatal. Agric. Biotechnol.* **2021,** *34,* 0–6.

Sharma, N.; Nehru, B. Curcumin Affords Neuroprotection and Inhibits α-Synuclein Aggregation in Lipopolysaccharide-Induced Parkinson's Disease Model. *Inflammopharmacology* **2018,** *26* (2), 349–360.

Singh, N. A.; Mandal, A. K. A.; Khan, Z. A. Potential Neuroprotective Properties of Epigallocatechin-3-Gallate (egcg). *Nutr. J.* **2016,** *15* (1), 1–17.

Singh, S. K.; Srivastav, S.; Castellani, R. J.; Plascencia-Villa, G.; Perry, G. Neuroprotective and Antioxidant Effect of *Ginkgo biloba* Extract Against ad and Other Neurological Disorders. *Neurotherapeutics* **2019,** *16* (3), 666–674.

Singhal, A.; Bangar, O.; Naithani, V. Medicinal Plants with a Potential to Treat Alzheimer and Associated Symptoms. *Int. J. Nutr. Pharmacol. Neurol. Dis.* **2012,** *2* (2), 84.

Sofia, K.; A, J.; Sneha, S. Plants as a Promising Source for the Treatment of Parkinson Disease: A Systematic Review. In *IP International Journal of Comprehensive and Advanced Pharmacology*; IP Innovative Publication, 2021, p 13052.

Tai, Y. H.; Lin, Y. Y.; Wang, K. C.; Chang, C. L.; Chen, R. Y.; Wu, C. C.; Cheng, I. H. Curcuminoid Submicron Particle Ameliorates Cognitive Deficits and Decreases Amyloid Pathology in Alzheimer's Disease Mouse Model. *Oncotarget* **2018,** *9* (12), 10681.

Taridi, N. M.; Yahaya, M. F.; Teoh, S. L.; Latiff, A. A.; Ngah, W. Z. W.; Das, S.; Mazlan, M. Tocotrienol Rich Fraction (TRF) Supplementation Protects Against Oxidative DNA Damage and Improves Cognitive Functions in Wistar Rats. *Clin. Therapeut.* **2011,** 1*62* (02), 1–2.

Tonda-Turo, C.; Origlia, N.; Mattu, C.; Accorroni, A.; Chiono, V. Current Limitations in the Treatment of Parkinson's and Alzheimer's Diseases: State-of-the-Art and Future Perspective of Polymeric Carriers. *Curr. Med. Chem.* **2018,** *25* (41), 5755–5771.

Tseng, Y. T.; Jong, Y. J.; Liang, W. F.; Chang, F. R.; Lo, Y. C. The Water Extract of *Liuwei dihuang* Possesses Multi-Protective Properties on Neurons and Muscle Tissue against Deficiency of Survival Motor Neuron Protein. *Phytomedicine* **2017,** *34,* 97–105.

Wang, H.; Jiang, T.; Li, W.; Gao, N.; Zhang, T. Resveratrol Attenuates Oxidative Damage Through Activating Mitophagy in an In Vitro Model of Alzheimer's Disease. *Toxicol. Lett.* **2018,** *282,* 100–108.

Wang, J.; Li, L.; Wang, Z.; Cui, Y.; Tan, X.; Yuan, T.; Liu, Q.; Liu, Z.; Liu, X. Supplementation of Lycopene Attenuates Lipopolysaccharide-Induced Amyloidogenesis and Cognitive Impairments via Mediating Neuroinflammation and Oxidative Stress. *J. Nutr. Biochem.* **2018,** *56,* 16–25.

Weydert, C. J.; Cullen, J. J. Measurement of Superoxide Dismutase, Catalase and Glutathione Peroxidase in Cultured Cells and Tissue. *Nat. Protocol.* **2010,** *5* (1), 51–66.

Yamazaki, Y.; Zhao, N.; Caulfield, T. R.; Liu, C. C.; Bu, G. Apolipoprotein E and Alzheimer Disease: Pathobiology and Targeting Strategies. *Nat. Rev. Neurol.* **2019,** *15* (9), 501–518.

Yin, Q.; Ma, Y.; Hong, Y.; Hou, X.; Chen, J.; Shen, C.; Sun, M.; Shang, Y.; Dong, S.; Zeng, Z. Lycopene Attenuates Insulin Signaling Deficits, Oxidative Stress, Neuroinflammation, and Cognitive Impairment in Fructose-Drinking Insulin Resistant Rats. *Neuropharmacology* **2014,** *86,* 389–396.

Yu, L.; Wang, W.; Pang, W.; Xiao, Z.; Jiang, Y.; Hong, Y. Dietary Lycopene Supplementation Improves Cognitive Performances in Tau Transgenic Mice Expressing p3011 Mutation via Inhibiting Oxidative Stress and Tau Hyperphosphorylation. *J. Alzheimers Dis.* **2017,** *57* (2), 475–482.

Zaky, A.; Bassiouny, A.; Farghaly, M.; El-Sabaa, B. M. A. Combination of Resveratrol and Curcumin is Effective against Aluminum Chloride-Induced Neuroinflammation in Rats. *J. Alzheimers Dis.* **2017,** *60* (S1), S221–S235.

Zeng, W.; Zhang, W.; Lu, F.; Gao, L.; Gao, G. Resveratrol Attenuates MPP+-Induced Mitochondrial Dysfunction and Cell Apoptosis via AKT/GSK-3β Pathway in SN4741 Cells. *Neurosci. Lett.* **2017,** *637,* 50–56.

CHAPTER 8

NUTRACEUTICAL ANTIOXIDANTS IN THE PREVENTION AND TREATMENT OF DIABETES MELLITUS

NEHA PANCHABHAI[1], HARSHAD JADHAV[2],
SANJIRI DILIP SHELAR[3], AMEY SUKHIA[1], NAYAN A. GUJARATHI[4],
and RAJ K. KESERVANI[5]

[1]*N.D.M.V.P. College of Pharmacy, Nashik, Maharashtra, India*

[2]*Department of Pharmaceutical Analysis, National Institute of Pharmaceutical Education and Research, S.A.S Nagar, Mohali, Punjab, India*

[3]*Department of Pharmaceutical Sciences and Technology, Institute of Chemical Technology, Matunga, Mumbai, Maharashtra, India*

[4]*Shri Vile Parle Kelavani Mandal's Institute of Pharmacy, Dhule, Maharashtra, India*

[5]*Faculty of B. Pharmacy, CSM Group of Institutions, Prayagraj, Uttar Pradesh, India*

ABSTRACT

Diabetes mellitus is a major cause of long-term illness and premature mortality. Moreover, changes in lifestyle and lack of improvement in healthcare contribute to it. Diabetes is classified into two major types according to the pathogenesis of the disease and not the treatment: type I diabetes and type II diabetes. Type I is an autoimmune disorder, while type II is characterized by insufficient synthesis and secretion of insulin. Hyperglycemia

Antioxidants as Nutraceuticals. Nayan A. Gujarathi, Raj K. Keservani, Rajesh K. Kesharwani, Bhushan R. Rane, Yogeeta Sameer Goyal (Eds.)

and glucotoxicity caused by diabetes mellitus are responsible for increased oxidative stress, thereby leading to injury to body cells and tissues and dysfunction or even death of β-cells. Therefore, it is crucial to maintain the antioxidant levels in diabetic patients. Nutraceuticals play an important role as antioxidants. This chapter includes information about the antioxidant nutraceuticals used to treat diabetes mellitus.

8.1 DIABETES MELLITUS

Diabetes implies "to pass through," while mellitus means "honey" (sweetness) in Greek. Diabetes is a leading cause of long-term illness as well as premature mortality. The death rate due to diabetes exceeds the deaths caused by HIV AIDS. In 2019, around a million deaths were attributed to diabetes alone. According to WHO, the number of diabetic patients has increased from 100 million to 422 million in the past 30 years. Its prevalence has risen more tremendously in underdeveloped and developing countries than in high-income, developed countries. Lack of improvement in healthcare and lifestyle change are major reasons for an increase in diabetes mellitus, especially in urban areas.

Diabetes mellitus is a metabolic disorder and is characterized by hyperglycemia (higher blood glucose level than normal) caused by either a defect in insulin secretion by β-cells, its action, or both (Alam et al., 2014). Diabetes is also associated with other complications such as retinopathy, nephropathy, and neuropathy. Chronic hyperglycemia can affect, dysfunction, and damage or even cause failure of organs like eyes, nerves, blood vessels, kidneys, and the heart (Maraschin et al., 2010; Report of the Expert Committee on the Diagnosis and Classification of Diabetes Mellitus, 1997). There are a series of processes that can occur when the disease is developed, from pancreatic β-cells destruction with insulin deficiency to insulin resistance (Rane et al., 2012).

8.1.1 PATHOPHYSIOLOGY OF DIABETES

To understand the disorder, it is essential to know the pathophysiology of diabetes.

Blood glucose regulation and pathophysiology of diabetes:

1. Regulation of blood glucose: Insulin is a polypeptide chain of 51 amino acids. It consists of chains A and B that are connected by

disulfide bridges. In case of high blood glucose levels, insulin is released by β cells of islets of Langerhans. Insulin then binds to the tyrosine kinase insulin receptor's β subunit to promote the β subunit autophosphorylation. Insulin signals the liver to convert excess available glucose to glycogen and triggers adipose/skeletal muscle cells to translocate the glucose transporter to the cell surface and take more glucose (Pessin and Saltiel, 2000). If there is low blood glucose concentration, the α cells release glucagon, which sends a signal to the liver for converting glycogen to glucose. This process maintains the homeostasis of sugar levels in the body (Fig. 8.1).

2. In diabetes, the blood glucose levels are high either due to irregularity in the synthesis or the secretion of insulin or insulin resistance. The first case with irregular synthesis/secretion of insulin refers to type I diabetes, while the latter is for type II diabetes.

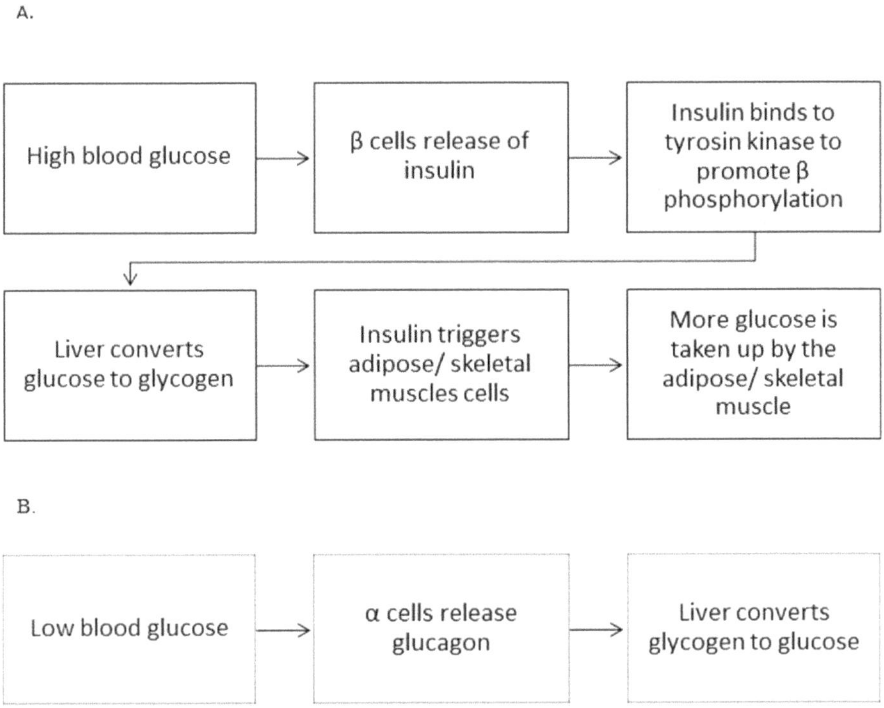

FIGURE 8.1 Normal regulation of blood glucose.

8.1.2 TYPES OF DIABETES

Diabetes can be classified according to the pathogenesis of the disease:

1. Type I diabetes: This type of diabetes is also called juvenile-onset diabetes and insulin-dependent diabetes. Type I diabetes is an autoimmune disorder, whose onset happens in childhood and initial adulthood. In type I diabetes, T cells, CD4+, CD8+, and macrophages are activated to destroy the beta cells (Phillips et al., 2009). Fulminant type I diabetes mellitus causes quick and complete destruction of beta cells. Few patients suffer from less-common autoimmune type I diabetes called idiopathic diabetes. Patients suffering from idiopathic diabetes lack insulin production. They are also prone to ketoacidosis (Phillips et al., 2009).
2. Type II diabetes: This type is characterized by inadequate synthesis and secretion of insulin. Type II diabetes accounts for almost 90% of worldwide diabetes cases. It can be further categorized into diabetes without obesity and diabetes with obesity. In patients with diabetes without obesity, additionally to a production and release deficiency of insulin, there is insulin resistance at the post-receptor level. In contrast, in obese type II diabetes patients, there is an alteration in cell receptors that causes resistance to endogenous insulin, and it is associated with abdominal fat distribution (Maraschin et al., 2010).
3. Gestational diabetes and other diabetes mellitus: Gestational diabetes happens to a pregnant woman and is resolved at the end of the gestational period.
4. Maturity-onset diabetes, also called M.O.D.Y., is a monogenic type of diabetes. There is a significantly less population diagnosed with this type of diabetes (Vikram et al., 2014).

8.1.3 OXIDATIVE STRESS IN DIABETES MELLITUS

Primary sources of diabetes-related oxidative stress are generally considered to be hyperglycemia and glucotoxicity. Oxidative stress pathways represent a crucial link between cell tissue damage and high glucose levels. These trials noted a crucial role of hyperglycemia in tissue damage.

The development and complications of diabetes can be linked to oxidative stress in patients with diabetes (Saeidnia and Abdollahi, 2013; Sarmento et al., 2013), where the reactive oxygen species (ROS) level exceeds the antioxidant level. Oxidative stress leads to an imbalance between the production of free radicals and an antioxidation defense system. This leads to injury to body cells and tissues and cell death or dysfunction (Varga et al., 2015). Long-term hyperglycemia roots in the generation of ROS, specifically during the glycosylation step of glucose oxidation. The generated ROS then damages the β cells and causes impairment of insulin release and resistance (Karunakaran and Park, 2013; Vikram et al., 2014). Similarly, blood glucose levels can rise if the antioxidant concentration is lower, leading to increased diabetes complications and insulin resistance risk. Therefore, insulin resistance and beta cell function can be improved by supplementing antioxidants (Vikram et al., 2014).

8.2 NUTRACEUTICALS

It is tough to differentiate between nutrients, food additives, and drugs. Independent of the matrix in which it is delivered, a dietary supplement can sometimes be food-like and other times drug-like (Serrano et al., 2018).

The term "nutraceutical" was coined from two words, "nutrition" and "pharmaceutical," by Stephen DeFelice. According to him, a nutraceutical is "a food that provides medical, prevention and treatment of a disease and medical benefits" (Kalra, 2003). Nutraceuticals have both therapeutic potential and the nutrition that they provide. Nutraceuticals can also be defined as a functional food that is used for the prevention and treatment of disease(s) or disorder(s) (Kalra, 2003; Keservani et al., 2010a; Keservani et al., 2010b; Keservani et al., 2017; Keservani et al., 2020).

Nutraceutical products are extracted from various sources like herbal products and different supplements extracted from diets and nutrients (Kalra, 2003), and based on that, they can be divided into three main categories: dietary supplements, nutrients, and herbals.

Herbals are obtained from plant sources. Different herbals such as Aloe vera gel are used as anti-inflammatory and emollient. Garlic acts as an antibacterial agent and also has anti-fungal activity. Lavender, ginger, and parsley are other examples of herbals used to prevent chronic diseases and improve health (Serrano et al., 2018). Nutrients have nutritional standards and are naturally present in our diets, such as polysaccharides, vitamins, minerals, and fatty acids. They are often used for the inhibition and treatment of diabetes mellitus, cancer, osteoarthritis, obesity, and osteoporosis (Kumar and Kumar, 2015).

Dietary fibers are categorized into soluble and insoluble dietary fibers. Soluble dietary fibers perform bowel functions. They also regulate the cholesterol levels in the body and help maintain sugar levels in the blood of a patient suffering from diabetes mellitus. Pectin and gums present in vegetables, fruits, and vegetables are soluble dietary fibers. Insoluble dietary fibers cause rapid passage of food ingredients from the intestine, avoiding constipation symptoms. They are also used for colon and diverticular disorders. Insoluble dietary fibers include whole-wheat flour, nuts, potatoes, etc.

The other natural food sources used as nutraceuticals are probiotics, prebiotics, antioxidants, polyunsaturated fatty acids, spices, and flavonoids (Ghani et al., 2019; Keservani and Sharma, 2014; Keservani et al., 2016a; Keservani et al., 2016b).

Diabetes and nutraceuticals: Diabetes is most common in people who use saturated fats. The progression of diabetes can be delayed by prohibiting trans and saturated fats from the diet. Moreover, nutraceuticals can also help to delay the disease progression. One of the nutraceuticals, R-lipoic acid, acts as an antioxidant, and because of its natural antioxidant coenzyme function, it decreases pyruvate and serum lactate levels in diabetes mellitus.

8.3 NUTRACEUTICALS USED AS ANTIOXIDANTS IN THE TREATMENT OF DIABETES

Following are the examples of antioxidants used as nutraceuticals and their mechanism of action given in Table 8.1.

8.3.1 ZINC

Insulin is stored in beta cells of the pancreas as a hexamer with two zinc ions. During beta-cell de-granulation, insulin is released into the portal venous system. More than 300 enzymes have zinc as their cofactor. Zinc is essential in antioxidant defense in type II diabetes mellitus patients, carbohydrate metabolism, and insulin action (Chausmer, 1998). In diabetes, there is increased oxidative stress, and zinc is a constituent of superoxide dismutase, an important antioxidant enzyme (Simon and Taylor, 2001). Zinc causes the reduction and neutralization of free radicals (Prasad, 2008). Some studies indicate a correlation between diabetes and hypozincemia (Garg et al., 1994) and hyperzincuria (Pidduck et al., 1970). As per a few studies, zinc supplementation can improve mice's fasting glucose and fasting insulin levels (Simon and Taylor, 2001).

TABLE 8.1 Nutraceuticals and Their Mechanism of Actions as an Anti-Diabetic.

Nutraceuticals	Mechanism of action as an anti-diabetic
Zinc	• Reduction and neutralization of free radicles • Reduction of oxidative stress • Increase in glutathione oxidase activity • Enhancement in glucose transport into cells • Conversion of pro-insulin to insulin
Curcuma longa	• Prevent hydrolysis of starch into glucose by inhibiting amylase enzyme • Inhibiting reactive oxygen species (ROS) • Abolish myristate-13, thapsigargin, phorbol-12, and acetate-induced generation of ROS • Normalization of levels of lipid peroxidation markers • Inhibition of increased TBARS and protein carbonyl levels
Chromium	• Enhancement in the activity of insulin • Alteration of carbohydrate, protein, and lipid metabolism
Magnesium	• Acting as a co-factor for vital metabolic processes for proteins and antioxidant enzymes • Preservation of adipocyte insulin sensitivity • Helps to reduce pathological complications of diabetes • Reduction of age-related macular degeneration
α-Lipoic Acid	• Inhibition and scavenging of ROS • Protection of the retina from ischemia caused by diabetes • Reduction of diabetic neuropathy
Selenium	• Mimics insulin activity • Reduction in lipid peroxidation • Induction of dephosphorylation and inactivation of insulin signaling enzymes
Vitamin E	• Scavenging reactive oxygen species • Inhibition protein kinase C • Prevention of the development of acellular capillaries • Reduction of catalase and sod1 enzyme activity
Flavonol	• Enhancing activation and expression of AMP-activated cellular protein • Regulation of caspase-3 activities • Increase synthesis and secretion of insulin from cells • Promote absorption of glucose by activating protein kinase C and some PI3K pathways • Production of new glucose transporters

Zinc can strive with copper and iron for binding sites on the cell membrane. The copper and iron ions produce lipid peroxides. If these metals are replaced by zinc in the plasma membrane, lipid peroxidation can be prevented (Oteiza, 2012).

According to several published studies, zinc controls the free radical production of neuronal cells in type II diabetic patients. It also inhibits N-methyl-D-aspartate receptors (NMDA) that play a role in calcium transportation. Therefore, NMDA receptors are activated in zinc deficiency, and intracellular calcium concentration increases. These conditions activate NADPH-oxidase and nitric oxide synthase, producing reactive oxygen and nitrogen species (Oteiza, 2012). Preclinical studies in diabetic mice reported that malondialdehyde concentration decreases while the metallothionein gene transcription in peripheral nerves is stimulated due to zinc supplementation (Liu et al., 2014). Therefore, zinc supplementation has the ability to reduce the oxidative stress and improve peripheral neuropathy caused by diabetes.

A study conducted by Zhu et al. (2013) suggested that zinc increases glutathione peroxidase enzyme activity and reduces nitric acid and malondialdehyde in diabetic rats. The authors observed that zinc could prevent damage to pancreatic tissues and improve liver function. Zinc enhances glucose transport into cells by promoting phosphorylation of insulin receptors. (Miao et al., 2013; Capdor et al., 2013). Moreover, zinc takes part in insulin secretion and action. It acts as a cofactor in the conversion of proinsulin, an inactive form of insulin, to the active form of insulin. Higher serum concentrations of zinc improved the insulin sensitivity of patients who have type II diabetes and acted against chronic hyperglycemia (Vashum et al., 2014).

8.3.2 CURCUMA LONGA

Curcuma longa is a rhizomatous herbaceous plant and is a member of the ginger family. The main part of curcuma longa is the rhizomes. The most active components of Curcuma longa are curcuminoids, which include curcumin, dimethoxy curcumin, and bisdemethoxycurcumin (Jena et al., 2017; Kocaadam and Şanlier, 2017; Lobo et al., 2009). Chemically curcuminoids are polyphenolic and mostly nontoxic. They have many applications in biological activities (Srivilai et al., 2017; Tyagi et al., 2015), like immunosuppressants production, apoptosis, and suppression of neurotoxic factors in alveolar monocytes and macrophages. Curcuma longa is famous for its safety profile antioxidant and anti-inflammatory activities (Kunnumakkara et al., 2017; Perrone et al., 2015; Pivari et al., 2019; Pulido-Moran et al., 2016). Curcumin has a role in many molecular pathways because of its structure. The structure of curcumin enables it to have many molecular targets. Curcuma longa inhibits amylase enzyme activities which is the common enzyme for the hydrolysis of starch into glucose. Natural curcuminoid bisdemethoxycurcumin inhibits a-glucosidase enzyme activities. In major diseases like diabetes mellitus, curcumin acts as an antioxidant by inhibiting ROS, reduces hyperglycemia, acts as an anti-inflammatory, and also inhibits the systemic complications caused by diabetes mellitus like hypertension, dyslipidemia, neuropathy, and nephropathy (Liang et al., 2020; Stanić, 2017).

As mentioned earlier, there are increased ROS levels in diabetes. Increased glucose levels cause glycation of proteins, oxidation of glucose, and polyol metabolism oxidation. Moreover, these changes further help increasing the ROS levels and cause modification of DNA, lipids, and proteins by oxidative chemical mechanisms. There are several mechanisms by which curcumin acts as an antioxidant.

1. Curcumin abolishes myristate-13, thapsigargin, phorbol-12, and acetate-induced generation of ROS by inhibiting PKC activity and entry of Ca2+ (Balasubramanyam et al., 2003).
2. Due to the blocking of ROS formation, cellular apoptosis takes place because of the blocking of apoptotic changes like caspase-3 activation, mitochondrial cytochrome c release, DNA fragmentation, JNK activation, and cleavage of PARP in blastocysts, ESC-B5 cells, and G2 cells (human hepatoma) (Chan et al., 2005; Hsuuw et al., 2005).
3. Normalization of levels of lipid peroxidation markers like vitamin C, SODC, circulatory lipid peroxidation, and vitamin E and antioxidant enzymatic activities due to oral administration of curcumin (Balamurugan et al., 2009; Mahesh et al., 2005).
4. In diabetic rats, curcumin inhibited an increase in thiobarbituric acid reactive substances (TBARS) and protein carbonyl levels and also reversed the activity of enzymes (Suryanarayana et al., 2007).

8.3.3 CHROMIUM

Chromium is an essential mineral and has a beneficial role in insulin secretion. Chromium is considered a vital factor for enhancing the activity of insulin. It affects lipid, protein, and carbohydrate metabolism. Diabetic patients have a deficiency of chromium (Lau et al., 2008). It is observed that there is an increment in insulin sensitivity and enhanced glucose tolerance due to chromium. A randomized trial was arranged for chromium supplementation effects on insulin and glucose response in healthy individuals and diabetic patients. The results indicated a noteworthy improvement in the level of glucose in diabetic patients and not in healthy volunteers (Althuis et al., 2002). However, the American Diabetes Association believes that the benefit of chromium supplementation has inconclusive evidence (American Diabetes Association, 2007).

8.3.4 MAGNESIUM

Magnesium is an alkaline earth metal and is one of the most abundant intracellular divalent cations (Giménez-Mascarell et al., 2018). It is part of many vital metabolic processes like blood glucose and blood pressure regulation, DNA synthesis, RNA expression, muscle and nerve signaling, and ATP-dependent biochemical reactions (Gröber et al., 2015). Therefore, magnesium deficiency is responsible for abnormalities, including impaired development, insulin resistance, glucose tolerance, and lipid metabolism (Zhang et al., 2018). Additionally, the important pathophysiological features that are seen in diabetes mellitus are dysfunctioning of pancreatic beta and insulin resistance (Palacios et al., 2019). Several studies showed an association between diabetes and low magnesium levels causing diabetic nephropathy, macrovascular disease, and neuropathy (Zhang et al., 2018). These associations are due to the role of magnesium as a cofactor in proteins and enzymes with antioxidant, anti-apoptotic, and anti-inflammatory activities. Although the mechanism for magnesium's effect on the development of diabetes is unclear, some studies showed a correlation between magnesium deficiency, an increase in the risk of insulin resistance, and the risk of hyperinsulinemia. Magnesium deficiency also affects the antioxidant system and lipid metabolism, which leads to metabolic diseases.

The clinical and animal data suggest that magnesium also preserves adipocyte insulin sensitivity (Bo and Pisu, 2008). Diets rich in magnesium decrease diabetes risk and improve insulin sensitivity. One of the body parts most prone to oxidative damage is the retina of the eye. The reason behind this is that the retina has many polyunsaturated fatty acids situated in the outer membranes of photoreceptors, and polyunsaturated fatty acids can be oxidized easily (Evans and Henshaw, 2008). A study on age-related eye disease investigated a reduction in risk progression of age-related macular degeneration by about 25% after the supplementation of magnesium.

8.3.5 β-LIPOIC ACID

It is a naturally occurring powerful antioxidant. α-Lipoic acid possesses ROS scavenging activity. It causes the quenching of several radicals when in the oxidized state and acts as an ROS scavenger. Dihydrolipoic acid and α-lipoic acid work in redox with an electron-donating molecule and oxidized form. Together, they cause the regeneration of antioxidants like vitamin C, glutathione, and vitamin E. They are also responsible for the chelation of transition metals (Ashwlayan, 2018). Diabetes mellitus causes ischemic injury to the retina and thereby visual loss. α-Lipoic acid protects the retina from in vitro and in vivo ischemia-reperfusion injuries caused by diabetes mellitus. In clinical trials review of α-lipoic acid, there was a positive effect of α-lipoic acid against diabetic neuropathy treatment on disease progression and the existing acute symptoms (Ziegler et al., 1999).

8.3.6 SELENIUM

Selenium is an essential element. It has gained importance due to the identification of selenoenzymes, which have catalytic potential and clarification of events in selenoprotein biosynthesis (Flohé et al., 2000; Köhrl et al., 2000). The biological role of selenium was not known for a long time. The element gained importance when Keshan disease (endemic cardiomyopathy caused due to extreme selenium deficiency) was documented. Selenium deficiency could also lead to an increase in viral infections due to mutation induction in the DNA of the virus (Beck et al., 2001). In central Africa, selenium and iodine deficiency are responsible for myxoedematous cretinism (Dumont et al., 1994). Nowadays, selenium is considered as a powerful catalytic element that constitutes the active center of 20 eukaryotic proteins, with some having antioxidant properties.

8.3.6.1 ROLE OF SELENIUM IN INSULIN RESISTANCE

Selenium possesses antioxidant properties due to selenium-dependent glutathione peroxidases (Burk, 2002; Rayman, 2000). Moreover, in some experimental models, inorganic selenium, that is, selenate mimics insulin activity. Due to these reasons, selenium can prevent the development of diabetes (Mueller and Pallauf, 2006; Stapleton, 2000).

Few studies have proved that selenium can effectively reduce insulin resistance index and fasting insulin concentration (Alizadeh et al., 2012; Bahmani et al., 2016; Farrokhian et al., 2016). As described earlier, selenium possesses insulin-mimetic action and is an effective antioxidant. This is because insulin signaling and secretion relate to the cellular redox state of selenium (Mao and Teng, 2013; Steinbrenner, 2013).

According to Steinbrenner et al.'s study, Sepp1 acts as a selenium donor; thus, it protects islets of Langerhans by antioxidation. Sepp1 donates selenium to carry out selenoprotein function (e.g., Gpx), thereby protecting the cell membrane from oxidative damage. The selenium donor, Sepp1, is found in cells secreting glucagon, but there is dysregulation of Sepp1 expression in beta cells during elevated glucose concentration. The dysregulation leads to reduced antioxidant properties and causes endocrine dysfunction. Zou et al. observed that selenium treatment leads to a decrease in lipid peroxidation. The activity of essential antioxidants like GPx, catalase, and superoxide dismutase increased due to selenium supplementation. Pancreatic beta cells have less protection against antioxidants because of ROS concentration in insulin signal pathways. These pancreatic cells have higher expression of Sepp1 and lower expression of GPx selenoproteins. These studies indicate that the redox state of pancreatic beta cells is also regulated by selenium (Lei and Vatamaniuk, 2011; Steinbrenner, 2013).

However, in some cases, selenium can dysregulate the redox state (Labunskyy et al., 2011; Wang et al., 2014). Hydrogen peroxide is an essential enzyme for insulin signaling. In some cases, when antioxidant selenium-dependent enzymes are overexpressed, hydrogen peroxide is removed. This action of selenium on hydrogen peroxide results in the induction of dephosphorylation and inactivation of insulin signaling enzymes. The deactivation of insulin-signaling enzymes leads to a change in insulin action (Steinbrenner, 2013; Wang et al., 2014; Zhou et al., 2013).

8.3.7 VITAMIN E

Vitamin E refers to a structurally similar tocopherols and tocotrienols group found in nature, each of which has four homologs, and α -tocopherol is the most prevalent vitamin E in the food and plasma, as well as the most physiologically active form. Vitamin E may be found in vegetable oils, lipids, nuts, almonds, and sunflower seeds. According to the Food and Nutrition Board (FNB) of the Institute of Medicine of the National Academies (United States), the recommended daily amount of vitamin E for women and men over 14 years of age is 22.4 IU (15 mg of alpha-tocopherol) (Medicine, 1997).

Vitamin E is a lipid-soluble antioxidant. It minimizes oxidative stress and protects cell membranes from oxidative damage by scavenging ROS. Vitamin E's antioxidant properties make it a strong option for research into antioxidant benefits against chronic illnesses including diabetes, cancer, age-related cataracts, and, more recently, COVID-19 adjuvant treatment.

α-Tocopherol has also been demonstrated to inhibit protein kinase C thereby altering cell signaling and acting as ligands for the transcription factor peroxisome proliferator-activated receptor-γ. However, it has been shown that vitamin E's major function in vivo is as a scavenger of lipid peroxyl radicals, and that this function likely underlies vitamin E's effects on pathways of cell signaling (Pazdro and Burgess, 2010; Traber, 2007). Figure 8.2 describes the roles of vitamin E in diabetes mellitus.

8.3.7.1 ROLE OF VITAMIN E IN DIABETIC NEPHROPATHY

Diabetic nephropathy is supposed to be a major complication seen in diabetes patients. Diabetes is known to harm several organs and tissues, including the kidney, peripheral nerves, brain, eye, and pancreas. Few reports by Koya et al. (2003) and Obrosova et al. (2003), showed that antioxidants like α-lipoic acid and vitamin C, may help to avoid diabetic nephropathy. In animal studies, vitamin E administration was observed to decrease oxidative stress in diabetic rat glomeruli (Koya et al., 2003). Supplementation of vitamin E (1000 IU/kg diet) for four weeks following streptozotocin-induced diabetes led to a substantial decrease in oxidative stress when compared to diabetic rats on a control diet. Vitamin E appears to aid diabetic animals' renal function, according to Farvid et al. (2005).

8.3.7.2 ROLE OF VITAMIN E IN DIABETES RETINOPATHY

Diabetic retinopathy is the most prevalent diabetic consequence, and it impedes the vision of many diabetic patients (Negi and Vernon, 2003). Previous research has indicated that antioxidants can help to protect the retina in people with diabetes (Kowluru and Chan, 2007). Vitamin E is used to prevent or reduce the progression of retinal degeneration due to pericyte ghosts and acellular capillaries. Vitamin E has been shown to prevent the development of acellular capillaries in diabetes-induced mice when coupled with vitamin C (Kowluru et al., 2001).

However, many studies did not show any link between vitamin E intake and the retinopathy severity in diabetes when studied in humans (Mayer-Davis et al., 1998; Millen et al., 2004). As a result, at the levels found in these trials, vitamin E standing from food or supplementation is not sufficient to protect diabetic retinas from the severity of oxidative stress generated by the disease.

In experimental diabetes, vitamin E protects against macromolecule damage, particularly lipid peroxidation. Vitamin E also protects the pancreas,

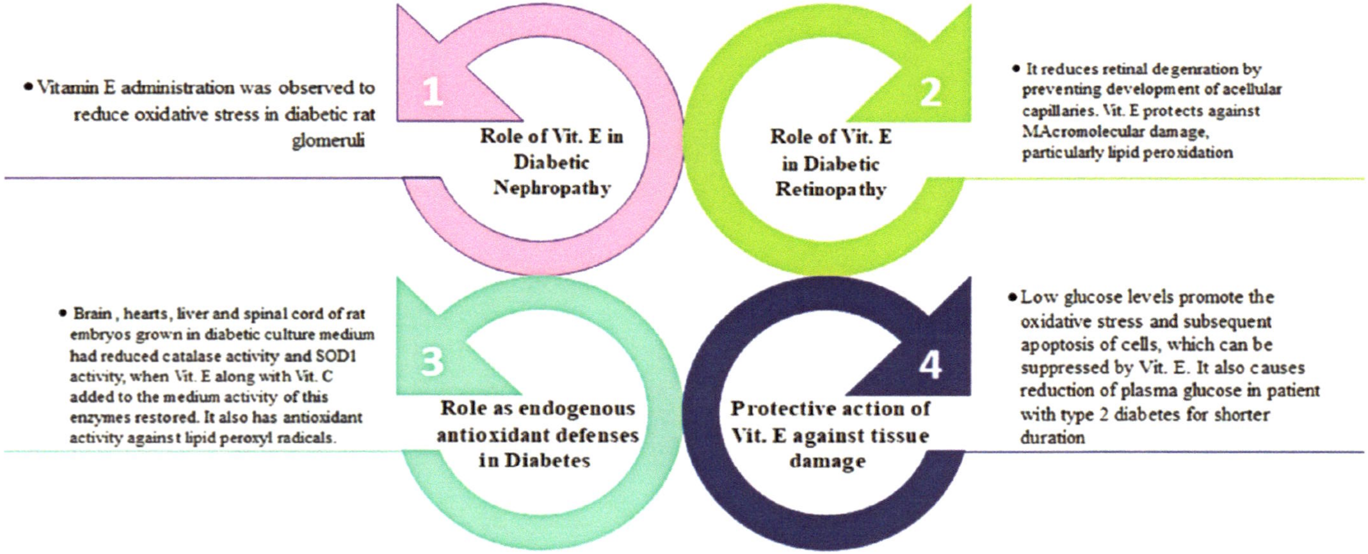

FIGURE 8.2 Role of vitamin E against diabetes mellitus.

kidneys, eyes, and nervous system in animals from diabetes consequences. Clinical evidence suggests that there is a possibility of vitamin E to protect diabetic humans from lipid peroxidation and also protein oxidation but to a lesser extent. Optimizing vitamin E supplementation through diet or dose as prescribed may help to reduce the progression of diabetes-related tissue damage, but further research is needed before definitive conclusions can be drawn (Pazdro and Burgess, 2010).

8.3.7.3 ROLE OF VITAMIN AS ENDOGENOUS ANTIOXIDANT DEFENSES IN DIABETES

Diabetes is a condition where maintaining the antioxidant defense system is of special relevance. The activity and transcription of antioxidant defense enzymes in diabetic patients have been studied in clinical investigations. For example, in a study by Chiarelli et al., supplementation of vitamin E for three months showed no change in enzyme activity in human fibroblasts, which were grown in either high or standard glucose conditions. However, similar studies by Gokkusu et al. (2001) reported that patients with type II diabetes mellitus showed an increase in activity of SOD1 and GPx.

Two preclinical studies in diabetic rats exhibited lower GSH, vitamin E, and GPx levels in the lens and kidney. Moreover, the study also showed a decrease in catalase and SOD1 activity when associated with the control rats (Kutlu et al., 2005; Sindhu et al., 2004). Insulin treatment or treatment with antioxidants seemed to normalize the trends from the above study.

The brain, hearts, liver, and spinal cord of rat embryos grown in diabetic culture medium had reduced catalase activity and SOD1 activity than those produced in control media (Zaken et al., 2001).

After adding vitamins E and C in the diabetic culture media, SOD1 and catalase activity were restored. Furthermore, it was discovered that a diet supplemented by vitamin E exhibited higher activity of SOD1 compared to a regular diet (Kinalski et al., 2000).

Overall, most information on vitamin E's effect on endogenous antioxidant defenses suggests that this nutrient can help normalize the dysregulation produced by diabetes. For lipid peroxyl radicals, vitamin E can operate as a scavenging antioxidant and preserve the integrity of the membrane and minimize damage due to high glucose levels, which is the cause of dysregulation of antioxidant defense.

8.3.7.4 PROTECTIVE ACTION OF VITAMIN E AGAINST TISSUE DAMAGE IN DIABETES

Type I diabetes is linked with progressive β-cells degeneration due to an autoimmune response. These events result in the depletion of β-cells, leading to type I diabetes (Robertson et al., 2003). However, chemically induced diabetes in animals showed the role of oxidative stress as one of the prime causes of diabetes, and after the administration of inducer, that is, streptozotocin, the antioxidants prevent or slow down the complications in the pancreas (Takatori et al., 2004). Type II diabetes is usually triggered due to insulin unresponsiveness to β-cells. In type II diabetes, functional β-cells are often retained for some time and start depleting over disease progression, leading to diminished insulin secretion (Ihara et al., 1999). This appears to be because of the induction of oxidative stress in the pancreas due to the disease state. Oxidative stress depletes insulin secretion through many mechanisms, including increased β-cells death and dysfunction in insulin transcriptional regulation through PDX-1 and MafA (Tanaka et al., 2002). Low glucose levels promote oxidative stress and subsequent apoptosis of cells, which can be suppressed by vitamin E (Cai et al., 2007). In addition, treatment with antioxidants like α-lipoic acid has increased insulin sensitivity in type II diabetes subjects. Several other studies with animal models also suggested the use of vitamin E along with other antioxidants as a promising option to exert pancreatic protective effects, as described in a review by Pazdro and Burgess, 2010. However, vitamin E supplementation resulted in reduction of plasma glucose in patients with type II diabetes for a shorter duration (Pazdro and Burgess, 2010).

8.3.8 FLAVONOL

Flavonols are found in grapes, berries, kale, lettuce, and onion. They have a structure of carbon ring with unsaturation at carbon 2-3, oxidizing at C4, and hydroxylated at C3.

8.3.8.1 KAEMPFEROL

Apples, beans, broccoli, tea, grapes, onions, kale, spinach, tomatoes, and potatoes are high in 3,4,5,7-tetrahydroxyflavone (Calderon-Montano et al., 2011), which is a nontoxic flavonoid. Kaempferol has anti-inflammatory, antioxidant, anti-microbial, and anticancer properties (Chen and Chen, 2013). Kaempferol extracts from a particular variety of leaves alleviate glycemia and increase absorption of glucose in the same way that insulin does (An et al., 2011, p. 2). In vitro experiments have shown that treating cells with 10M kaempferol inhibits apoptosis and increases cell viability (Jorge et al., 2004). Kaempferol has several antidiabetic properties, including enhancing activation and expression of AMP-activated cellular protein, regulation of caspase-3 activities which lowers cellular death, and increased synthesis and insulin secretion from cells (Zhang et al., 2011). Furthermore, it promotes the absorption of glucose by activating protein kinase C and some PI3K pathways, as well as the production of new glucose transporters (Zanatta et al., 2008). Oral kaempferol treatment raised fasting blood glucose levels, reduced HbA1c levels in serum, and increased insulin resistance. Kaempferol also modulated the AMPK activation thereby inhibiting the PPAR genetic expression (Sharma et al., 2019). Furthermore, the flavonoid alleviated diabetes mellitus in STZ-induced mice in two ways. Firstly, it promotes glucose metabolism of skeletal muscle and secondly by hindering gluconeogenesis in the liver (Alkhalidy et al., 2018). In another work, kaempferol suppressed Rho A/ Rhokinase-mediated pro-inflammatory signaling in RPTEC and NRK-52E cells, reducing diabetic nephropathy (Sharma et al., 2019).

8.3.9 FLAVANONES

Flavanones are also called di-hydroflavones. These compounds possess a saturated oxidized carbon ring. Citrus fruits contain flavanones; hence are known for antioxidant properties and free radical scavenging (Panche et al., 2016).

8.3.9.1 HESPERIDIN

It is a 5,7,3'-trihydroxy-4'-methoxyflavanone. Hesperidin is prevalent in fruits like lemons, cherries, and tomatoes (Parhiz et al., 2015). Hesperidin and glycoside of hesperidin have antioxidant, vascular, neuroprotective, anti-allergic, anti-inflammatory, and anticarcinogenic activity (Visnagri et al., 2014). Moreover, after including supplementation of hesperidin in the diet of db/db C56BL6 mice, it was found to assist in regulating the glycolytic liver enzyme activity and gluconeogenesis, and improve hyperglycemia (Jung et al., 2004). The study showed that hesperidin was effective in the animals used as it boosted fecal excretion of triglyceride and blocked enzymes that metabolize fats which improved lipid metabolism. Upregulating PPAR.

and translocation of GLUT, the flavanone efficiently reduced levels of blood glucose (Agrawal et al., 2014). In diabetic rats induced with STZ, G6Pase was reduced due to hesperidin administration, which had an effect on glucose transporter membrane protein resulting in reduction in export of glucose (Akiyama et al., 2009). Administration of hesperidin at a dose of 10 g/kg meal lowers glucose levels due to modification in enzymes that regulate glucose (Akiyama et al., 2009). Hesperidin and hesperetin, when taken jointly, have diverse consequences on glucose metabolism, lipid metabolism, and lower cholesterol levels (Vinayagam and Xu, 2015). In a study, hesperidin showed positive control on Klotho/FGF-23 pathway in STZ-induced DM rats thereby preventing and treating damage to the kidney and liver because of diabetes (Dokumacioglu et al., 2019).

8.3.9.2 NARINGENIN

Naringenin is profusely present in fruits like tomatoes, grapefruits, and oranges. These are saturated oxidized aglycone (5,7,4'-Trihydroxyflavanone) (Hasanein and Fazeli, 2014). It contains various properties, including antidiabetic, anti-inflammatory, anticancer, antimutagenic properties, and most importantly antioxidant activity (Hasanein and Fazeli, 2014). The antidiabetic and anti-obesity properties of naringenin and glycoside of naringenin have been reported (Zygmunt et al., 2010). Naringenin replicates the impact of insulin by lowering its secretion in liver cells, according to in vitro research (van Acker et al., 2000). This flavonoid (25 mg/kg) inhibited alpha-glucosidase activity in diabetic rats, delaying carbohydrate absorption and lowering postprandial levels of blood glucose (Priscilla et al., 2014). This flavanone causes upregulation of GLUT4 in type II diabetes and also regulates the hepatic enzyme expression that are part of glycolysis and gluconeogenesis (Pu et al., 2012; Singh et al., 2018). Naringenin was discovered to limit glucose uptake in an everted rat intestinal sleeve by blocking the co-transporter of sodium-glucose in the gut (Li et al., 2006). In diabetic rat models, the injection of naringenin has a variety of effects: The flavonoid reduced plasma glucose levels in STZ-induced diabetic rats; it increased insulin sensitivity in fructose-fed insulin resistance rats; and it helped reduce insulin resistance in H.F.D. mice (Choi et al., 1991; Kannappan and Anuradha, 2010; Mulvihill et al., 2009). Diabetic rats were treated for 45 days with 25 mg/kg of Naringenin. The results showed a decrease in peroxidation of the lipid membrane, hyperinsulinemia, improvement in hepatic indicators, hyperglycemia, corrected lipid profile abnormalities, and increased antioxidant activity. Antioxidant and anti-apoptotic activities characterized the desired effects of naringenin in diabetes-induced rats, indicating that naringenin can prevent diabetic retinopathy as well as neurodegeneration caused by diabetes (Al-Dosari et al., 2017).

8.3.10 FLAVONES

When compared to flavonols, flavones (Annadurai et al., 2012) lack hydroxylation at carbon three and have a ketone group at carbon 4 and an unsaturated carbon ring at Carbon 2–3. Flowers, leaves, and fruits are all known to manufacture them (Panche et al., 2016).

8.3.10.1 APIGENIN

The phytoestrogen glycogen 5,7,4'-trihydroxyflavone is predominantly present in almonds, oregano, chamomile, spinach, garlic, vine, oranges, and tea (Panda and Kar, 2007). The oral dose of apigenin for 10 days in diabetic rats resulted in the decrease of hepatic antioxidants like superoxide dismutase, glutathione, and catalase. Apigenin theory results in reduction in glucose 6-phosphatase activity and also lowers the serum cholesterol and hyperglycemia (Rauter et al., 2010). In STZ-induced rats, apigenin showed considerable action against hyperglycemia when administered with a dose of 4 mg/kg (Kim et al., 2007). The therapy of this flavone inhibited NF-B activation, which prevented induced apoptosis (Zang et al., 2006). Apigenin's impact is 200 times stronger than metformin. Apigenin therapy increased GLUT4 translocation, implying that it has a blood glucose-lowering impact (Hossain et al., 2014). There is an increase in AMPK phosphorylation in hepatocytes due to apigenin. Apigenin injection has many advantages including reduction in ROS generation, lipid peroxidation, cellular DNA damage and protein carboxylation, and reversed cell apoptosis in STZ-induced rats which improved oxidative damage to the pancreatic cells and apigenin even inhibited TGF-1-MAPK-fibronectin and MAPK-NF-B-TNF signaling in diabetic nephropathy by caused by diabetes (Malik et al., 2017; Wang et al., 2017).

8.3.10.2 WOGONIN

It is a flavonoid with structure of 5,7-dihydroxy-8-methoxy flavone. Wogonin is derived from Scutellaria baicalensis roots (Huynh et al., 2017). Similar to other nutraceuticals, wogonin has anti-inflammatory, neuroprotective, antibacterial, antiviral, and antioxidant properties (Tai et al., 2005). This flavonoid triggers PPAR and AMPK thereby impacting insulin sensitivity, lipid metabolism, and blood glucose (Bak et al., 2014). Vascular inflammation caused due to high glucose induction was reduced by pretreatment of Wogonin (Ku and Bae, 2015). The anti-inflammatory and anti-oxidative activity of Wogonin were reported to reduce diabetic cardiomyopathy in preclinical research (Khan et al., 2016).

8.3.11 ANTHOCYANINS

Figure 8.3 briefly describes the anthocyanins used in diabetes mellitus.

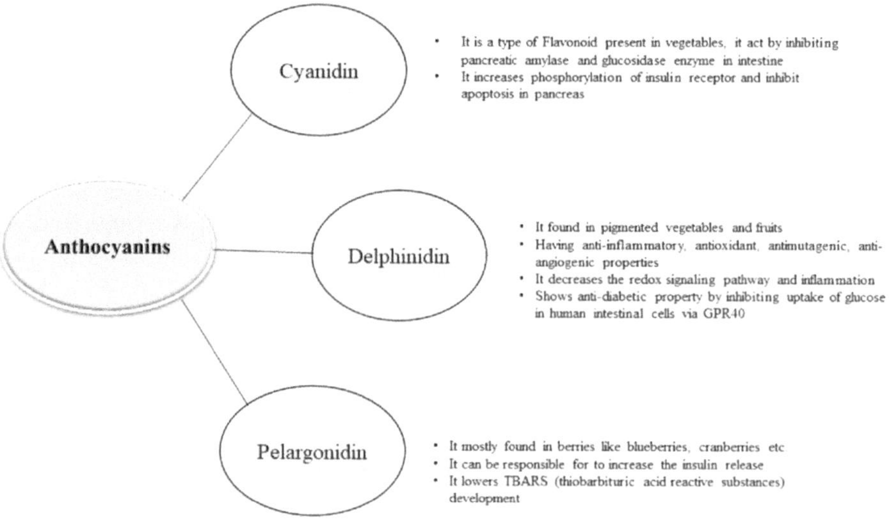

FIGURE 8.3 Anthocyanins used in the treatment of diabetes.

8.3.11.1 CYANIDIN

It is a type of flavonoid and is present in vegetables, plant-based diets, and crops (Akkarachiyasit et al., 2010). Cyanidin has a antidiabetic action as it inhibits the pancreatic amylase and glucosidase enzymes in the intestine (Nizamutdinova et al., 2009). This flavonoid can increase phosphorylation of insulin receptors and inhibit apoptosis in the pancreas according to a study carried out in STZ-induced diabetic rats (Nasri et al., 2011). C3G, a common anthocyanidin in diet, protects hepatocytes from being damaged by oxidative stress and also enhances the antioxidant effect (Zhu et al., 2012).

8.3.11.2 DELPHINIDIN

Delphinidin, an anthocyanin present in pigmented vegetables and fruits, sweet potatoes, tomato, red onion, berries, grapes, red cabbage, carrots, and eggplant (Ko et al., 2015). Anti-inflammatory, antioxidant, antimutagenic, and anti-angiogenic properties are all present in it (Lim and Song, 2017). Delphinidin was found to attenuate damage of endothelial cells caused due to diabetes (Bertuglia et al., 1995). Diabetes-induced mice were administered delphinidin with a dose of 100 mg per kg and showed reduced glycation of HbA1c and albumin rate (Gharib et al., 2013). There was increased insulin resistance in high-fat-fed mice because cyanidin and delphinidin decreased the redox signaling pathway and inflammation (Daveri et al., 2018). Delphinidin's antidiabetic action is owed to its ability to inhibit glucose uptake in human intestinal cells via GPR40 (Hidalgo et al., 2017).

8.3.11.3 PELARGONIDIN

Pelargonidin is a flavonoid found in blueberries, cranberries, and raspberries (Mazza, 2005). Pelargonidin therapy helps lower oxidative stress and hyperglycemia (Roy et al., 2008). This type of anthocyanin lowers TBARS development (Nasri et al., 2011). Pelargonidin-3-galactoside and pelargonidin were responsible for increasing insulin released in one in vitro research (Jayaprakasam et al., 2005).

8.3.12 RESVERATROL

Resveratrol is a naturally occurring component in many plants like berries (blueberries and cranberries), peanuts, Japanese knotweed, and grapes. It belongs to a non-flavonoid group of polyphenols. Resveratrol is one of the major constituents of grape skin, with a concentration of 50–100 μg per gram, while its concentration in red wine is around 0.1–14 mg/L (Mark et al., 2005; Pervaiz, 2003). Plants produce it in reaction to injury or fungal attack. Resveratrol has been shown to have anti-inflammatory activity as it counteracts effects induced by TNF alpha. Resveratrol is also known to decline mRNA expression and secrete plasminogen activator inhibitor-1(PAI1), IL-1, IL-6, IL-8, and MCP-1. The function of beta cells is also increased as resveratrol inhibits phosphodiesterase (PDE) activity. By reducing PDE activity, resveratrol improves pancreatic cell function. It also prevents beta-cell malfunction. In T2DM, cAMP is responsible for the production of insulin (incretin-stimulated) and glucose.

The enzyme PDE can degrade cAMP. Therefore, regulating the activity of P.D.E. is important. Resveratrol acts as inhibitor of PDE but are still investigated for its PDE inhibitor activity in beta cells. Using these polyphenols in beta-cell lines and human islets increased intracellular cAMP levels. Resveratrol is a direct PDE inhibitor that reduces PDE activity in pancreatic beta-cells. In one of the studies, PDE expression significantly reduced human and mice cells that were treated with curcumin and resveratrol, notably PDE10A, PDE3B, and PDE8A which are involved in the signaling of insulin (Rouse et al., 2014). In addition, resveratrol and curcumin therapy inhibited PDE activity in pancreatic cells in a significant way. Because PDE inhibition hindered cAMP breakdown, resveratrol and curcumin therapy led to an increase in intracellular cAMP levels. As a result, there was activation of signaling pathways and increased beta cell function and insulin secretion (Rouse et al., 2014). Resveratrol is also responsible for increased fatty acid oxidation and mobilization, increased apoptosis, and lipolysis. It also accounts for decreased adipogenesis and lipogenesis.

8.3.13 VITAMIN D FOR DIABETES MELLITUS

8.3.13.1 VITAMIN D'S IMPACT ON GLYCEMIC CONTROL

Anti-inflammatory effects of vitamin D are present. The production of cytokines is decreased by vitamin D, which aids in minimizing chronic inflammation (Christakos and Liu, 2004). Vitamin D enhances insulin action through the human insulin receptor gene expression and thus enhance the production of the insulin receptor. Insulin receptor protein is found in many cells' outer membranes and connects to circulating insulin in the blood (*Stimulation by 1, 25-dihydroxy vitamin* D_3 *of Insulin Receptor Expression and Insulin Responsiveness for Glucose Transport in U-937 Human Promonocytic Cells*, n.d.). The presence and connection helps in the transcription of the human insulin gene resulting in insulin hormone production (Dunlop et al., 2005). Additionally, vitamin D affects fatty acid oxidation by raising the expression of the peroxisome proliferator-activated receptor delta (PPAR-δ) gene (Dunlop et al., 2005).

Two of the many complicated processes that regulate insulin production are calcium influx and calcium outflux. Furthermore, vitamin D has the primary calcium regulator activity which indirectly influences secretion of insulin. Vitamin D receptors are found on beta cells of the pancreas, which enhance vitamin D action as per the glucose levels, causing insulin secretion (*Immunohistochemical Localization of the 1,25(O.H.)2D3 Receptor and Calbindin D28k in Human and Rat Pancreas | American Journal of Physiology-Endocrinology and Metabolism*, n.d.). The ability of the 1-alpha hydroxylase enzyme to activate vitamin D is highlighted by its presence in pancreatic B cells (*Immunohistochemical Localization of the 1,25(O.H.)2D3 Receptor and Calbindin D28k in Human and Rat Pancreas | American Journal of Physiology-Endocrinology and Metabolism*, n.d.). Vitamin D's active form, calcitriol, speeds up proinsulin conversion to insulin. Vitamin D receptors are thought to take part in the homeostasis of glucose in skeletal muscle tissue. Hyperglycemia causes non-enzymatic glycosylation of hemoglobin, which is known as hemoglobin A1c (HbA1c). It is hard to determine glycemic control if it is affected by short-term medications against diabetes mellitus. Seven hundred forty-seven diabetic patients with the therapy of vitamin D were compared to 627 patients taking a placebo in a randomized clinical trial post-meta-analysis study (Hu et al., 2019), which concluded that the short-term vitamin D treatment was observed to be effective in preventing an increase in HbA1c (Hu et al., 2019).

Another randomized control trial was conducted by Khan et al. (2018) compared patients with type II diabetes mellitus. Patients taking metformin and oral vitamin D formed one group compared with patients prescribed only metformin (Khan et al., 2018). The results showed that patients administering metformin with vitamin D showed a greater reduction than the other group after 3 months. The scientists discovered that taking vitamin D supplements reduces insulin resistance after studying the meta-analysis. In the same way, insulin secretion was improved (Hu et al., 2019). Vitamin D triggers L-type calcium channels in β cells in islets of Langerhans, which are accountable for insulin release (*A Highly Energetic Process Couples Calcium Influx through L-Type Calcium Channels to Insulin Secretion in Pancreatic β-Cells | American Journal of Physiology-Endocrinology and Metabolism*, n.d.). The peroxisome proliferator-activated receptor delta (PPAR) gene regulates fatty acid metabolism and plays a role in insulin resistance; thus, vitamin D therapy reduces insulin resistance (*Stimulation by 1, 25-Dihydroxyvitamin* D_3 *of Insulin Receptor Expression and Insulin Responsiveness for Glucose Transport in U-937 Human Promonocytic*

Cells, n.d., p. 3). The levels of glucose and insulin in the body can both be used to identify insulin resistance.

Vitamin D supplement effects varies depending on ethnicity. Because of a binding protein variation of this vitamin, Middle Eastern participants got better results than Asians (Li et al., 2018). People who get less sun exposure because they wear a particular type of clothes are more likely to have insufficient vitamins, and when given vitamin D supplements, they have a better response. The problem was not just that they lacked vitamin D; antidiabetic medication and food control were also responsible for the results.

8.3.13.2 EFFECT OF VITAMIN D ON DIABETIC PERIPHERAL NEUROPATHY

This is a frequent nerve condition caused by diabetes that significantly impacts the quality of life of patients. It might range from minor neuropathy to excruciating agony. It is the most common reason for a diabetic foot that can lead to amputation of limbs. Several studies have discovered a reverse link between the level of vitamin D and the nerve condition and the fact that levels of vitamin D in normal individuals are higher than the patients with diabetic peripheral neuropathy (Shillo et al., 2019). Clinical experiments that looked at this vitamin as a potent analgesic found that administration of a high intramuscular dose of vitamin D resulted in relieving discomfort.

Furthermore, oral supplementation of vitamin D increases nerve function and aids wound healing in diabetic foot ulcers and ulcers (Shehab et al., 2015). Vitamin D protects neurons by regulating neurotrophin levels (proteins that promote neuron survival, growth, and function) and calcium homeostasis in neurons (Garcion et al., 2002).

A trial of 67 patients with diabetic peripheral neuropathy who received 40,000 IU of vitamin D weekly found improvement in symptoms, as well as a drop in interleukin-6 (IL-6) and an increase in interleukin-10 (IL-10) (Karonova et al., 2020). Another study indicated that supplementing with vitamin D reduces pain associated with the reduction of semi-synthetic opioids.

With a rise of 1 ng/mL of 25-hydroxy vitamin D [25(O.H.)-D], there is an increase in the frequency of nerve conduction by 2.2% (Alamdari et al., 2015). Higher levels of IL-6 and TNF-alpha, as well as lower IL-10 levels, are linked to an increase in HbA1c (Colotta et al., 2017). Vitamin D has also been shown to reduce IL-6 and TNF-alpha and increase IL-10 (Colotta et al., 2017). Patients taking high doses of this had a substantial benefit (Colotta et al., 2017).

8.3.13.3 VITAMIN D'S EFFECT ON DIABETIC NEPHROPATHY

Despite the use of therapeutic medicines, chronic kidney disease (CKD) is increasing with diabetes duration (*Diabetes and CKD in the United States Population, 2009–2014 | American Society of Nephrology*, n.d.). When an active form of Vitamin D3 is administered with a short-term dose, it reduces urine albumin excretion significantly compared to placebo in a meta-analysis; however, long-term treatment did not affect GFR (Borst et al., 2013). Vitamin D is thought to protect the kidneys when taken in high doses. In one randomized control trial with diabetic nephropathy patients, there was a reduction in urine albumin levels with enough vitamin D3 administration (Joergensen et al., 2015). Li et al. discovered that vitamin D's active form inhibits the renin-angiotensin system (RAS) by suppressing the release of renin. Vitamin D supplementation can assist in avoiding hypertension.

8.3.13.4 VITAMIN D'S EFFECT ON DIABETIC RETINOPATHY

Oxidative stress in the retina is responsible for diabetic retinopathy. This happens when the retina is subjected to an elevated amount of polyunsaturated fatty acids, glucose oxidation, and an increase in oxygen uptake (Anderson et al., 1984). Oxidative stress is a condition when antioxidants and free radicals are out of balance, causing tissue damage. In both direct and indirect ways, hyperglycemia induces oxidative stress. Auto-oxidation during glucose metabolism causes a direct impact (*The Pathobiology of Diabetic Complications | Diabetes | American Diabetes Association*, n.d.). The secondary effect is caused by advanced glycation end-products (AGEs). AGEs wreak havoc on retinal blood vessels, stiffening them and reducing their flexibility. Nitric oxide (NO) synthase is activated by AGEs, and diacylglycerol triggers NADPH oxidase and protein kinase C thereby producing ROS (Zhang et al., 2017). In diabetic retinopathy, the inactivation of SOD and catalase enzymes play an important role (King et al., 1998).

SOD, glutathione peroxidase (GPx), and glutathione reductase (GR) are some of the antioxidant enzymes that are involved in ROS detoxification that vitamin D can boost (Alvarez et al., 2014). Both reduced glutathione and GR are produced due to this. It also promotes the activity of (SOD-2) superoxide dismutase 2, which is vitamin D's important mechanism for protection against oxidative stress. When the levels of vitamin D increase,

GPx, and GR activity decreases while it is the opposite in SOD activity. An increase in the vitamin D level increases the activity of SOD in diabetes mellitus. Vitamin D acts as an immunomodulator as it limits translocation of nuclear factor kappa B, which reduces apoptosis and inflammatory reactions (Alvarez et al., 2014). Respiratory activity and integrity of mitochondria against oxidative stress are also regulated by vitamin D. As a result, diabetic retinopathy progression can be slowed down with the administration of vitamin D. The available research still does not guarantee the activity of vitamin D in diabetic retinopathy yet.

8.4 CONCLUSION

Nutraceuticals are abundantly found in natural products like vegetables and fruits and therefore possess nil or minimum toxicity. Administering nutraceutical antioxidants can prevent and even control diabetes as discussed in the chapter. All the nutraceutical antioxidants have their specific actions against oxidative stress in diabetes. The dose regimen is yet to be discovered for many nutraceuticals. Few conditions that arise due to diabetes like diabetic retinopathy, diabetic nephropathy, tissue damage, etc., can be controlled by some of the nutraceutical antioxidants. Vitamins E and D play an important role in diabetic nephropathy and retinopathy. Nevertheless, the need for determining the importance of nutraceuticals in the treatment of diabetes mellitus is urgent and significant.

KEYWORDS

- **kaempferol**
- **naringenin**
- **delphinidin**
- **nutraceutical**
- **antioxidants**
- **hyperglycemia**
- **diabetes mellitus**

REFERENCES

Agrawal, Y. O.; Sharma, P. K.; Shrivastava, B.; Ojha, S.; Upadhya, H. M.; Arya, D. S.; Goyal, S. N. Hesperidin Produces Cardioprotective Activity via PPAR-γ Pathway in Ischemic Heart Disease Model in Diabetic Rats. *PloS One* **2014,** *9* (11), e111212. https://doi.org/10.1371/journal.pone.0111212.

Akiyama, S.; Katsumata, S.; Suzuki, K.; Nakaya, Y.; Ishimi, Y.; Uehara, M. Hypoglycemic and Hypolipidemic Effects of Hesperidin and Cyclodextrin-Clathrated Hesperetin in Goto-Kakizaki Rats with Type 2 Diabetes. *Biosci. Biotechnol. Biochem.* **2009,** *73* (12), 2779–2782. https://doi.org/10.1271/bbb.90576.

Akkarachiyasit, S.; Charoenlertkul, P.; Yibchok-anun, S.; Adisakwattana, S. Inhibitory Activities of Cyanidin and Its Glycosides and Synergistic Effect with Acarbose against Intestinal α-Glucosidase and Pancreatic α-Amylase. *Int. J. Mol. Sci.* **2010,** *11* (9), 3387–3396. https://doi.org/10.3390/ijms11093387.

Alam, U.; Asghar, O.; Azmi, S.; Malik, R. A. Chapter 15 - General Aspects of Diabetes Mellitus. In *Handbook of Clinical Neurology*; Zochodne, D. W., Malik, R. A., Eds.; Diabetes and the Nervous System; Elsevier, 2014; vol 126, pp 211–222. https://doi.org/10.1016/B978-0-444-53480-4.00015-1.

Alamdari, A.; Mozafari, R.; Tafakhori, A.; Faghihi-Kashani, S.; Hafezi-Nejad, N.; Sheikhbahaei, S.; Naderi, N.; Ebadi, M.; Esteghamati, A. An Inverse Association between Serum Vitamin D Levels with the Presence and Severity of Impaired Nerve Conduction Velocity and Large Fiber Peripheral Neuropathy in Diabetic Subjects. *Neurol. Sci.* **2015,** *36* (7), 1121–1126. https://doi.org/10.1007/s10072-015-2207-0.

Al-Dosari, D. I.; Ahmed, M. M.; Al-Rejaie, S. S.; Alhomida, A. S.; Ola, M. S. Flavonoid Naringenin Attenuates Oxidative Stress, Apoptosis and Improves Neurotrophic Effects in the Diabetic Rat Retina. *Nutrients* **2017,** *9* (10), 1161. https://doi.org/10.3390/nu9101161.

Alizadeh, M.; Safaeiyan, A.; Ostadrahimi, A.; Estakhri, R.; Daneghian, S.; Ghaffari, A.; Gargari, B. P. Effect of L-Arginine and Selenium Added to a Hypocaloric Diet Enriched with Legumes on Cardiovascular Disease Risk Factors in Women with Central Obesity: A Randomized, Double-Blind, Placebo-Controlled Trial. *Ann. Nutr. Metab.* **2012,** *60* (2), 157–168. https://doi.org/10.1159/000335470.

Alkhalidy, H.; Moore, W.; Wang, Y.; Luo, J.; McMillan, R. P.; Zhen, W.; Zhou, K.; Liu, D. The Flavonoid Kaempferol Ameliorates Streptozotocin-Induced Diabetes by Suppressing Hepatic Glucose Production. *Molecules* **2018,** *23* (9), 2338. https://doi.org/10.3390/molecules23092338.

Althuis, M. D.; Jordan, N. E.; Ludington, E. A.; Wittes, J. T. Glucose and Insulin Responses to Dietary Chromium Supplements: A Meta-Analysis. *Am. J. Clin. Nutr.* **2002,** *76* (1), 148–155. https://doi.org/10.1093/ajcn/76.1.148.

Alvarez, J. A.; Chowdhury, R.; Jones, D. P.; Martin, G. S.; Brigham, K. L.; Binongo, J. N.; Ziegler, T. R.; Tangpricha, V. Vitamin D Status Is Independently Associated with Plasma Glutathione and Cysteine Thiol/Disulphide Redox Status in Adults. *Clin. Endocrinol. (Oxf.)* **2014,** *81* (3), 458–466. https://doi.org/10.1111/cen.12449.

American Diabetes Association. Nutrition Recommendations and Interventions for Diabetes: A Position Statement of the American Diabetes Association. *Diabetes Care* **2007,** *30* Suppl 1, S48–S65. https://doi.org/10.2337/dc07-S048.

An, G.; Gallegos, J.; Morris, M. E. The Bioflavonoid Kaempferol Is an Abcg2 Substrate and Inhibits Abcg2-Mediated Quercetin Efflux. *Drug Metab. Dispos. Biol. Fate Chem.* **2011,** *39* (3), 426–432. https://doi.org/10.1124/dmd.110.035212.

Anderson, R. E.; Rapp, L. M.; Wiegand, R. D. Lipid Peroxidation and Retinal Degeneration. *Curr. Eye Res.* **1984,** *3* (1), 223–227. https://doi.org/10.3109/02713688408997203.

Annadurai, T.; Muralidharan, A. R.; Joseph, T.; Hsu, M. J.; Thomas, P. A.; Geraldine, P. Antihyperglycemic and Antioxidant Effects of a Flavanone, Naringenin, in Streptozotocin–Nicotinamide-Induced Experimental Diabetic Rats. *J. Physiol. Biochem.* **2012,** *68* (3), 307–318. https://doi.org/10.1007/s13105-011-0142-y.

Bahmani, F.; Kia, M.; Soleimani, A.; Asemi, Z.; Esmaillzadeh, A. Effect of Selenium Supplementation on Glycemic Control and Lipid Profiles in Patients with Diabetic Nephropathy. *Biol. Trace Elem. Res.* **2016,** *172* (2), 282–289. https://doi.org/10.1007/s12011-015-0600-4.

Bak, E. J.; Kim, J.; Choi, Y. H.; Kim, J. H.; Lee, D. E.; Woo, G. H.; Cha, J. H.; Yoo, Y. J. Wogonin Ameliorates Hyperglycemia and Dyslipidemia via PPARα Activation in Db/Db Mice. *Clin. Nutr.* **2014,** *33* (1), 156–163. https://doi.org/10.1016/j.clnu.2013.03.013.

Balamurugan, A. N.; Akhov, L.; Selvaraj, G.; Pugazhenthi, S. Induction of Antioxidant Enzymes by Curcumin and Its Analogues in Human Islets: Implications in Transplantation. *Pancreas* **2009,** *38* (4), 454–460. https://doi.org/10.1097/MPA.0b013e318196c3e7.

Balasubramanyam, M.; Koteswari, A. A.; Kumar, R. S.; Monickaraj, S. F.; Maheswari, J. U.; Mohan, V. Curcumin-Induced Inhibition of Cellular Reactive Oxygen Species Generation: Novel Therapeutic Implications. *J. Biosci.* **2003,** *28* (6), 715–721. https://doi.org/10.1007/BF02708432.

Beck, M. A.; Nelson, H. K.; Shi, Q.; Van Dael, P.; Schiffrin, E. J.; Blum, S.; Barclay, D.; Levander, O. A. Selenium Deficiency Increases the Pathology of an Influenza Virus Infection. *F.A.S.E.B. J. Off. Publ. Fed. Am. Soc. Exp. Biol.* **2001,** *15* (8), 1481–1483.

Bertuglia, S.; Malandrino, S.; Colantuoni, A. Effects of the Natural Flavonoid Delphinidin on Diabetic Microangiopathy. *Arzneimittelforschung* **1995,** *45* (4), 481–485.

Bo, S.; Pisu, E. Role of Dietary Magnesium in Cardiovascular Disease Prevention, Insulin Sensitivity and Diabetes. *Curr. Opin. Lipidol.* **2008,** *19* (1), 50–56. https://doi.org/10.1097/MOL.0b013e3282f33ccc.

Borst, M. H. de; Hajhosseiny, R.; Tamez, H.; Wenger, J.; Thadhani, R.; Goldsmith, D. J. A. Active Vitamin D Treatment for Reduction of Residual Proteinuria: A Systematic Review. *J. Am. Soc. Nephrol.* **2013,** *24* (11), 1863–1871. https://doi.org/10.1681/ASN.2013030203.

Burk, R. F. Selenium, an Antioxidant Nutrient. *Nutr. Clin. Care Off. Publ. Tufts Univ.* **2002,** *5* (2), 75–79. https://doi.org/10.1046/j.1523-5408.2002.00006.x.

Cai, Y.; Martens, G. A.; Hinke, S. A.; Heimberg, H.; Pipeleers, D.; Van de Casteele, M. Increased Oxygen Radical Formation and Mitochondrial Dysfunction Mediate Beta Cell Apoptosis under Conditions of AMP-Activated Protein Kinase Stimulation. *Free Radic. Biol. Med.* **2007,** *42* (1), 64–78. https://doi.org/10.1016/j.freeradbiomed.2006.09.018.

Calderon-Montano, J. M.; Burgos-Moron, E.; Perez-Guerrero, C.; Lopez-Lazaro, M. A Review on the Dietary Flavonoid Kaempferol. *Mini-Rev. Med. Chem.* **2011,** *11* (4), 298–344.

Capdor, J.; Foster, M.; Petocz, P.; Samman, S. Zinc and Glycemic Control: A Meta-Analysis of Randomised Placebo Controlled Supplementation Trials in Humans. *J. Trace Elem. Med. Biol. Organ Soc. Miner. Trace Elem. GMS* **2013,** *27* (2), 137–142. https://doi.org/10.1016/j.jtemb.2012.08.001.

Chan, W. H.; Wu, H. J.; Hsuuw, Y. D. Curcumin Inhibits R.O.S. Formation and Apoptosis in Methylglyoxal-Treated Human Hepatoma G2 Cells. *Ann. N. Y. Acad. Sci.* **2005,** *1042* (1), 372–378. https://doi.org/10.1196/annals.1338.057.

Chausmer, A. B. Zinc, Insulin and Diabetes. *J. Am. Coll. Nutr.* **1998,** *17* (2), 109–115. https://doi.org/10.1080/07315724.1998.10718735.

Chen, A. Y.; Chen, Y. C. A Review of the Dietary Flavonoid, Kaempferol on Human Health and Cancer Chemoprevention. *Food Chem.* **2013,** *138* (4), 2099–2107. https://doi.org/10.1016/j.foodchem.2012.11.139.

Choi, J. S.; Yokozawa, T.; Oura, H. Improvement of Hyperglycemia and Hyperlipemia in Streptozotocin-Diabetic Rats by a Methanolic Extract of Prunus Davidiana Stems and Its Main Component, Prunin. *Planta Med.* **1991,** *57* (03), 208–211. https://doi.org/10.1055/s-2006-960075.

Christakos, S.; Liu, Y. Biological Actions and Mechanism of Action of Calbindin in the Process of Apoptosis. *J. Steroid Biochem. Mol. Biol.* **2004,** *89–90*, 401–404. https://doi.org/10.1016/j.jsbmb.2004.03.007.

Colotta, F.; Jansson, B.; Bonelli, F. Modulation of Inflammatory and Immune Responses by Vitamin D. *J. Autoimmun.* **2017,** *85*, 78–97. https://doi.org/10.1016/j.jaut.2017.07.007.

Daveri, E.; Cremonini, E.; Mastaloudis, A.; Hester, S. N.; Wood, S. M.; Waterhouse, A. L.; Anderson, M.; Fraga, C. G.; Oteiza, P. I. Cyanidin and Delphinidin Modulate Inflammation and Altered Redox Signaling Improving Insulin Resistance in High Fat-Fed Mice. *Redox Biol.* **2018,** *18*, 16–24. https://doi.org/10.1016/j.redox.2018.05.012.

Dokumacioglu, E.; Iskender, H.; Musmul, A. Effect of Hesperidin Treatment on α-Klotho/FGF-23 Pathway in Rats with Experimentally-Induced Diabetes. Biomed. *Biomed. Pharmacother.* **2019,** *109* (Suppl 1), 1206–1210. https://doi.org/10.1016/j.biopha.2018.10.192.

Dumont, J. E.; Corvilain, B.; Contempre, B. The Biochemistry of Endemic Cretinism: Roles of Iodine and Selenium Deficiency and Goitrogens. *Mol. Cell. Endocrinol.* **1994,** *100* (1–2), 163–166. https://doi.org/10.1016/0303-7207(94)90297-6.

Dunlop, T. W.; Väisänen, S.; Frank, C.; Molnár, F.; Sinkkonen, L.; Carlberg, C. The Human Peroxisome Proliferator-Activated Receptor δ Gene Is a Primary Target of 1α,25-Dihydroxyvitamin D3 and Its Nuclear Receptor. *J. Mol. Biol.* **2005,** *349* (2), 248–260. https://doi.org/10.1016/j.jmb.2005.03.060.

Evans, J. R.; Henshaw, K. Antioxidant Vitamin and Mineral Supplements for Preventing Age-Related Macular Degeneration. *Cochrane Database Syst. Rev.* **2008,** (1), CD000253. https://doi.org/10.1002/14651858.CD000253.pub2.

Farrokhian, A.; Bahmani, F.; Taghizadeh, M.; Mirhashemi, S. M.; Aarabi, M. H.; Raygan, F.; Aghadavod, E.; Asemi, Z. Selenium Supplementation Affects Insulin Resistance and Serum Hs-CRP in Patients with Type 2 Diabetes and Coronary Heart Disease. *Horm. Metab. Res.* **2016,** *48* (4), 263–268. https://doi.org/10.1055/s-0035-1569276.

Flohé, L.; Andreesen, J. R.; Brigelius-Flohé, R.; Maiorino, M.; Ursini, F. Selenium, the Element of the Moon, in Life on Earth. *IUBMB Life* **2000,** *49* (5), 411–420. https://doi.org/10.1080/152165400410263.

Garcion, E.; Wion-Barbot, N.; Montero-Menei, C. N.; Berger, F.; Wion, D. New Clues about Vitamin D Functions in the Nervous System. *Trends Endocrinol. Metab.* **2002,** *13* (3), 100–105. https://doi.org/10.1016/S1043-2760(01)00547-1.

Garg, V. K.; Gupta, R.; Goyal, R. K. Hypozincemia in Diabetes Mellitus. *J. Assoc. Physicians India* **1994,** *42* (9), 720–721.

Ghani, U.; Naeem, M.; Rafeeq, H.; Imtiaz, U.; Amjad, A.; Ullah, S.; Rehman, A.; Qasim, F. A Novel Approach towards Nutraceuticals and Biomedical Applications. *Sch. Int. J. Biochem.* **2019,** *02* (10), 245–252. https://doi.org/10.36348/SIJB.2019.v02i10.001.

Gharib, A.; Faezizadeh, Z.; Godarzee, M. Treatment of Diabetes in the Mouse Model by Delphinidin and Cyanidin Hydrochloride in Free and Liposomal Forms. *Planta Med.* **2013,** *79* (17), 1599–1604. https://doi.org/10.1055/s-0033-1350908.

Giménez-Mascarell, P.; Schirrmacher, C. E.; Martínez-Cruz, L. A.; Müller, D. Novel Aspects of Renal Magnesium Homeostasis. *Front. Pediatr.* **2018,** *6,* 77.

Gökkusu, C.; Palanduz, S.; Ademoğlu, E.; Tamer, S. Oxidant and Antioxidant Systems in Niddm Patients: Influence of Vitamin E Supplementation. *Endocr. Res.* **2001,** *27* (3), 377–386. https://doi.org/10.1081/erc-100106015.

Gröber, U.; Schmidt, J.; Kisters, K. Magnesium in Prevention and Therapy. *Nutrients* **2015,** *7* (9), 8199–8226. https://doi.org/10.3390/nu7095388.

Hasanein, P.; Fazeli, F. Role of Naringenin in Protection against Diabetic Hyperalgesia and Tactile Allodynia in Male Wistar Rats. *J. Physiol. Biochem.* **2014,** *70* (4), 997–1006. https://doi.org/10.1007/s13105-014-0369-5.

Hidalgo, J.; Teuber, S.; Morera, F. J.; Ojeda, C.; Flores, C. A.; Hidalgo, M. A.; Núñez, L.; Villalobos, C.; Burgos, R. A. Delphinidin Reduces Glucose Uptake in Mice Jejunal Tissue and Human Intestinal Cells Lines through FFA1/GPR40. *Int. J. Mol. Sci.* **2017,** *18* (4), 750. https://doi.org/10.3390/ijms18040750.

Hsuuw, Y. D.; Chang, C. K.; Chan, W. H.; Yu, J. S. Curcumin Prevents Methylglyoxal-Induced Oxidative Stress and Apoptosis in Mouse Embryonic Stem Cells and Blastocysts. *J. Cell. Physiol.* **2005,** *205* (3), 379–386. https://doi.org/10.1002/jcp.20408.

Hu, Z.; Chen, J.; Sun, X.; Wang, L.; Wang, A. Efficacy of Vitamin D Supplementation on Glycemic Control in Type 2 Diabetes Patients: A Meta-Analysis of Interventional Studies. *Medicine (Baltimore)* **2019,** *98* (14), e14970. https://doi.org/10.1097/MD.0000000000014970.

Huynh, D. L.; Sharma, N.; Kumar Singh, A.; Singh Sodhi, S.; Zhang, J.-J.; Mongre, R. K.; Ghosh, M.; Kim, N.; Ho Park, Y.; Kee Jeong, D. Anti-Tumor Activity of Wogonin, an Extract from Scutellaria Baicalensis, through Regulating Different Signaling Pathways. *Chin. J. Nat. Med.* **2017,** *15* (1), 15–40. https://doi.org/10.1016/S1875-5364(17)30005-5.

Ihara, Y.; Toyokuni, S.; Uchida, K.; Odaka, H.; Tanaka, T.; Ikeda, H.; Hiai, H.; Seino, Y.; Yamada, Y. Hyperglycemia Causes Oxidative Stress in Pancreatic Beta-Cells of G.K. Rats, a Model of Type 2 Diabetes. *Diabetes* **1999,** *48* (4), 927–932. https://doi.org/10.2337/diabetes.48.4.927.

Jayaprakasam, B.; Vareed, S. K.; Olson, L. K.; Nair, M. G. Insulin Secretion by Bioactive Anthocyanins and Anthocyanidins Present in Fruits. *J. Agric. Food Chem.* **2005,** *53* (1), 28–31. https://doi.org/10.1021/jf049018+.

Jena, S.; Ray, A.; Banerjee, A.; Sahoo, A.; Nasim, N.; Sahoo, S.; Kar, B.; Patnaik, J.; Panda, P. C.; Nayak, S. Chemical Composition and Antioxidant Activity of Essential Oil from Leaves and Rhizomes of Curcuma Angustifolia Roxb. *Nat. Prod. Res.* **2017,** *31* (18), 2188–2191. https://doi.org/10.1080/14786419.2017.1278600.

Joergensen, C.; Tarnow, L.; Goetze, J. P.; Rossing, P. Vitamin D Analogue Therapy, Cardiovascular Risk and Kidney Function in People with Type 1 Diabetes Mellitus and Diabetic Nephropathy: A Randomized *Trial. Diabet. Med.* **2015,** *32* (3), 374–381. https://doi.org/10.1111/dme.12606.

Jorge, A. P.; Horst, H.; de Sousa, E.; Pizzolatti, M. G.; Silva, F. R. M. B. Insulinomimetic Effects of Kaempferitrin on Glycaemia and on 14C-Glucose Uptake in Rat Soleus Muscle. *Chem. Biol. Interact.* **2004,** *149* (2–3), 89–96. https://doi.org/10.1016/j.cbi.2004.07.001.

Jung, U. J.; Lee, M.-K.; Jeong, K.-S.; Choi, M.-S. The Hypoglycemic Effects of Hesperidin and Naringin Are Partly Mediated by Hepatic Glucose-Regulating Enzymes in C57BL/KsJ-Db/Db Mice. *J. Nutr.* **2004,** *134* (10), 2499–2503. https://doi.org/10.1093/jn/134.10.2499.

Kalra, E. K. Nutraceutical-Definition and Introduction. *AAPS PharmSci* **2003,** *5* (3), 27–28. https://doi.org/10.1208/ps050325.

Kannappan, S.; Anuradha, C. V. Naringenin Enhances Insulin-Stimulated Tyrosine Phosphorylation and Improves the Cellular Actions of Insulin in a Dietary Model of Metabolic Syndrome. *Eur. J. Nutr.* **2010,** *49* (2), 101–109. https://doi.org/10.1007/s00394-009-0054-6.

Karonova, T.; Stepanova, A.; Bystrova, A.; Jude, E. B. High-Dose Vitamin D Supplementation Improves Microcirculation and Reduces Inflammation in Diabetic Neuropathy Patients. *Nutrients* **2020,** *12* (9), 2518. https://doi.org/10.3390/nu12092518.

Karunakaran, U.; Park, K.-G. A Systematic Review of Oxidative Stress and Safety of Antioxidants in Diabetes: Focus on Islets and Their Defense. *Diabetes Metab. J.* **2013,** *37* (2), 106–112. https://doi.org/10.4093/dmj.2013.37.2.106.

Keservani, R. K.; Kesharwani, R. K.; Sharma, A. K.; Vyas, N.; Chadoker, A. Nutritional Supplements: An Overview. Int. J. Curr. Pharm. Rev. Res. **2010b,** *1* (1), 59–75.

Keservani, R. K.; Kesharwani, R. K.; Vyas, N.; Jain, S.; Raghuvanshi, R.; Sharma, A. K. Nutraceutical and Functional Food as Future Food: A Review. *Der Pharmacia Lettre* **2010a,** *2* (1), 106–116.

Keservani, R. K.; Sharma, A. K. Flavonoids: Emerging Trends and Potential Health Benefits. *J. Chinese Pharm. Sci.* **2014,** *23* (12), 815.

Keservani, R. K.; Sharma, A. K.; Kesharwani, R. K. Nutraceutical and Functional Foods for Cardiovascular Health. In *Food Process Engineering*; Apple Academic Press, CRC Press, 2016a; pp 291–312, pp 257–278. ISBN: 9781771884020.

Keservani, R. K.; Sharma, A. K.; Kesharwani, R. K. Medicinal Effect of Nutraceutical Fruits for the Cognition and Brain Health. *Scientifica* **2016b,** *2016,* 3109254. DOI:10.1155/2016/3109254.

Keservani, R. K.; Sharma, A. K.; Kesharwani, R. K. An Overview and Therapeutic Applications of Nutraceutical and Functional Foods. *Rec. Adv. Drug Deliv. Technol.* **2017,** 160–201. ISBN: 9781522507543.

Keservani, R. K.; Sharma, A. K.; Kesharwani, R. K. Eds.; In *Nutraceuticals and Dietary Supplements: Applications in Health Improvement and Disease Management*; CRC Press, 2020; pp 1–342. ISBN: 9781771888738.

Khan, S.; Zhang, D.; Zhang, Y.; Li, M.; Wang, C. Wogonin Attenuates Diabetic Cardiomyopathy through Its Anti-Inflammatory and Anti-Oxidative Properties. *Mol. Cell. Endocrinol.* **2016,** *428*, 101–108. https://doi.org/10.1016/j.mce.2016.03.025.

Kim, E. K.; Kwon, K. B.; Song, M. Y.; Han, M. J.; Lee, J. H.; Lee, Y. R.; Lee, J. H.; Ryu, D. G.; Park, B. H.; Park, J. W. Flavonoids Protect Against Cytokine-Induced Pancreatic β-Cell Damage Through Suppression of Nuclear Factor KB Activation. *Pancreas* **2007,** *35* (4), e1. https://doi.org/10.1097/mpa.0b013e31811ed0d2.

Kinalski, M.; Sledziewski, A.; Telejko, B.; Zarzycki, W.; Kinalska, I. Lipid Peroxidation and Scavenging Enzyme Activity in Streptozotocin-Induced Diabetes. *Acta Diabetol.* **2000,** *37* (4), 179–183. https://doi.org/10.1007/s005920070002.

King, H.; Aubert, R. E.; Herman, W. H. Global Burden of Diabetes, 1995-2025: Prevalence, Numerical Estimates, and Projections. *Diabetes Care* **1998,** *21* (9), 1414–1431. https://doi.org/10.2337/diacare.21.9.1414.

Ko, H.; Jeong, M. H.; Jeon, H.; Sung, G. J.; So, Y.; Kim, I.; Son, J.; Lee, S.; Yoon, H. G.; Choi, K. C. Delphinidin Sensitizes Prostate Cancer Cells to TRAIL-Induced Apoptosis, by Inducing DR5 and Causing Caspase-Mediated HDAC3 Cleavage. *Oncotarget* **2015,** *6* (12), 9970–9984. https://doi.org/10.18632/oncotarget.3667.

Kocaadam, B.; Şanlier, N. Curcumin, an Active Component of Turmeric (Curcuma Longa), and Its Effects on Health. *Crit. Rev. Food Sci. Nutr.* **2017,** *57* (13), 2889–2895. https://doi.org/10.1080/10408398.2015.1077195.

Köhrl, J.; Brigelius-Flohé, R.; Böck, A.; Gärtner, R.; Meyer, O.; Flohé, L. Selenium in Biology: Facts and Medical Perspectives. *Biol. Chem.* **2000,** *381* (9–10), 849–864. https://doi.org/10.1515/BC.2000.107.

Kowluru, R. A.; Chan, P. S. Oxidative Stress and Diabetic Retinopathy. *Exp. Diabetes Res.* **2007,** *2007*, 43603. https://doi.org/10.1155/2007/43603.

Kowluru, R. A.; Tang, J.; Kern, T. S. Abnormalities of Retinal Metabolism in Diabetes and Experimental Galactosemia. VII. Effect of Long-Term Administration of Antioxidants on the Development of Retinopathy. *Diabetes* **2001,** *50* (8), 1938–1942. https://doi.org/10.2337/diabetes.50.8.1938.

Ku, S. K.; Bae, J. S. Baicalin, Baicalein and Wogonin Inhibits High Glucose-Induced Vascular Inflammation in Vitro and in Vivo. *B.M.B. Rep.* **2015,** *48* (9), 519–524. https://doi.org/10.5483/BMBRep.2015.48.9.017.

Kumar, K.; Kumar, S. Role of Nutraceuticals in Health and Disease Prevention: A Review. South Asian *J. Food Technol. Environ.* **2015,** *1*, 116–121. https://doi.org/10.46370/sajfte.2015.v01i02.02.

Kunnumakkara, A. B.; Bordoloi, D.; Padmavathi, G.; Monisha, J.; Roy, N. K.; Prasad, S.; Aggarwal, B. B. Curcumin, the Golden Nutraceutical: Multitargeting for Multiple Chronic Diseases. *Br. J. Pharmacol.* **2017,** *174* (11), 1325–1348. https://doi.org/10.1111/bph.13621.

Kutlu, M.; Naziroğlu, M.; Simşek, H.; Yilmaz, T.; Sahap Kükner, A. Moderate Exercise Combined with Dietary Vitamins C and E Counteracts Oxidative Stress in the Kidney and Lens of Streptozotocin-Induced Diabetic-Rat. *Int. J. Vitam. Nutr. Res.* **2005,** *75* (1), 71–80. https://doi.org/10.1024/0300-9831.75.1.71.

Labunskyy, V. M.; Lee, B. C.; Handy, D. E.; Loscalzo, J.; Hatfield, D. L.; Gladyshev, V. N. Both Maximal Expression of Selenoproteins and Selenoprotein Deficiency Can Promote Development of Type 2 Diabetes-like Phenotype in Mice. *Antioxid. Redox Signal.* **2011,** *14* (12), 2327–2336. https://doi.org/10.1089/ars.2010.3526.

Lau, F. C.; Bagchi, M.; Sen, C. K.; Bagchi, D. Nutrigenomic Basis of Beneficial Effects of Chromium(III) on Obesity and Diabetes. *Mol. Cell. Biochem.* **2008,** *317* (1–2), 1–10. https://doi.org/10.1007/s11010-008-9744-2.

Lei, X. G.; Vatamaniuk, M. Z. Two Tales of Antioxidant Enzymes on β Cells and Diabetes. *Antioxid. Redox Signal.* **2011,** *14* (3), 489–503. https://doi.org/10.1089/ars.2010.3416.

Li, J. M.; Che, C. T.; Lau, C. B. S.; Leung, P. S.; Cheng, C. H. K. Inhibition of Intestinal and Renal Na+-Glucose Cotransporter by Naringenin. *Int. J. Biochem. Cell Biol.* **2006,** *38* (5), 985–995. https://doi.org/10.1016/j.biocel.2005.10.002.

Li, X.; Liu, Y.; Zheng, Y.; Wang, P.; Zhang, Y. The Effect of Vitamin D Supplementation on Glycemic Control in Type 2 Diabetes Patients: A Systematic Review and Meta-Analysis. *Nutrients* **2018,** *10* (3), 375. https://doi.org/10.3390/nu10030375.

Liang, Y.; Zhu, B.; Li, S.; Zhai, Y.; Yang, Y.; Bai, Z.; Zeng, Y.; Li, D. Curcumin Protects Bone Biomechanical Properties and Microarchitecture in Type 2 Diabetic Rats with Osteoporosis via the TGFβ/Smad2/3 Pathway. *Exp. Ther. Med.* **2020,** *20* (3), 2200–2208. https://doi.org/10.3892/etm.2020.8943.

Lim, W.; Song, G. Inhibitory Effects of Delphinidin on the Proliferation of Ovarian Cancer Cells via PI3K/AKT and ERK 1/2 MAPK Signal Transduction. *Oncol. Lett.* **2017,** *14* (1), 810–818. https://doi.org/10.3892/ol.2017.6232.

Liu, F.; Ma, F.; Kong, G.; Wu, K.; Deng, Z.; Wang, H. Zinc Supplementation Alleviates Diabetic Peripheral Neuropathy by Inhibiting Oxidative Stress and Upregulating Metallothionein in Peripheral Nerves of Diabetic Rats. *Biol. Trace Elem. Res.* **2014,** *158* (2), 211–218. https://doi.org/10.1007/s12011-014-9923-9.

Lobo, R.; Prabhu, K. S.; Shirwaikar, A.; Shirwaikar, A. Curcuma Zedoaria Rosc. (White Turmeric): A Review of Its Chemical, Pharmacological and Ethnomedicinal Properties. *J. Pharm. Pharmacol.* **2009,** *61* (1), 13–21. https://doi.org/10.1211/jpp/61.01.0003.

Mahesh, T.; Balasubashini, M. S.; Menon, V. P. Effect of Photo-Irradiated Curcumin Treatment Against Oxidative Stress in Streptozotocin-Induced Diabetic Rats. *J. Med. Food* **2005,** *8* (2), 251–255. https://doi.org/10.1089/jmf.2005.8.251.

Malik, S.; Suchal, K.; Khan, S. I.; Bhatia, J.; Kishore, K.; Dinda, A. K.; Arya, D. S. Apigenin Ameliorates Streptozotocin-Induced Diabetic Nephropathy in Rats via MAPK-NF-KB-TNF-α and TGF-B1-MAPK-Fibronectin Pathways. *Am. J. Physiol.-Ren. Physiol.* **2017,** *313* (2), F414–F422. https://doi.org/10.1152/ajprenal.00393.2016.

Mao, J.; Teng, W. The Relationship between Selenoprotein P and Glucose Metabolism in Experimental Studies. *Nutrients* **2013,** *5* (6), 1937–1948. https://doi.org/10.3390/nu5061937.

Maraschin, J. de F.; Murussi, N.; Witter, V.; Silveiro, S. P. Diabetes Mellitus Classification. *Arq. Bras. Cardiol.* **2010,** *95* (2), e40–e46. https://doi.org/10.1590/s0066-782x2010001200025.

Mark, L.; Nikfardjam, M. S. P.; Avar, P.; Ohmacht, R. A Validated HPLC Method for the Quantitative Analysis of Trans-Resveratrol and Trans-Piceid in Hungarian Wines. *J. Chromatogr. Sci.* **2005,** *43* (9), 445–449. https://doi.org/10.1093/chromsci/43.9.445.

Mayer-Davis, E. J.; Bell, R. A.; Reboussin, B. A.; Rushing, J.; Marshall, J. A.; Hamman, R. F. Antioxidant Nutrient Intake and Diabetic Retinopathy: The San Luis Valley Diabetes Study. *Ophthalmology* **1998,** *105* (12), 2264–2270. https://doi.org/10.1016/S0161-6420(98)91227-1.

Mazza, G. Compositional and Functional Properties of Saskatoon Berry and Blueberry. *Int. J. Fruit Sci.* **2005,** *5* (3), 101–120. https://doi.org/10.1300/J492v05n03_10.

Miao, X.; Sun, W.; Fu, Y.; Miao, L.; Cai, L. Zinc Homeostasis in the Metabolic Syndrome and Diabetes. *Front. Med.* **2013,** *7* (1), 31–52. https://doi.org/10.1007/s11684-013-0251-9.

Millen, A. E.; Klein, R.; Folsom, A. R.; Stevens, J.; Palta, M.; Mares, J. A. Relation between Intake of Vitamins C and E and Risk of Diabetic Retinopathy in the Atherosclerosis Risk in Communities Study. *Am. J. Clin. Nutr.* **2004,** *79* (5), 865–873. https://doi.org/10.1093/ajcn/79.5.865.

Mueller, A. S.; Pallauf, J. Compendium of the Antidiabetic Effects of Supranutritional Selenate Doses. In Vivo and in Vitro Investigations with Type II Diabetic Db/Db Mice. *J. Nutr. Biochem.* **2006,** *17* (8), 548–560. https://doi.org/10.1016/j.jnutbio.2005.10.006.

Mulvihill, E. E.; Allister, E. M.; Sutherland, B. G.; Telford, D. E.; Sawyez, C. G.; Edwards, J. Y.; Markle, J. M.; Hegele, R. A.; Huff, M. W. Naringenin Prevents Dyslipidemia, Apolipoprotein B Overproduction, and Hyperinsulinemia in LDL Receptor–Null Mice

With Diet-Induced Insulin Resistance. *Diabetes* **2009,** *58* (10), 2198–2210. https://doi.org/10.2337/db09-0634.

Nasri, S.; Roghani, M.; Baluchnejadmojarad, T.; Rabani, T.; Balvardi, M. Vascular Mechanisms of Cyanidin-3-Glucoside Response in Streptozotocin-Diabetic Rats. *Pathophysiol.* **2011,** *18* (4), 273–278. https://doi.org/10.1016/j.pathophys.2011.03.001.

Negi, A.; Vernon, S. A. An Overview of the Eye in Diabetes. *J. R. Soc. Med.* **2003,** *96* (6), 266–272.

Nizamutdinova, I. T.; Jin, Y. C.; Chung, J. I.; Shin, S. C.; Lee, S. J.; Seo, H. G.; Lee, J. H.; Chang, K. C.; Kim, H. J. The Anti-Diabetic Effect of Anthocyanins in Streptozotocin-Induced Diabetic Rats through Glucose Transporter 4 Regulation and Prevention of Insulin Resistance and Pancreatic Apoptosis. *Mol. Nutr. Food Res.* **2009,** *53* (11), 1419–1429. https://doi.org/10.1002/mnfr.200800526.

Oteiza, P. I. Zinc and the Modulation of Redox Homeostasis. *Free Radic. Biol. Med.* **2012,** *53* (9), 1748–1759. https://doi.org/10.1016/j.freeradbiomed.2012.08.568.

Palacios, O. M.; Kramer, M.; Maki, K. C. Diet and Prevention of Type 2 Diabetes Mellitus: Beyond Weight Loss and Exercise. *Expert Rev. Endocrinol. Metab.* **2019,** *14* (1), 1–12. https://doi.org/10.1080/17446651.2019.1554430.

Panche, A. N.; Diwan, A. D.; Chandra, S. R. Flavonoids: An Overview. *J. Nutr. Sci.* **2016,** *5*, e47. https://doi.org/10.1017/jns.2016.41.

Panda, S.; Kar, A. Apigenin (4',5,7-Trihydroxyflavone) Regulates Hyperglycaemia, Thyroid Dysfunction and Lipid Peroxidation in Alloxan-Induced Diabetic Mice. *J. Pharm. Pharmacol.* **2007,** *59* (11), 1543–1548. https://doi.org/10.1211/jpp.59.11.0012.

Parhiz, H.; Roohbakhsh, A.; Soltani, F.; Rezaee, R.; Iranshahi, M. Antioxidant and Anti-Inflammatory Properties of the Citrus Flavonoids Hesperidin and Hesperetin: An Updated Review of Their Molecular Mechanisms and Experimental Models. *Phytother. Res.* **2015,** *29* (3), 323–331. https://doi.org/10.1002/ptr.5256.

Pazdro, R.; Burgess, J. R. The Role of Vitamin E and Oxidative Stress in Diabetes Complications. *Mech. Ageing Dev.* **2010,** *131* (4), 276–286. https://doi.org/10.1016/j.mad.2010.03.005.

Perrone, D.; Ardito, F.; Giannatempo, G.; Dioguardi, M.; Troiano, G.; Lo Russo, L.; De Lillo, A.; Laino, L.; Lo Muzio, L. Biological and Therapeutic Activities, and Anticancer Properties of Curcumin (Review). *Exp. Ther. Med.* **2015,** *10* (5), 1615–1623. https://doi.org/10.3892/etm.2015.2749.

Pervaiz, S. Resveratrol: From Grapevines to Mammalian Biology. *FASEB. J.* **2003,** *17* (14), 1975–1985. https://doi.org/10.1096/fj.03-0168rev.

Pessin, J. E.; Saltiel, A. R. Signaling Pathways in Insulin Action: Molecular Targets of Insulin Resistance. *J. Clin. Invest.* **2000,** *106* (2), 165–169. https://doi.org/10.1172/JCI10582.

Phillips, J. M.; Parish, N. M.; Raine, T.; Bland, C.; Sawyer, Y.; De La Peña, H.; Cooke, A. Type 1 Diabetes Development Requires Both CD4+ and CD8+ T Cells and Can Be Reversed by Non-Depleting Antibodies Targeting Both T Cell Populations. *Rev. Diabet. Stud.* **2009,** *6* (2), 97–103. https://doi.org/10.1900/RDS.2009.6.97.

Pidduck, H. G.; Wren, P. J.; Evans, D. A. Hyperzincuria of Diabetes Mellitus and Possible Genetical Implications of This Observation. *Diabetes.* **1970,** *19* (4), 240–247. https://doi.org/10.2337/diab.19.4.240.

Pivari, F.; Mingione, A.; Brasacchio, C.; Soldati, L. Curcumin and Type 2 Diabetes Mellitus: Prevention and Treatment. *Nutrients* **2019,** *11* (8), 1837. https://doi.org/10.3390/nu11081837.

Prasad, A. S. Zinc in Human Health: Effect of Zinc on Immune Cells. *Mol. Med.* **2008,** *14* (5–6), 353–357. https://doi.org/10.2119/2008-00033.Prasad.
Priscilla, D. H.; Roy, D.; Suresh, A.; Kumar, V.; Thirumurugan, K. Naringenin Inhibits α-Glucosidase Activity: A Promising Strategy for the Regulation of Postprandial Hyperglycemia in High Fat Diet Fed Streptozotocin Induced Diabetic Rats. *Chem. Biol. Interact.* **2014,** *210,* 77–85. https://doi.org/10.1016/j.cbi.2013.12.014.
Pu, P.; Gao, D. M.; Mohamed, S.; Chen, J.; Zhang, J.; Zhou, X.-Y.; Zhou, N.-J.; Xie, J.; Jiang, H. Naringin Ameliorates Metabolic Syndrome by Activating AMP-Activated Protein Kinase in Mice Fed a High-Fat Diet. *Arch. Biochem. Biophys.* **2012,** *518* (1), 61–70. https://doi.org/10.1016/j.abb.2011.11.026.
Pulido-Moran, M.; Moreno-Fernandez, J.; Ramirez-Tortosa, C.; Ramirez-Tortosa, Mc. Curcumin and Health. *Molecules* **2016,** *21* (3), 264. https://doi.org/10.3390/molecules21030264.
Rane, B. R.; Gujarathi, N. A; Patel, J. K. Biodegradable Anionic Acrylic Resin based Hollow Microspheres of Moderately Water Soluble Drug Rosiglitazone Maleate: Preparation and In Vitro Characterization. *Drug Dev. Ind. Pharm.* **2012**, *38* (12), 1460–1469. https://doi.org/10.3109/03639045.2011.653811.
Rauter, A. P.; Martins, A.; Borges, C.; Mota-Filipe, H.; Pinto, R.; Sepodes, B.; Justino, J. Antihyperglycaemic and Protective Effects of Flavonoids on Streptozotocin–Induced Diabetic Rats. *Phytother. Res.* **2010,** *24* (S2), S133–S138. https://doi.org/10.1002/ptr.3017.
Rayman, M. P. The Importance of Selenium to Human Health. *Lancet Lond. Engl.* **2000,** *356* (9225), 233–241. https://doi.org/10.1016/S0140-6736(00)02490-9.
Report of the Expert Committee on the Diagnosis and Classification of Diabetes Mellitus. *Diabetes Care* **1997,** *20* (7), 1183–1197. https://doi.org/10.2337/diacare.20.7.1183.
Robertson, R. P.; Harmon, J.; Tran, P. O.; Tanaka, Y.; Takahashi, H. Glucose Toxicity in Beta-Cells: Type 2 Diabetes, Good Radicals Gone Bad, and the Glutathione Connection. *Diabetes* **2003,** *52* (3), 581–587. https://doi.org/10.2337/diabetes.52.3.581.
Rouse, M.; Younès, A.; Egan, J. M. Resveratrol and Curcumin Enhance Pancreatic β-Cell Function by Inhibiting Phosphodiesterase Activity. *J. Endocrinol.* **2014,** *223* (2), 107–117. https://doi.org/10.1530/JOE-14-0335.
Roy, M.; Sen, S.; Chakraborti, A. S. Action of Pelargonidin on Hyperglycemia and Oxidative Damage in Diabetic Rats: Implication for Glycation-Induced Hemoglobin Modification. *Life Sci.* **2008,** *82* (21), 1102–1110. https://doi.org/10.1016/j.lfs.2008.03.011.
Saeidnia, S.; Abdollahi, M. Toxicological and Pharmacological Concerns on Oxidative Stress and Related Diseases. *Toxicol. Appl. Pharmacol.* **2013,** *273* (3), 442–455. https://doi.org/10.1016/j.taap.2013.09.031.
Sarmento, R. A.; Silva, F. M.; Sbruzzi, G.; Schaan, B. D.; Almeida, J. C. de. Antioxidant Micronutrients and Cardiovascular Risk in Patients with Diabetes: A Systematic Review. *Arq. Bras. Cardiol.* **2013,** *101* (3), 240–248. https://doi.org/10.5935/abc.20130146.
Serrano, A.; Ros, G.; Nieto, G. Bioactive Compounds and Extracts from Traditional Herbs and Their Potential Anti-Inflammatory Health Effects. *Med. Basel Switz.* **2018,** *5* (3), E76. https://doi.org/10.3390/medicines5030076.
Sharma, D.; Gondaliya, P.; Tiwari, V.; Kalia, K. Kaempferol Attenuates Diabetic Nephropathy by Inhibiting RhoA/Rho-Kinase Mediated Inflammatory Signalling. *Biomed. Pharmacother.* **2019,** *109,* 1610–1619. https://doi.org/10.1016/j.biopha.2018.10.195.
Shehab, D.; Al-Jarallah, K.; Abdella, N.; Mojiminiyi, O. A.; Mohamedy, H. A. Prospective Evaluation of the Effect of Short-Term Oral Vitamin D Supplementation on Peripheral

Neuropathy in Type 2 Diabetes Mellitus. *Med. Princ. Pract.* **2015,** *24* (3), 250–256. https://doi.org/10.1159/000375304.

Shillo, P.; Selvarajah, D.; Greig, M.; Gandhi, R.; Rao, G.; Wilkinson, I. D.; Anand, P.; Tesfaye, S. Reduced Vitamin D Levels in Painful Diabetic Peripheral Neuropathy. *Diabet. Med.* **2019,** *36* (1), 44–51. https://doi.org/10.1111/dme.13798.

Simon, S. F.; Taylor, C. G. Dietary Zinc Supplementation Attenuates Hyperglycemia in Db/Db Mice. *Exp. Biol. Med.* **2001,** *226* (1), 43–51. https://doi.org/10.1177/153537020122600107.

Sindhu, R. K.; Koo, J. R.; Roberts, C. K.; Vaziri, N. D. Dysregulation of Hepatic Superoxide Dismutase, Catalase and Glutathione Peroxidase in Diabetes: Response to Insulin and Antioxidant Therapies. *Clin. Exp. Hypertens.* **2004,** *26* (1), 43–53. https://doi.org/10.1081/ceh-120027330.

Singh, A. K.; Raj, V.; Keshari, A. K.; Rai, A.; Kumar, P.; Rawat, A.; Maity, B.; Kumar, D.; Prakash, A.; De, A.; Samanta, A.; Bhattacharya, B.; Saha, S. Isolated Mangiferin and Naringenin Exert Antidiabetic Effect via PPARγ/GLUT4 Dual Agonistic Action with Strong Metabolic Regulation. *Chem. Biol. Interact.* **2018,** *280*, 33–44. https://doi.org/10.1016/j.cbi.2017.12.007.

Srivilai, J.; Phimnuan, P.; Jaisabai, J.; Luangtoomma, N.; Waranuch, N.; Khorana, N.; Wisuitiprot, W.; Scholfield, C. N.; Champachaisri, K.; Ingkaninan, K. Curcuma Aeruginosa Roxb. Essential Oil Slows Hair-Growth and Lightens Skin in Axillae; a Randomised, Double Blinded Trial. Phytomedicine**2017,** *25*, 29–38. https://doi.org/10.1016/j.phymed.2016.12.007.

Stanić, Z. Curcumin, a Compound from Natural Sources, a True Scientific Challenge – A Review. *Plant Foods Hum. Nutr.* **2017,** *72* (1), 1–12. https://doi.org/10.1007/s11130-016-0590-1.

Stapleton, S. R. Selenium: An Insulin-Mimetic. *Cell. Mol. Life Sci.* **2000,** *57* (13–14), 1874–1879. https://doi.org/10.1007/PL00000669.

Steinbrenner, H. Interference of Selenium and Selenoproteins with the Insulin-Regulated Carbohydrate and Lipid Metabolism. *Free Radic. Biol. Med.* **2013,** *65*, 1538–1547. https://doi.org/10.1016/j.freeradbiomed.2013.07.016.

Suryanarayana, P.; Satyanarayana, A.; Balakrishna, N.; Kumar, P. U.; Reddy, G. B. Effect of Turmeric and Curcumin on Oxidative Stress and Antioxidant Enzymes in Streptozotocin-Induced Diabetic Rat. *Med. Sci. Monit.* **2007,** *13* (12), BR286–BR292.

Tai, M. C.; Tsang, S. Y.; Chang, L. Y. F.; Xue, H. Therapeutic Potential of Wogonin: A Naturally Occurring Flavonoid. *C.N.S. Drug Rev.* **2005,** *11* (2), 141–150. https://doi.org/10.1111/j.1527-3458.2005.tb00266.x.

Takatori, A.; Ishii, Y.; Itagaki, S.; Kyuwa, S.; Yoshikawa, Y. Amelioration of the Beta-Cell Dysfunction in Diabetic A.P.A. Hamsters by Antioxidants and A.G.E. Inhibitor Treatments. *Diabetes Metab. Res. Rev.* **2004,** *20* (3), 211–218. https://doi.org/10.1002/dmrr.428.

Tanaka, Y.; Tran, P. O. T.; Harmon, J.; Robertson, R. P. A Role for Glutathione Peroxidase in Protecting Pancreatic β Cells against Oxidative Stress in a Model of Glucose Toxicity. *Proc. Natl. Acad. Sci. U. S. A.* **2002,** *99* (19), 12363–12368. https://doi.org/10.1073/pnas.192445199.

Tyagi, S.; Ammerman, N. C.; Li, S. Y.; Adamson, J.; Converse, P. J.; Swanson, R. V.; Almeida, D. V.; Grosset, J. H. Clofazimine Shortens the Duration of the First-Line Treatment Regimen for Experimental Chemotherapy of Tuberculosis. *Proc. Natl. Acad. Sci. U. S. A.* **2015,** *112* (3), 869–874. https://doi.org/10.1073/pnas.1416951112.

van Acker, F. A. A.; Schouten, O.; Haenen, G. R. M. M.; van der Vijgh, W. J. F.; Bast, A. Flavonoids Can Replace α-Tocopherol as an Antioxidant. *FEBS Lett.* **2000,** *473* (2), 145–148. https://doi.org/10.1016/S0014-5793(00)01517-9.

Vashum, K. P.; McEvoy, M.; Milton, A. H.; Islam, M. R.; Hancock, S.; Attia, J. Is Serum Zinc Associated with Pancreatic Beta Cell Function and Insulin Sensitivity in Pre-Diabetic and Normal Individuals? Findings from the Hunter Community Study. *PloS One* **2014,** *9* (1), e83944. https://doi.org/10.1371/journal.pone.0083944.

Vikram, A.; Tripathi, D. N.; Kumar, A.; Singh, S. Oxidative Stress and Inflammation in Diabetic Complications. *Int. J. Endocrinol.* **2014,** *2014*, e679754. https://doi.org/10.1155/2014/679754.

Vinayagam, R.; Xu, B. Antidiabetic Properties of Dietary Flavonoids: A Cellular Mechanism Review. *Nutr. Metab.* **2015,** *12* (1), 60. https://doi.org/10.1186/s12986-015-0057-7.

Visnagri, A.; Kandhare, A. D.; Chakravarty, S.; Ghosh, P.; Bodhankar, S. L. Hesperidin, A Flavanoglycone Attenuates Experimental Diabetic Neuropathy via Modulation of Cellular and Biochemical Marker to Improve Nerve Functions. *Pharm. Biol.* **2014,** *52* (7), 814–828. https://doi.org/10.3109/13880209.2013.870584.

Wang, N.; Yi, W. J.; Tan, L.; Zhang, J. H.; Xu, J.; Chen, Y.; Qin, M.; Yu, S.; Guan, J.; Zhang, R. Apigenin Attenuates Streptozotocin-Induced Pancreatic β Cell Damage by Its Protective Effects on Cellular Antioxidant Defense. *Vitro Cell. Dev. Biol. Anim.* **2017,** *53* (6), 554–563. https://doi.org/10.1007/s11626-017-0135-4.

Wang, X.; Zhang, W.; Chen, H.; Liao, N.; Wang, Z.; Zhang, X.; Hai, C. High Selenium Impairs Hepatic Insulin Sensitivity through Opposite Regulation of R.O.S. *Toxicol. Lett.* **2014,** *224* (1), 16–23. https://doi.org/10.1016/j.toxlet.2013.10.005.

Zaken, V.; Kohen, R.; Ornoy, A. Vitamins C and E Improve Rat Embryonic Antioxidant Defense Mechanism in Diabetic Culture Medium. *Teratology* **2001,** *64* (1), 33–44. https://doi.org/10.1002/tera.1045.

Zanatta, L.; Rosso, Â.; Folador, P.; Figueiredo, M. S. R. B.; Pizzolatti, M. G.; Leite, L. D.; Silva, F. R. M. B. Insulinomimetic Effect of Kaempferol 3-Neohesperidoside on the Rat Soleus Muscle. *J. Nat. Prod.* **2008,** *71* (4), 532–535. https://doi.org/10.1021/np070358+.

Zang, M.; Xu, S.; Maitland-Toolan, K. A.; Zuccollo, A.; Hou, X.; Jiang, B.; Wierzbicki, M.; Verbeuren, T. J.; Cohen, R. A. Polyphenols Stimulate AMP-Activated Protein Kinase, Lower Lipids, and Inhibit Accelerated Atherosclerosis in Diabetic LDL Receptor–Deficient Mice. *Diabetes* **2006,** *55* (8), 2180–2191. https://doi.org/10.2337/db05-1188.

Zhang, Z.; Ding, Y.; Dai, X.; Wang, J.; Li, Y. Epigallocatechin-3-Gallate Protects pro-Inflammatory Cytokine Induced Injuries in Insulin-Producing Cells through the Mitochondrial Pathway. *Eur. J. Pharmacol.* **2011,** *670* (1), 311–316. https://doi.org/10.1016/j.ejphar.2011.08.033.

Zhang, W.; Li, P.; Guo, X.; Huang, Q. Role of Moesin, Src, and R.O.S. in Advanced Glycation End Product-Induced Vascular Endothelial Dysfunction. *Microcirculation* **2017,** *24* (3), e12358. https://doi.org/10.1111/micc.12358.

Zhang, Y.; Li, Q.; Xin, Y.; Lv, W.; Ge, C. Association between Serum Magnesium and Common Complications of Diabetes Mellitus. *Technol. Health Care* **2018,** *26* (S1), 379–387. https://doi.org/10.3233/THC-174702.

Zhou, J.; Huang, K.; Lei, X. G. Selenium and Diabetes--Evidence from Animal Studies. *Free Radic. Biol. Med.* **2013,** *65*, 1548–1556. https://doi.org/10.1016/j.freeradbiomed.2013.07.012.

Zhu, K.; Nie, S.; Li, C.; Huang, J.; Hu, X.; Li, W.; Gong, D.; Xie, M. Antidiabetic and Pancreas-Protective Effects of Zinc Threoninate Chelate in Diabetic Rats May Be Associated with Its Antioxidative Stress Ability. *Biol. Trace Elem. Res.* **2013,** *153* (1–3), 291–298. https://doi.org/10.1007/s12011-013-9675-y.

Zhu, W.; Jia, Q.; Wang, Y.; Zhang, Y.; Xia, M. The Anthocyanin Cyanidin-3-O-β-Glucoside, A Flavonoid, Increases Hepatic Glutathione Synthesis and Protects Hepatocytes against Reactive Oxygen Species during Hyperglycemia: Involvement of a CAMP–PKA-Dependent Signaling Pathway. *Free Radic. Biol. Med.* **2012,** *52* (2), 314–327. https://doi.org/10.1016/j.freeradbiomed.2011.10.483.

Ziegler, D.; Reljanovic, M.; Mehnert, H.; Gries, F. A. Alpha-Lipoic Acid in the Treatment of Diabetic Polyneuropathy in Germany: Current Evidence from Clinical Trials. Exp. Clin. Endocrinol. Diabetes Off. *J. Ger. Soc. Endocrinol. Ger. Diabetes Assoc.* **1999,** *107* (7), 421–430. https://doi.org/10.1055/s-0029-1212132.

Zygmunt, K.; Faubert, B.; MacNeil, J.; Tsiani, E. Naringenin, a Citrus Flavonoid, Increases Muscle Cell Glucose Uptake via A.M.P.K. *Biochem. Biophys. Res. Commun.* **2010,** *398* (2), 178–183. https://doi.org/10.1016/j.bbrc.2010.06.048.

PART III

FUNCTIONAL FOODS RICH IN ANTIOXIDANTS

CHAPTER 9

ANTIOXIDANTS-RICH FOOD SOURCES OF NUTRACEUTICAL AND FUNCTIONAL FOODS

SUJIT ARUN DESAI[1], PREETI KHULBE[2], YUVRAJ DILIP DANGE[1], SATWASHILA KADAM[3], and MEENAKSHI JAISWAL[4]

[1]*Annasaheb Dange College of D Pharmacy, Ashta Sangli, Maharashtra, India*

[2]*Gyan Vihar School of Pharmacy, Suresh Gyan Vihar University, Gyan Vihar Marg, Jagatpura, Jaipur, Rajasthan, India*

[3]*Womens College of Pharmacy, Peth-Vadgaon, Maharashtra, India*

[4]*Department of Pharmacy, Guru Ghasidas Central University, Koni, Bilaspur, Chhattisgarh, India*

ABSTRACT

This chapter aims to clarify how food, particularly for elderly people, and brain functioning are related. This includes the relationship between food color, flavor, scent, and nutritional adequacy or the connection between antioxidants and neurodegenerative disorders. The impact of these disorders on olfaction was also investigated. By suppressing acetylcholinesterase, other comparable treatments based on the foods' herbs, spices, and antioxidants were considered a prospective management for diseases. Antioxidants are crucial to maintain the physiology of the vital organs as well as for the prevention of cancer and cardiovascular disorders. The topic promotes the health of the elderly through dietary intake frequency and patterns. Ultimately, it was examined how the food sector, the press, and technology affect the new elderly generation.

Antioxidants as Nutraceuticals. Nayan A. Gujarathi, Raj K. Keservani, Rajesh K. Kesharwani, Bhushan R. Rane, Yogeeta Sameer Goyal (Eds.)

9.1 INTRODUCTION

With some definitions and disclaimers related to the title, this section provides an overview of the methodology used to create it.

9.1.1 HEALTH

It seems logical to incorporate neuro-cellular with humoral differences—which together make up the temporal aspects of physiology—that would result in the consensus of divisions in time (Halberg et al., 1960); it suggests that young or elderly persons, males or females, have different physiological rhythms that might be described and measured in terms of health and disease. Such age and gender differences may facilitate the detection and quantification of rhythmic alterations that mark the transformation from a healthy person to one having conspicuous and hidden disorders.

9.1.2 ELDERLY INDIVIDUALS

Sequential changes among the two or more states are frequently difficult to determine because of the experiment design, which recurrently focuses on the duration of the study and required results, as well as confounding factors like the inclusion/exclusion features of the applicants to clinical trials, for example, body mass index and health definitions.

9.1.3 ANTIOXIDANTS IN FOOD

Antioxidants, which are either organic or inorganic food preservatives, serve to protect food from "farm to plate" and to prevent oxidative deterioration during processing and storage. Due to their high stability and low volatility, antioxidants help to preserve the amount of nutrients, texture, color, taste, freshness, functionality, aroma, and appeal to end-users, even the elderly, ceteris paribus. Both food additives and dietary supplements (Keservani et al., 2010a; Keservani et al., 2010b; Keservani et al., 2017; Keservani et al., 2020) include antioxidants; hence, it is important to measure the amount of these substances in human fluids and tissues (Franco et al., 2017). *Aronia melanocarpa*, a fruit that is commonly found in foods like jams, purees, and juices, is a lesser-known source of antioxidants than those listed in reference

(Griffiths et al., 2016). It contains high quantities of polyphenols and other antioxidants (Singh et al., 2017).

Since they play a role in intricate metabolism with signaling processes, antioxidants are crucial in favor of both animal and plant life. Phytoalexins, such as isoflavonoid structures, are produced by them in response to microbial and fungal disease invasion to protect plants (Ahuja et al., 2012). It is crucial to study the mechanisms associated with, for example, microglia senescence, with neural aging to develop nutritional therapies, such as multifunctional foods and plant nutrients that may improve our understanding of aberrant aging and the beginning of neurodegenerative disorders (Wu et al., 2016).

Excellent reviews (>100; 2015–2017 Medline searches as well as other sources) on free radicals and related subjects that affect human health included (Lobo et.al., 2010), however, conflicting results may emerge and have an impact on health awareness campaigns, like resveratrol (Vang et al., 2011), because of a variety of factors which include study design, inadequate statistical analysis, the environment of cohorts, the follow-up time, conditions laid down, etc. The blind should not lead the blind, the current human gut metabolism in response to a "normal" diet or one that may be modified or controlled by dietary antioxidants medicines, including such flavonoids (Keservani and Sharma, 2014; Keservani et al., 2016a; Keservani et al., 2016b), carotenoids, etc., with an emphasis on gut-brain interactions, is an area of research that is becoming more and more active. This overview concentrated on elderly people's health, whose prevalence of neurological illnesses is increasing. As more structural information is gathered from natural compounds with antioxidant, anti-inflammatory, and anti-amyloidogenic capabilities, novel synthetic structures are becoming more and more feasible (Hiremathad et.al., 2017). These brand-new synthetic compounds could eventually be used to treat conditions like Alzheimer's disease. The simplest definition of a food antioxidant is a scavenger of "free" radicals, which have chemical structures that have at least one unpaired electron and can cause genetic and cellular changes due to their highly reactive state. Examples of these radicals include the hydroxyl (HO•) radical, hydroperoxyl (HOO•), alkyloxyl (ROO•), and superoxide (ROO•). As would be expected, a balance between potential cellular/tissue distress and the benefits of radicals required for regular intra- and intercellular signaling actions must be found. It provides a thorough examination of dietary antioxidants and the four million radicals produced each day (Griffiths et al., 2016). In fact, Lavoisier discovered the oxidation of food in 1775 and first described it a few years later (Lavoisier et al., 1775). He used it as a source of body heat in addition to energy for mobility.

9.2 NUTRITION

This phrase describes something that is consumed. It also includes behaviors related to the time along with frequency of mealtimes, which is the responsibility of caregivers toward a patient's squat dietary/nutrient ingestion (Lin et al., 2010). These behaviors include perceptive of when to "give in" or else "step in" with the patient at mealtime (Keller, 2007), especially in hospitals and nursing homes (Keller et al., 2007), with constrained dietary intake with potential positive changes to prolonged existence (Hufeland et al., 2022; Weindruch et al., 1996). Such measures are taken in an effort to maximize the number of "years to life" also "life to years" that can be gained, as well as the advantages to the physical with mental health outcomes that form the core of this message. At first glance, it seems logical to look into whether biological and chronological aging (Cornelissen et al., 2016) is closely related to changes in the microflora, digestive enzymes, and transporters for such absorption of food products, microelements (minerals, vitamins, etc.), as from gastrointestinal tract; malfunction of internal organs, as the heart and kidney; as well as possible drug-food/herbal interactions (PGPs).

9.3 FOOD AND AGRICULTURE

The progression and evolution of food and water contribute significantly to health from the past to the present. The ability to eat healthily can be improved by a greater awareness of food gathering, storage, preservation practices, and cultures. In contrast to the present trend, tradition, price, and availability all played a role in limiting food production in Britain in the 1950s. The interface involving man, microbes, as well as food was present during the Paleolithic period (Selhub et al., 2014), about 10,000 years ago, according to Stein (1993) (Stein et al., 2010), before more complex farming or the conversion from collecting and hunting with "plant breeding" programs in Neolithic times took place. The "Mediterranean diet" of today includes starchy foods like bread, pasta, olive oil, fish, seeds, almonds, legumes, and cereal grains. The N-3 fatty acids found in the Mediterranean diet have an impact on brain development and changes, especially in terms of neurogenesis and neuroplasticity, and they also impact cognition, mood, and behavior (Crupi et al., 2013). Both the lifespan of their residents, such as Cretans, and the comparatively high intake of foods produced from plants that are antioxidants are notable. South America contributes to the development of foods that are anti-inflammatory and healthy, thanks to its diverse and plentiful plant life (Mocchegiani et al., 2014).

Climate change poses a threat to food security, necessitating the discovery of alternative crops/foods for human consumption in drought-affected areas. One such crop is the Prosopis tree pod, which pre-Columbian humans harvested in the ABC countries and later used to make alcohol, syrup, flour, and other products (Schmeda-Hirschmann et al., 2015). As might be expected in an abiotic stress, these foods contain considerable antioxidant content. Although it is clear that the average lifetime of human existence has increased through time, its importance for antagonistic pleiotropy, planned death, or inherent reasons for mortality has not yet been thoroughly understood. According to Halberg's group's Natick experiments, adequate food intake is crucial, but limiting calorie consumption may lengthen life by causing weight loss through the timing of nutritional intake (Graeber et al., 2022).

9.4 ANTIOXIDANTS AND FOOD

Memantine may be supplemented through vitamin D, an antioxidant along with neurosteroidal hormone by means of preventive characteristics, in interventions, particularly with prodromal cognitive impairment (Singh et al., 2022). Dietary nutrients are necessary for brain function, and target organs like the brain's regions—which need omega-3 polyunsaturated fatty acids (Bourre et al., 2006) and vitamins B, E, and D—are implied in the description of functional foods and molecules. A review of nutrient intake, and central nervous system systems, including potential neuroprotective effects by dietary components is given in Bourre (Caracciolo et al., 2014). It shows huge improved awareness of the ecology and how dietary choices affect cognitive decline. If nutritional patterns employing functional foods to promote the health of the elderly in fastidious can be standardized and predicted with sufficient accuracy, it might lead to significant developmental studies on immune coordination, which have shown the importance of antioxidants in maintaining a healthy balance between the generation of free radicals and oxidative stress, which worsens with aging. How the immune system responds to antioxidant intake may be another indicator of health or disease (Evans et al., 2000). When combined with food restriction on, for instance, a balanced diet, aerobic exercise in humans raises superoxide dismutase thresholds and reinforces the antioxidant defensive reaction, offering medical benefits together with reducing the chance for metabolic syndrome, insulin resistance, or rather cardiovascular diseases (Everitt et al., 2006). Toxicities brought on by the interaction among amino acids with sugars present a risk in food preparation. It frequently happens when high-starch foods, including potatoes, root vegetables, and sometimes even bread, when fried, roasted, or baked at high heat (above 120 °C). It can be enhanced by choosing plant products with fewer precursors, using cooking ingredients that lessen acrylamide synthesis, reducing the physical conditions of cooking, etc. Depending on their place of origin, food pollutants might potentially be risk factors for unhealthy eating. For instance, the mycotoxinochratoxin A, which is prevalent in grape pomaces used during plant nutritional supplement and food coloring, may be present. It has nephrotoxic and carcinogenic consequences (Moncalvo et al., 2016). Lipoic acid or its reduced version enhances the levels of reduced glutathione by enhancing the production of acetylcholine, chelating redox-active metal complexes, reducing hydroxyl radicals, and scavenging reactive oxygen species. Heavy metals (Wilson et al., 2017) may also be eliminated from aquatic nutrient-fed horticulture systems of such compounds (ROS). The R-alpha monomer may be utilized to treat dementias such as Alzheimer's disease (Wilson et al., 2017). It is amazing that both plants and mammals naturally have this enantiomer. Because iron plays a significant part in the creation of neurotransmitters and the transportation of oxygen to the brain, it has a previously unknown function that has implicated neurodegenerative illnesses in the elderly. Human neurological disorders may be prevented with treatments that reduce iron levels (Henning et al., 2010).

9.5 SPICES AND FRAGRANT HERBS

A spice is defined by Griffiths et al. (2016) as any grain, fruit, rhizome, root, snarl, resin, berry, blossom, and stigma, as well as vegetable content that's also customarily used for seasoning and adds sweetness or savory flavors, various colors, or preserves food. A spice can also be a cosmetic product, a natural remedy, or just a vegetable (Griffiths et al., 2016). Coriander, fennel, mustard, cinnamon, mace, clove, saffron, ginger, asafetida, bay leaf oil, cloves, fenugreek, turmeric, poppy seed, pomegranate, red Chile, sesame seed, and other spices are among the many types of spices. Chaat masala, a type of spice blend, is present in many nations (Pakistan and India). Leafy green plant components known as herbs are used to season food or as a garnish. Thyme, sage, oregano, parsley, dill, marjoram, chives, rosemary, mint, lemon grass, and other herbs are examples of aromatic herbs. Of course, fresh, dried, or paste forms of spices and herbs are employed. According to reports, the total phenolic content and antioxidant capability are both still present in the processed end product, with some phenolics being less degraded than others (Lage et al., 2006). For example, the total phenolic content of many herbs and spices is unaltered.

9.6 SPECIFIC ORGAN SYSTEMS AND ANTIOXIDANTS

9.6.1 THE POTENTIAL OF HEPATOPROTECTIVE DIETARY ANTIOXIDANTS TO TREAT ALZHEIMER'S DISEASE

Senile plaques with neurofibrillary tangles were found in the cerebral cortex with one Auguste Deter, a 51-year-old Darmstadt woman who displayed characteristic dementia signs in 1901. Researchers have been looking for a cure for a very long time. Alzheimer's disease is a word Kraepelin created to describe the condition that Alois Alzheimer identified in 1906 (Cai et al., 2016). Because of its antioxidant properties and suppression of hepatic oxidative stress and having more than 5 Ka, berberine, a protoberberine category of benzylisoquinoline alkaloids found in *Berberis vulgaris* and many other plants, has been used in Chinese medicine (Bagchi et al., 2000). It is asserted that it protects against a variety of ailments. The watchword is to prevent unsupported statements, such as those about tea that might not be supported by evidence caution. However, it has been demonstrated to delay neurofibrillary tangle formation, reduce oxidative stress, and attenuate hyperphosphorylation and cytostatic caused by Calyculin A of the microtubule-related protein tau. It may be fruitful to screen plants for these alkaloids, especially if ingestion is associated with low liver or other organ damage. In addition to the grape seed proanthocyanidin extract mentioned above, which has elevated bioavailability and protects against liver and kidney damage (Milk Thistle: et al., 2022), *Silybum marianum*, also known as milk thistle, is occasionally consumed in the pastis, a medicinal herb that had long been utilized as a treatment for hepatoprotection. Numerous liver conditions characterized by functional impairment or progressive necrosis have been treated with it. Antioxidant and anti-inflammatory actions, cell permeability modulation, membrane stabilization, acceleration of liver regeneration, and avoidance of collagen deposition are only a few of its special hepatoprotective qualities.

9.6.2 RENO-PROTECTIVE DIETARY ANTIOXIDANTS

It is observed that in late-stage renal disease, blood isoflavonoids accumulate due to nutritional soy intake, which is higher in patients compared to healthy individuals with normal kidney function. However, both unconjugated and sulfated levels are significantly different compared to healthy subjects, and food effects may vary depending on the disease (Ho et al., 2015). Specific definitions of functional foods are required, and the effects of food can change depending on the ailment. Following up on 96,196 women from the Women's Health Initiative Program showed that 240 of them developed renal cell cancer, which (as indicated by a food frequency questionnaire) was negatively linked with lycopene (Galli et al., 2004). When hemodialysis patients were compared to healthy controls, plasma levels of carboxyethyl-hydroxychramans increased in one more example of abridged renal function, but it would seem that the antioxidant status remained the same. Obviously, additional investigation is required.

9.6.3 CARDIOVASCULAR DISEASE AND NUTRITIONAL ANTIOXIDANTS

Fiber, a necessary dietary component, may assist in reducing the risk of getting various cancers. For instance, 35,000 menopausal women (aged 55–69) who completed a 127-item dietary regularity questionnaire over 20 years ago discovered that whole-grain cereals strong in antioxidants or fiber were highly preventative for myocardial infarction (Mendoza-Nunez et al., 2009). Elevated levels of lipoperoxide were connected to high blood pressure in a case-control study of elderly Mexicans. Plasma concentrations of anti-oxidant enzymes, total antioxidants, and lipoperoxide were also examined (Mulvad et al., 1996). Interestingly, the incidences of myocardial infarction, cardiac disease, and arteriosclerosis are low among Greenlander Inuits who consume marine foods. Autopsies on people who later died in Nuuk and Ilulissat generally indicated high amounts of omega-3 fatty acids within adipose tissue with high levels of selenium in the liver (Liu et al., 2003). Intake of vegetables (carotenoids) was inversely correlated with coronary heart disease risk according to both a questionnaire about food frequency and just a putative randomly selected case encompassing over 22,000 male clinicians between both the ages of 40 and 84 (Pantavos et al., 2014), which is coherent with many studies on the subject.

9.6.4 BREAST CANCER AND NUTRITIONAL ANTIOXIDANTS

Based on dietary frequency questionnaire and estimates of the antioxidants flavonoids, selenium, carotenoids, including vitamins E, C, as well as A, the incidence of breast tumor was determined in a probable Rotterdam research of over 3200 people, aged 55 and older, followed it up for a median of 17 years. High antioxidant levels were linked to a decreased incidence of this malignancy. The Cancer Institute in Chennai, India found that reduced antioxidant intake (lutein, zeaxanthin, green-yellow foods) was linked to higher malignancies for both breast cancer patients and controls. Functional foods meant to reduce oxidative stress for patients with advanced breast cancer were also reported; however, the trial was tiny and probably lacked statistical power (Nkondjock et al., 2014). Similar results have been reported for cancer of any source or breast cancer, although not always (Do et al., 2003; Gaudet et al., 2004; Genkinger et al., 2004; Hjartaker et al., 2015; Meydani et al., 2002; Ahn et al., 2005) due to potential antioxidant heterogeneity (Peresadina et al., 2004). Consumption of isoflavones combined with selenium boosted the clinical signs of people with hypertension, and heart disease, along with lipid metabolism that may have been related to antioxidants, as per a Russian abstract of an investigation by Peresadina et al. (2004) (Norton et al., 2014).

9.6.5 FACTORS INFLUENCING FEEDING THE ELDERLY

Dietary nutrients have multifaceted, multifactorial, and chemosensory effects on the health of individuals of every age. Biological, natural antioxidants, chronobiology, ecology, culture, religion, eating patterns, memory loss, and dietary habits are a few of these aspects. They also include the consumption of organic foods and herbal remedies (Sharma et al., 2020; Rane et al., 2020a; Rane et al., 2020b; Rane et al., 2020c) (such as phytoalexins, phytochemicals, carotenoids, spices, and fragrant herbs), as well as marketing hype and commercialization. In addition to breastfeeding and home care, infants are fed through a variety of feeding methods, including intra- and intravenous and tube feeding. Nutrients such as omega-3 fatty acids and vitamins such as B12 and B6 are delivered intravenously and through the nose via mouth and nose. Food must undoubtedly appeal to older people in terms of presentation, texture, color, flavor, and aroma, as long as their sensory function is unimpaired (Dunne et al., 2004). Benefits from non-traditional foods and plants are possible (Liu et al., 2001); however, the phytochemical effects differ depending on whether they are consumed alone or in combination with other foods (Green et al., 2015). The sensation of sweetness and bitterness in the mouth is referred to as flavor. However, there are risks associated with the brain's "reward" regions, such as obesity and metabolic syndrome (Watson et al., 2002), even though hyperphagia, or hunger, in dementia patients can result in either overeating or undereating due to a complex process. Fruit aroma volatiles, for instance, vary depending on the species and variation. These volatiles could include phenolic chemicals (even in strawberries; Noguer et al., 2012) aliphatic esters, such as those found in strawberries, and even in wine without alcohol (EL-Hadi et al., 2013), sesquiterpenes, etc. (Luevano-Contreras et al., 2010).

9.7 FOOD COLOR, THE BRAIN, AND DIETARY SUFFICIENCY

In the context of food coloring as a desirable aspect for consumers and dietary acceptability, there are four key themes:

1. Progress in areas beyond the scope of this review, such as the utilization of solar power with photosynthesis.
2. Early history of food coloring (Shamina et al., 2007).
3. The use of natural regulatory food colorants locally and globally, which eliminates the need for potentially dangerous dyes, sometimes not primarily for safety reasons.
4. The use of food coloring as a chemical additive (Alessandri et al., 2004).

9.8 DIETARY SUFFICIENCY, BRAIN FUNCTION, AND FOOD FLAVOR

The role of flavor in dietary composition is discussed in this section (q.v. Griffiths et al. (Griffiths et al., 2016 Brogggio et al., 2001)) with a more targeted intervention action. Various examples show the finding that gustatory (tasting) interruption was experiential agnosia during mild Alzheimer's disease, trying to suggest a dissociation of olfactory as well as gustatory thresholds at a central level, from a trial of a variety of dishes that made up a typical diet in Alzheimer's disease subjects (Ogawa et al., 2017) According to Ansoleaga et al. (2013), significant neuronal brain loss, such as that brought on by Alzheimer's disease, is typically thought to have an impact on gustatory function, but it's unclear whether this is true of the tangential transmission of sensory input commencing taste receptors (saline, sour, sugary, and bitter) to gustatory neurofibers. Functional foods may be involved in this pathological process because the expression of olfactory and gustatory chemoreceptors in the human brain differs in Parkinson's as well as Alzheimer's disease response (Lang et al., 2006). Both the frontal cortex and the entorhinal cortex exhibit dysregulation of these receptor subtypes.

9.9 PROSPECTIVE FUNCTION OF FUNCTIONAL FOODS MEANT FOR PREVENTION OF NEURODEGENERATION

Some dietary components produced from plants, including such functional foods (Kundu et al., 2013), have been proposed as prospective targets for the management of Alzheimer's disease. Alzheimer's disease and other neurological conditions are treated with acetylcholinesterase inhibitors (AD). Functional foods can be either natural or manufactured, and may contain either recognized or unidentified biologically active ingredients, and help with both dietary needs and enhancing health and wellness. These foods have clinically proven health advantages for the prevention, management, and chronic disease treatment. The words "clinically demonstrated and not hypothetical" and "documented," which refer to studies that have been appropriately published in the scientific literature, and "related to intact species and therefore not ex vivo as in cell culture" are all keys to the candidate food in this definition of functional foods.

9.10 DISCUSSION

9.10.1 GENERAL

This overview aimed to clarify how the brain works in connection to nutritional intake, particularly in elderly people. It started with some earliest examples of food, feeding, health, and food antioxidants, the development of agriculture as well as plant breeding, the restructuring of the food source for nutrition, and factors directly referencing the needs of the elderly with regard to food color, aroma, and flavor, as well as how the brain functioned to ensure dietary sufficiency. Prior to going into greater detail on dietary antioxidants, the advantages of functional foods were described. Herbal antioxidants, such as spices and aromatic herbs, then came next. We have also given a quick overview of the vast field of antioxidants in relation to cancer, cardiovascular disease, liver, kidney, and digestive system disorders.

9.10.2 HEALTH PROMOTION

This useful, up-to-date information was thought to be missing an essential component of health promotion (Itharat et al., 2017; Keller et al., 2007; Buttar et al. 2005), such as obesity (Aoi et al., 2009), including exercise (Lachat et al., 2006), the latter of which was thought to be outside the purview of this overview. In order to change a bad social impact into a positive one in the case of Japan, a brief discourse that has previously been examined as social therapy (Arai et al., 2011) has been incorporated into the conversation here, potentially establishing a model for the rest of the world to follow (158). Practitioners may argue that this is “much ado about nothing” (Wilson et al., 2017) and that "we want some guidance to help the older person now.” Epidemiological evidence-based recommendations for healthy eating aim to incorporate serving frequency and patterns may vary by nation. The US Department of Agriculture then proposed the Food Guide Pyramid, which is utilized by groups in the Republic of Ireland, for example, but which exhibits significant variation—those who are more impoverished have extra health issues. This was in response to Sweden implementing a health food promotion program known as matpyramid (O’Connor et al., 2017). This has been replaced by the more user-friendly “My plate” method, which calls for consuming 30% grains, 40% vegetables, 10% fruits, and 20% proteins. However, disparities are linked to older people on a broad range of factors that have been examined in various ways, such as meta-analysis (Kaiser et al., 2011), implicit in food security, including social exclusion (Walsh et al., 2016, Bronfenbrenner et al., 2022), The human ecological framework (Krondl et al., 2008) includes its interconnected micro-, meso-, and macro-components as well as life-course-chronosystem (implicit in chronobiology, which has wider remit well beyond this overview) once lack of access to nutrition traders and low levels of income are important effects on dietary quality and wellness disparities, especially in elderly people.

9.11 CONCLUSIONS

This outline has covered a few important brain functions related to diet, as well as how foods might affect conditions like senile dementia, Alzheimer’s disease, and cardiovascular diseases. We have spoken about how older people experience food inequities within a social setting. To meet the welfare with nutritional requirements of the next generation of the older population, as well as to bring the disparate threads of progress together, further effort is required.

KEYWORDS

- aging
- diet
- olfactory function
- food flavor
- color
- scent
- dementia

REFERENCES

Ahn, J.; Gammon, M. D.; Santella, R. M.; Gaudet, M. M.; Britton, J. A.; Teitelbaum, S. L.; Terry, M. B.; Nowell, S.; Davis, W.; Garza, C.; Neugut, A. I.; Ambrosone, C. B. Associations between Breast Cancer Risk and the Catalase Genotype, Fruit and Vegetable Consumption, and Supplement Use. *Am. J. Epidemiol.* **2005,** *162* (10), 943–952.

Ahuja, I.; Kissen, R.; Bones, A. M. Phytoalexins in Defense against Pathogens. *Trends Plant Sci.* **2012,** *17* (2), 73–90.

Alessandri, J. M.; Guesnet, P.; Vancassel, S.; Astorg, P.; Denis, I.; Langelier, B.; Aïd, S.; Poumès-Ballihaut, C.; Champeil-Potokar, G.; Lavialle, M. Polyunsaturated Fatty Acids in the Central Nervous System: Evolution of Concepts and Nutritional Implications throughout Life. *Reprod. Nutr. Dev.* **2004,** *44* (6), 509–538.

Ansoleaga, B.; Garcia-Esparcia, P.; Llorens, F.; Moreno, J.; Aso, E.; Ferrer, I. Dysregulation of Brain Olfactory and Taste Receptors in AD, PSP and CJD, and AD-Related Model. *Neuroscience* **2013,** *248*, 369–382.

Aoi, W. Exercise and Food Factors. *Forum Nutr.* **2009,** *61*, 147–155.

Arai, H.; Ouchi, Y.; Yokode, M.; Ito, H.; Uematsu, H.; Eto, F.; Oshima, S.; Ota, K.; Saito, Y.; Sasaki, H.; Tsubota, K.; Fukuyama, H.; Honda, Y.; Iguchi, A.; Toba, K.; Hosoi, T.; Kita, T. Toward the Realization of a Better Aged Society: Messages from Gerontology and Geriatrics. *Geriatr. Gerontol. Int.* **2011,** *12* (1), 16–22.

Bagchi, D.; Bagchi, M.; Stohs, S. J.; Das, D. K.; Ray, S. D.; Kuszynski, C. A.; Joshi, S. S.; Pruess, H. G. Free Radicals and Grape Seed Proanthocyanidin Extract: Importance in Human Health and Disease Prevention. *Toxicology* **2000,** *148* (2-3), 187–197.

Bourre, J. M. Effects of Nutrients (in Food) on the Structure and Function of the Nervous System: Update on Dietary Requirements for Brain. Part 1: Micronutrients. *J. Nutr. Health Aging,* **2006,** *10* (5), 377–385.

Broggio, E.; Pluchon, C.; Ingrand, P.; Gil, R. [Taste Impairment in Alzheimer's Disease]. *Rev. Neurol.* **2001,** *157* (4), 409–413.

Buttar, H. S.; Li, T.; Ravi, N. Prevention of Cardiovascular Diseases: Role of Exercise, Dietary Interventions, Obesity and Smoking Cessation. *Exp. Clin. Cardiol.* **2005,** *10* (4), 229–249.

Cai, Z.; Wang, C.; Yang, W. Role of Berberine in Alzheimer's Disease. *Neuropsychiatr. Dis. Treat.* **2016,** *12*, 2509–2520.

Caracciolo, B.; Xu, W.; Collins, S.; Fratiglioni, L. Cognitive Decline, Dietary Factors and Gut–Brain Interactions. *Mech. Ageing Dev.* **2014,** *136–137*, 59–69.

Cornelissen, G.; Otsuka, K. Chronobiology of Aging: A Mini-Review. *Gerontology* **2016,** *63* (2), 118–128.

Crupi, R.; Marino, A.; Cuzzocrea, S. N-3 Fatty Acids: Role in Neurogenesis and Neuroplasticity. *Curr. Med. Chem.* **2013,** *20* (24), 2953–2963.

Do, M. H.; Lee, S. S.; Jung, P. J.; Lee, M. H. Intake of Dietary Fat and Vitamin in Relation to Breast Cancer Risk in Korean Women: A Case-Control Study. *J. Korean Med. Sci.* **2003,** *18* (4), 534.

Dunne, T. E.; Neargarder, S. A.; Cipolloni, P. B.; Cronin-Golomb, A. Visual Contrast Enhances Food and Liquid Intake in Advanced Alzheimer's Disease. *Clin. Nutr.* **2004,** *23* (4), 533–538.

El Hadi, M. A. M.; Zhang, F. J.; Wu, F. F.; Zhou, C. H.; Tao, J. Advances in Fruit Aroma Volatile Research. *Molecules* **2013,** *18* (7), 8200–8229.

Evans, W. J. Vitamin E, Vitamin C, and Exercise. *Am. J. Clin. Nutr.* **2000,** *72* (2), 647S652S.

Everitt, A. V.; Hilmer, S. N.; Brand-Miller, J. C.; Jamieson, H. A.; Truswell, A. S.; Sharma, A. P.; Mason, R. S.; Morris, B. J.; Couteur, D. G. L. Dietary Approaches That Delay Age-Related Diseases. *Clin. Interv. Aging* **2006,** *1* (1), 11–31.

Galli, F.; Floridi, A. G.; Floridi, A.; Buoncristiani, U. Accumulation of Vitamin E Metabolites in the Blood of Renal Failure Patients. *Clin. Nutr.* **2004,** *23* (2), 205–212.

Gaudet, M. M.; Britton, J. A.; Kabat, G. C.; Steck-Scott, S.; Eng, S. M.; Teitelbaum, S. L.; Terry, M. B.; Neugut, A. I.; Genkinger, J. M.; Platz, E. A.; Hoffman, S. C.; Comstock, G. W.; Helzlsouer, K. J. Fruit, Vegetable, and Antioxidant Intake and All-Cause, Cancer, and Cardiovascular Disease Mortality in a Community-Dwelling Population in Washington County, Maryland. *Am. J. Epidemiol.* **2004,** *160* (12), 1223–1233.

Graeber, R. C.; Gatty, R.; Halberg, F.; Levine, H. Human Eating Behavior: Preferences. Consumption Patterns, and Biorhythms [Online] 2022. https://apps.dtic.mil/sti/citations/ADA073571 accessedApr 21, 2022).

Green, E.; Jacobson, A.; Haase, L.; Murphy, C. Neural Correlates of Taste and Pleasantness Evaluation in the Metabolic Syndrome. *Brain Res.* **2015,** *1620*, 57–71.

Griffiths, K.; Aggarwal, B.; Singh, R.; Buttar, H.; Wilson, D.; De Meester, F. Food Antioxidants and Their Anti-Inflammatory Properties: A Potential Role in Cardiovascular Diseases and Cancer Prevention. *Diseases* **2016,** *4* (4), 28.

Henning, S. M.; Zhang, Y.; Seeram, N. P.; Lee, R. P.; Wang, P.; Bowerman, S.; Heber, D. Antioxidant Capacity and Phytochemical Content of Herbs and Spices in Dry, Fresh and Blended Herb Paste Form. *Int. J. Food Sci. Nutr.* **2010,** *62* (3), 219–225.

Hiremathad, A. A Review: Natural Compounds as Anti-Alzheimer´S Disease Agents. *Curr. Nutr. Food Sci.* **2017,** *13* (4), 247–254.

Hjartåker, A.; Knudsen, M. D.; Tretli, S.; Weiderpass, E. Consumption of Berries, Fruits and Vegetables and Mortality among 10,000 Norwegian Men Followed for Four Decades. *Euro. J. Nutr.* **2015,** *54* (4), 599–608.

Ho, W. J.; Simon, M. S.; Yildiz, V. O.; Shikany, J. M.; Kato, I.; Beebe-Dimmer, J. L.; Cetnar, J. P.; Bock, C. H. Antioxidant Micronutrients and the Risk of Renal Cell Carcinoma in the Women's Health Initiative Cohort. *Cancer* **2015,** *121* (4), 580–588.

Itharat, A.; Takahashi, T.; Singh, R. G.; Singh, R. B.; Krisentu, K.; Lobenberg, R.; Noguchi, H.; Jantan, I.; Istvan, T. G.; Wilson, D. W.; Shastun, S.; Buttar, H. S.; Elkilany, G.; Hristova, K.; Cornélissen, G.; Hussain, L.; Sulaeman, A.; Singh, M.; Srivastav, R. K. Holistic Approaches for Health Education and Health Promotion. *World Heart J.* **2017,** *9* (1), 81–96.

Kaiser, M. Food Security: An Ecological-Social Analysis to Promote Social Development. *J. Community Pract.* **2011,** *19* (1), 62–79.

Keller, H. H. Promoting Food Intake in Older Adults Living in the Community: A Review. *Appl. Physiol. Nutr. Metab.* **2007,** *32* (6), 991–1000.

Keller, H. H.; Edward, H. G.; Cook, C. Mealtime Experiences of Families with Dementia. *Am. J. Alzheimer's Dis.* **2007,** *21* (6), 431–438.

Keservani, R. K.; Sharma, A. K. Flavonoids: Emerging Trends and Potential Health Benefits. *J. Chinese Pharm. Sci.* **2014,** *23* (12), 815.

Keservani, R. K.; Kesharwani, R. K.; Vyas, N.; Jain, S.; Raghuvanshi, R.; Sharma, A. K. Nutraceutical and Functional Food as Future Food: A Review. *Der Pharmacia Lettre* **2010a,** *2* (1), 106–116.

Keservani, R. K.; Sharma, A. K.; Kesharwani, R. K. Nutraceutical and Functional Foods for Cardiovascular Health. In *Food Process Engineering*; Apple Academic Press, CRC Press, 2016a; pp 291–312, pp 257–278. ISBN: 9781771884020.

Keservani, R. K.; Sharma, A. K.; Kesharwani, R. K. Medicinal Effect of Nutraceutical Fruits for the Cognition and Brain Health. *Scientifica* 2016b, *2016*, 3109254. DOI: 10.1155/2016/3109254.

Keservani, R. K.; Sharma, A. K.; Kesharwani, R. K. An overview and therapeutic applications of nutraceutical and functional foods. In *Recent Advances in Drug Delivery Technology*, 2017; pp 160–201. ISBN: 9781522507543.

Keservani, R. K.; Sharma, A. K.; Kesharwani, R. K. Eds.; In *Nutraceuticals and Dietary Supplements: Applications in Health Improvement and Disease Management*; CRC Press, 2020; pp 1–342. ISBN: 9781771888738.

Keservani, R. K.; Kesharwani, R. K.; Sharma, A. K.; Vyas, N.; Chadoker, A. Nutritional Supplements: An Overview. *Int. J. Curr. Pharm. Rev. Res.* **2010b,** *1* (1), 59–75.

Krondl, M.; Coleman, P.; Lau, D. Helping Older Adults Meet Nutritional Challenges. *J. Nutr. Elderly* **2008,** *27* (3-4), 205–220.

Kundu, A.; Mitra, A. Flavoring Extracts of HemidesmusIndicus Roots and Vanilla Planifolia Pods Exhibit in Vitro Acetylcholinesterase Inhibitory Activities. *Plant Foods Human Nutr.* **2013,** *68* (3), 247–253.

Lachat, C.; Dehenauw, S.; van Camp, J.; Matthys, C.; Larondelle, Y.; Kolsteren, P. [A Review of the Nutritional Management Plans in the Member States of the European Union]. *Verhandelingen – Koninklijke Academie Voo rGeneeskunde Van Belgie* **2006,** *68* (1), 55–76.

Lage, J. M. M. 100 Years of Alzheimer's Disease (1906–2006). *J. Alzheimer's Dis.* **2006,** *9* (s3), 15–26.

Liu, R. H. Health Benefits of Fruit and Vegetables Are from Additive and Synergistic Combinations of Phytochemicals. *Am. J. Clin. Nutr.* **2003,** *78* (3), 517–520.

Liu, S.; Lee, I. M.; Ajani, U.; Cole, S. R.; Buring, J. E.; Manson, J. E. Intake of Vegetables Rich in Carotenoids and Risk of Coronary Heart Disease in Men: The Physicians' Health Study. *Int. J. Epidemiol.* **2001,** *30* (1), 130–135.

Lobo, V.; Patil, A.; Phatak, A.; Chandra, N. Free Radicals, Antioxidants and Functional Foods: Impact on Human Health. *Pharmacogn. Rev.* **2010,** *4* (8), 118–126.

Luevano-Contreras, C.; Chapman-Novakofski, K. Dietary Advanced Glycation End Products and Aging. *Nutrients* **2010,** *2* (12), 1247–1265.

Mendoza-Núñez, V. M.; Sánchez-Rodríguez, M. A.; Correa-Muñoz, E. Undernutrition and Oxidative Stress as Risk Factors for High Blood Pressure in Older Mexican Adults. *Ann. Nutr. Metab.* **2009,** *54* (2), 119–123.

Meydani, M. The Boyd Orr Lecture: Nutrition Interventions in Aging and Age-Associated Disease. *Proc. Nutr. Soc.* **2002,** *61* (2), 165–171.

Mocchegiani, E.; Costarelli, L.; Giacconi, R.; Malavolta, M.; Basso, A.; Piacenza, F.; Ostan, R.; Cevenini, E.; Gonos, E. S.; Monti, D. Micronutrient-Gene Interactions Related to Inflammatory/Immune Response and Antioxidant Activity in Ageing and Inflammation. A Systematic Review. *Mech. Ageing Dev.* **2014,** *136–137*, 29–49.

Moncalvo, A.; Marinoni, L.; Dordoni, R.; DusermGarrido, G.; Lavelli, V.; Spigno, G. Waste Grape Skins: Evaluation of Safety Aspects for the Production of Functional Powders and Extracts for the Food Sector. *Food Addit. Contam. Part A Chem. Anal. Control Expo. Risk Assess.* **2016,** *33* (7), 1116–1126.

Mulvad, G.; Pedersen, H. S.; Hansen, J. C.; Dewailly, E.; Jul, E.; Pedersen, M.; Deguchi, Y.; Newman, W. P.; Malcom, G. T.; Tracy, R. E.; Middaugh, J. P.; Bjerregaard, P. The Inuit Diet. Fatty Acids and Antioxidants, Their Role in Ischemic Heart Disease, and Exposure to Organochlorines and Heavy Metals. An International Study. *Arctic Med. Res.* **1996,** *55* (Suppl 1), 20–24.

Nkondjock, A.; Ghadirian, P. Intake of Specific Carotenoids and Essential Fatty Acids and Breast Cancer Risk in Montreal, Canada. *Am. J. Clin. Nutr.* **2004,** *79* (5), 857–864.

Noguer, M. A.; Cerezo, A. B.; Donoso Navarro, E.; Garcia-Parrilla, M. C. Intake of Alcohol-Free Red Wine Modulates Antioxidant Enzyme Activities in a Human Intervention Study. *Pharmacol. Res.* **2012,** *65* (6), 609–614.

Norton, J. E.; Wallis, G. A.; Spyropoulos, F.; Lillford, P. J.; Norton, I. T. Designing Food Structures for Nutrition and Health Benefits. *Ann. Rev. Food Sci. Technol.* **2014,** *5* (1), 177–195.

Ogawa, T.; Irikawa, N.; Yanagisawa, D.; Shiino, A.; Tooyama, I.; Shimizu, T. Taste Detection and Recognition Thresholds in Japanese Patients with Alzheimer-Type Dementia. *Auris Nasus Larynx* **2017,** *44* (2), 168–173.

Pantavos, A.; Ruiter, R.; Feskens, E. F.; de Keyser, C. E.; Hofman, A.; Stricker, B. H.; Franco, O. H.; Kiefte-de Jong, J. C. Total Dietary Antioxidant Capacity, Individual Antioxidant Intake and Breast Cancer Risk: The Rotterdam Study. *Int. J. Cancer* **2014,** *136* (9), 2178–2186.

Peresadina, V. R.; Dmitrievskaia, M. N.; Mal'tsev, G. I.; Pogozheva, A. V.; Vasil'ev, A. V. [The Use of Nutritional Antioxidants for the Correction of Metabolic Disorders of Cardiovascular Patients]. *VoprosyPitaniia* **2004,** *73* (3), 3–6.

Rane, B. R.; Bharath, M. S.; Patil, R. R.; Keservani, R. K.; Jain, A. S. Novel Approaches in Nutraceuticals, Chapter 11. In *Enhancing the Therapeutic Efficacy of Herbal Formulations through Novel Drug Delivery Systems*; Kesharwani, R. K.; Keservani, R. K.; Sharma, A. K., IGI Global International Publisher: Pennsylvania, USA, 2020b; pp 241–266. ISBN13: 9781799844532.

Rane, B. R.; Patil, A. S.; Keservani, R. K.; Jain, A. S. Novel Approaches in Herbal Formulation, Chapter 2. In *Enhancing the Therapeutic Efficacy of Herbal Formulations through Novel Drug Delivery Systems*; Kesharwani, R. K.; Keservani, R. K.; Sharma, A. K., IGI Global International Publisher: Pennsylvania, USA, 2020a; pp 43–68. ISBN13: 9781799844532.

Rane, B. R.; Tadavi, S. A.; Keservani, R. K. Naturopathy, Chapter 12. In *Herbal Product Development*; Sharma, A. K., Keservani, R. K., Gautam, S. P., Apple Academic Press, CRC Press, Taylor & Francis Group, 2020c; pp 321–347. ISBN: 9781771888776.

Vang, O.; Ahmad, N.; Baile, C. A.; Baur, J. A.; Brown, K.; Csiszar, A.; Das, D. K.; Delmas, D.; Gottfried, C.; Lin, H. Y.; Ma, Q. Y.; Mukhopadhyay, P.; Nalini, N.; Pezzuto, J. M.; Richard, T.; Shukla, Y.; Surh, Y. J.; Szekeres, T.; Szkudelski, T.; Walle,T.; Wu, J. M. What is New for An Old Molecule? Systematic Review and Recommendations on the use of Resveratrol. *PloS One*, **2011**,*6* (6), 19881.

Schmeda-Hirschmann, G.; Quispe, C.; Soriano, M.; Theoduloz, C.; Jiménez-Aspée, F.; Pérez, M.; Cuello, A.; Isla, M. Chilean Prosopis Mesocarp Flour: Phenolic Profiling and Antioxidant Activity. *Molecules* **2015,** *20* (4), 7017–7033.

Selhub, E. M.; Logan, A. C.; Bested, A. C. Fermented Foods, Microbiota, and Mental Health: Ancient Practice Meets Nutritional Psychiatry. *J. Physiol. Anthropol.* **2014,** *33* (1).

Shamina, A. Food Colours of Plant Origin. *CABI Rev.* **2007,** *2* (087).

Sharma, A. K.; Keservani, R. K.; Gautam, S. P. In *Herbal Product Development*; Apple Academic Press, CRC Press, Taylor & Francis Group, 2020; pp 1–376. ISBN: 9781771888776.

Singh, P.; Kesharwani, R. K.; Keservani, R. K. Antioxidants and Vitamins: Roles in Cellular Function and Metabolism. In *Sustained Energy for Enhanced Human Functions and Activity*; Academic Press, 2017; pp 385–407. ISBN: 9780128054130.

Singh, P.; Paul, V.; Dubey, R. Antioxidant Foods. *Int. J. Adv. Agric. Sci. Technol.* **2022,** *9* (4), 1–7.

Steinbach, S.; Hundt, W.; Vaitl, A.; Heinrich, P.; Förster, S.; Bürger, K.; Zahnert, T. Taste in Mild Cognitive Impairment and Alzheimer's Disease. *J. Neurol.* **2010,** *257* (2), 238–246.

Walsh, K.; Scharf, T.; Keating, N. Social Exclusion of Older Persons: A Scoping Review and Conceptual Framework. *Euro. J. Ageing* **2016,** *14* (1), 81–98.

Watson, R. Influence of Harvest Date and Light Integral on the Development of Strawberry Flavour Compounds. *J. Exp. Bot.* **2002,** *53* (377), 2121–2129.

Weindruch, R. The Retardation of Aging by Caloric Restriction: Studies in Rodents and Primates. *Toxicol. Pathol.* **1996,** *24* (6), 742–745.

Wilson, D.; Keith, G.; Harpal, B.; Ram, S.; Meester Fabien, D.; Agnieszka, W.; Toru, T. Therapy through Social Medicine: Cultivating Connections and Inspiring Solutions for Healthy Living. *AIMS Med. Sci.* **2017,** *4* (2), 131–150.

Wilson, D.; Nash, P.; Buttar, H.; Griffiths, K.; Singh, R.; De Meester, F.; Horiuchi, R.; Takahashi, T. The Role of Food Antioxidants, Benefits of Functional Foods, and Influence of Feeding Habits on the Health of the Older Person: An Overview. *Antioxidants* **2017,** *6* (4), 81.

Wu, Z.; Yu, J.; Zhu, A.; Nakanishi, H. Nutrients, Microglia Aging, and Brain Aging. *Oxid. Med. Cell. Longev.* **2016,** *2016*, 1–9.

CHAPTER 10

ANTI-STRESS FUNCTIONAL FOODS

NEELESH KUMAR MAURYA[1], LATIKA YADAV[2], PRATIBHA ARYA[3], ABHIJEET AHER[4], and NAYAN A. GUJARATHI[4]

[1]*Department of Home Science, P.K. University Shivpuri, Shivpuri, Madhya Pradesh, India*

[2]*Government Degree College, Punwarka, Saharanpur, Uttar Pradesh, India*

[3]*Institute of Home Science, Bundelkhand University, Jhansi, Uttar Pradesh, India*

[4]*Shri Vile Parle Kelavani Mandal's Institute of Pharmacy, Dhule, Maharashtra, India*

ABSTRACT

Stress is any external or internal pressure that causes an organism to react. Stress aids in the survival of organisms by compelling them to adapt to frequently changing environmental conditions. Intense stress prompts the body's fight-or-flight reflex. The adrenal glands release catecholamines such as adrenaline, norepinephrine, and cortisol in response. These chemicals increase heart rate, increase cerebral oxygen delivery, increase muscle blood vessel dilation, and raise blood glucose levels. They can lead to difficulty concentrating, mood swings, anxiety, frustration, and anxiousness. Chronic stress affects the brain's structure and functions. Persistently high levels of cytokines and stress chemical mediators in the brain during a stress state may also damage the parenchyma and cause neuronal death, contributing to the previously noted anatomical changes in the brain associated with chronic stress. There is abundant scientific evidence demonstrating a clear

Antioxidants as Nutraceuticals. Nayan A. Gujarathi, Raj K. Keservani, Rajesh K. Kesharwani, Bhushan R. Rane, Yogeeta Sameer Goyal (Eds.)

association between stress and food. Nutrients in foods contribute to the regulation of neurotransmitters with calming and relaxing characteristics. Various foods that produce serotonin and dopamine include beans, fruits and vegetables, green tea, chamomile tea, and red wine. These foods also contain antioxidants, such as zinc, selenium, magnesium, omega-3 fatty acids, and vitamins C and E. These neurotransmitters and antioxidants, naturally produced in a variety of fruits and vegetables, cereals, nuts and seeds, and beverages, aid in stress reduction and are discussed in this chapter for the benefits of mental health.

10.1 INTRODUCTION

"Stress" is a situation that disrupts the balance of a living entity with its environment. Numerous stressful situations occur in daily life, such as work pressure, examinations, mental and physical stress caused by trauma, surgery, and different health problems (Shahrajabian et al., 2021). The World Health Organization (WHO) defines stress as "the reaction that individuals may have when confronted with expectations and pressures that are out of proportion to their knowledge and abilities and that put their ability to cope to the test." It is not a pathological condition. Stress is any situation that impacts and creates discomfort in emotional or physical terms. Stress is the body's response to anything that requires one's attention or action (Khan et al., 2020).

10.2 STRESS

There are two primary categories of stress:

1. Acute stress
2. Chronic stress

10.2.1 ACUTE STRESS

Acute stress disorder (ASD) is a mental health condition that can develop immediately following a traumatic event. It can cause a variety of psychotic symptoms, and if left untreated, can lead to post-traumatic stress disorder (PTSD). ASD and PTSD have a strong relationship. Some people develop PTSD because of having ASD (Lefebvre et al., 2020).

10.2.1.1 ASD SYMPTOMS

ASD symptoms are classified into five categories. The symptoms occur when a person is unable to stop reliving a traumatic experience in their mind through flashbacks, recollections, or nightmares. This can happen when the individual is unable to stop thinking about the event (Kalmakis et al., 2020; Violanti et al., 2018).

1. Negative mood: Negative ideas, sorrow, and an overall poor attitude are all things that are not impossible to experience (Violanti et al., 2018).
2. Symptoms of dissociation: These symptoms can include a distorted sense of reality, a loss of awareness of one's surroundings, and an inability to recall details of the traumatic experience (Lefebvre et al., 2020; Kalmakis et al., 2020).
3. Symptoms of avoidance: People who are affected by these symptoms make a conscious effort to steer clear of any thoughts, feelings, people, or locations that are connected to the traumatic event (Violanti et al., 2018).
4. Arousal symptoms: Insomnia and other sleep problems, difficulty concentrating, and anger or violent behavior, either verbal or physical, are also potential indicators. The person might also feel tense or on guard, and they might give off the impression that they are troubled (Lefebvre et al., 2020; Kalmakis et al., 2020).

   People with ASD are further prone to having other mental health problems, such as anxiety and depression.
5. Symptoms of anxiety: Common symptoms are a sense of impending doom, overwhelming anxiety, inability to concentrate, and feelings of hopelessness, fatigue, restlessness, and anxious thoughts (Lefebvre et al., 2020; Kalmakis et al., 2020).
6. Depression: Acute stress depression disorder arising due to acute stress. Symptoms include persistent feelings of hopelessness, melancholy, or lethargy; outbursts of crying; loss of concentration in previously pleasurable activities; changes in appetite or weight loss or gain; and thoughts of suicide, self-harm, or both (Lefebvre et al., 2020; Violanti et al., 2018; Forresi et al., 2022).

10.2.2 CHRONIC STRESS

The physiological or psychological response that is generated by an internal or external stressor that lasts for a prolonged period is referred to as chronic stress. The same effect will be produced by the stressor regardless of whether it is physically present or remembered; this will cause a chronic stress response to be triggered. Although there are a wide variety of things that can be considered chronic stressors, most of them involve relatively long-lasting issues, conflicts, and threats that people face daily. "Neighborhood environment," "financial strain," "interpersonal stress," "job stress," and "caregiving" are some of the chronic stressors that have been discovered to be connected with disease and mortality (Seo, 2021; Loman and Schuttelaar, 2022).

10.2.2.1 CHRONIC STRESS IMPACTS ON THE HUMAN BODY

Common hazards and psychological demands, such as work deadlines, exams, and athletic competitions, can all provoke a state of tension. The physical symptoms of stress do not usually last long. Some people, on the other hand, are on high alert almost all the time. This is chronic tension. Chronic stress is caused by prolonged, persistent stress that affects various parts of the body as well as the mind. These are discussed in the below subheading (Loman and Schuttelaar, 2022).

10.3 STRESS AND BRAIN FUNCTION COMPLICATIONS

According to the findings of previous research, prolonged exposure to stress has a variety of negative effects on brain function. It has been revealed to interfere with synapse control, which can lead to a decrease in sociability and an avoidance of contact with other people. Stress can cause the death of brain cells and even a diminution in the total volume of the brain (Marsh et al., 2022). When an individual is under prolonged stress, the prefrontal cortex, the area of the brain responsible for memory and learning, decreases. Hormones, on the other hand, have been shown to have physiologic impacts on several CNS regions as well as a role in behavior and cognition. The idea that the brains of rodents can react to glucocorticoids was first postulated by McEwen in 1968 (Lupien et al., 2022). After that, the idea that stress might cause changes to the CNS became widely acknowledged. During this time, glucocorticoid receptors and mineralocorticoids were discovered for the first time. In comparison to the affinity that mineralocorticoids have for cortisol and corticosterone, glucocorticosteroid receptors have a 10% lower affinity for these two hormones. Except for the hippocampus, most of the receptors in the brain are glucocorticosteroid receptors.

It has been discovered that stress has several negative effects on the nervous system, one of which is the induction of structural changes in a variety of brain regions. Both losses of weight and brain tissue can be caused by stress. Structural alterations can affect a person's stress response as well as cognition and memory. The extent and severity of the changes, however, are influenced by the length and amount of stress. An altered brain structure can be the result of chronic stress, which can harm the nervous system. Therefore, it is extremely important to investigate the effects of stress on the nervous system (Lupien et al., 2022; de Kolet, 2022).

10.3.1 DESTRUCTIVE EFFECTS OF STRESS ON CNS FUNCTION

The CNS has both short-term and long-term memories. The frontal and parietal lobes govern short-term memory, while wide brain areas control long-term memory. The hippocampus has the most glucocorticosteroid receptors and the strongest stress response. Stress affects memory, according to research. The hippocampus's structure and function are altered by stress. Atrophic ankles, brain, neurogenesis abnormalities, and shrinking neurons and synapses change neuronal metabolism, hippocampal cell sensitivity to amino acids, or extracellular glutamate levels (Kim et al., 2015). Trauma and stress hormones affect memory. Stress causes hippocampal shrinkage and spatial memory loss in mice. High levels of glucocorticosteroids can cause memory loss and hippocampal atrophy. Hippocampal atrophy and memory problems occur in people with Cushing's disease (increased glucocorticoid secretion) or who take high doses of synthetic anti-inflammatory medicines. Per MRI, PTSD patients showed smaller hippocampi and lower verbal memory. Prolonged stress diminishes memory, but less stress increases memory. Stress is a significant barrier to learning.

Memory isn't always impaired by stress. Certain types of stress may boost memory. Imposed stimulation includes unfamiliarity, unpredictability, and life-threatening features. Temporarily, stress can increase brain function and memory. In some cases, stress improves memory. A written exam can temporarily boost memory, for example. This is connected to decreased cortisol in the saliva. Predicting stress can boost or hinder memory power. Stress and glucocorticoids increase animal and human memory. Learning and memory require glucocorticoids, not mineralocorticoids. Memory tests with stress or glucocorticoid injections damage humans and animals (Daskalakis et al., 2022).

10.3.2 STRESS AFFECTS COGNITION AND LEARNING

One form of mental activity is called cognition. Learning, making decisions, paying attention, and having good judgment are all components of cognition. Alterations in cognition brought on by stress are impacted by a wide variety of factors. Memory is formed in the brain via the amygdala and the temporal lobe. The alleviation of stress has a beneficial effect, in general, on the functioning of cognitive systems. Some of the physiological systems, such as the hypothalamus-pituitary-adrenal axis, the central neurotransmitter and neuropeptide systems, and the autonomic nervous system, are activated by stress, which in turn affects the neuronal circuits that are involved in the processing of data (Yaribeygi et al., 2017; Roustazade et al., 2022). The production and discharge of glucocorticoids are both triggered by stress. Glucocorticoids are lipophilic and can cross the blood-brain barrier; they have an impact on both short-term and long-term processing and cognition. It would appear that disorders in behavior, cognition, and mood are caused in the brain by stress. This is quite similar to what is found in people who suffer from depression and other mood disorders in addition to having cognitive issues. There is a connection, at a physiological level, between the effects of stress and mood-based cognitive impairments. There is a possibility that disruptions in these neuroendocrine, neuroamine, and neurodegenerative pathways are responsible for the stress-induced cognitive abnormalities in mice. It is critical to understand that depression is not always caused by an overactive physiological stress response. Catecholamines and glucocorticoids affect cognitive performance in both acute and chronic stress. Steroids alter gene expression, resulting in long-term effects, whereas adrenaline has only short-term effects. The cognitive decline caused by stress can be mitigated in a variety of different ways (Yaribeygi et al., 2017; Roustazade et al., 2022).

10.4 STRESS AFFECTS THE GASTROINTESTINAL SYSTEM

Stress delays digestion, slows stomach emptying, and accelerates colonic motility. Stress increases the large intestine's contraction and motility. Previous research demonstrates that CRH improves terminal GI tract mobility while decreasing proximal mobility. Corticotropin-releasing hormone 2 (CRH-2) receptors delay stomach emptying, while CRH-1 receptors affect the colon. CRH is a promising treatment for irritable bowel syndrome (IBS). Stress-induced serotonin increases colon motility. Stress on the mind and emotions both raise the sensitivity of the gut and activate mast cells in the mucosa. Stress stimulates the CNS, altering GI tract motility. Stress impacts the brain-intestinal axis. Studies relate stress to IBS, intestinal inflammation, and peptic ulcers. Intestinal bacteria numbers rise during GI stress (Yaribeygi et al., 2017; Sun et al., 2019).

10.5 STRESS AFFECTS THE RESPIRATORY SYSTEM

The respiratory system oxygenates cells and eliminates CO_2 waste. The air that humans breathe in travels from the nasal cavity, down the trachea, and into the bronchi. Bronchioles circulate oxygen to red blood cells. Stress and intense emotions can cause shortness of breath and fast breathing as the nasal-pulmonary airway constricts. Psychological stressors can exacerbate breathing problems for people with preexisting respiratory disorders like asthma and chronic obstructive pulmonary disease (COPD), which includes emphysema and chronic bronchitis. Acute stress has been shown in trials to precipitate asthma attacks. Stress-induced hyperventilation can trigger a panic attack in someone prone to it. Relaxation, breathing, and other cognitive behavioral approaches can be beneficial (Yaribeygi et al., 2017; Wiegman et al., 2020).

10.6 STRESS AFFECTS THE CARDIOVASCULAR SYSTEM

Organs are nourished and oxygenated by the heart and arteries. In the body's stress reaction, these two parts work together. Momentary or short-term stress, such as meeting deadlines, being trapped in traffic, or slamming on the brakes to prevent an accident, produces an increase in heart rate and greater heart muscle contractions. Adrenaline, noradrenaline, and cortisol act as messengers for these effects. The body recovers from these types of stresses. Long-term stress can damage the heart and blood vessels. High heart rate, stress hormones, and blood pressure are harmful. Stress causes hypertension, heart attacks, and strokes. Stress can cause inflammation in the circulatory system, especially in the coronary arteries. This may cause stress-related heart attacks. Stress can affect cholesterol levels (Yaribeygi et al., 2017; Daiber et al., 2019).

10.7 STRESS AFFECTS THE REPRODUCTIVE SYSTEM

Nerves affect the male reproductive system. Parasympathetic nerves rest while sympathetic nerves are stimulated. In male anatomy, the fight-or-flight response synthesizes testosterone and activates the sympathetic nervous system, causing arousal. Stress stimulates the adrenal glands to produce cortisol. Cortisol regulates blood pressure and normalizes the cardiovascular, circulatory, and reproductive systems. Excess cortisol can damage male reproductive biochemistry. Symptoms affect sexual desire (Yaribeygi et al., 2017). Chronic stress can cause a loss of sexual desire, or libido, and erectile dysfunction, or impotence. The reproduction system is also affected. Chronic stress can affect sperm production and maturation, resulting in infertility. Men who had two or more stressful life events in the past year reported decreased sperm motility and morphology. Infertility stress can weaken the immune system, causing illness. Testes, prostate, and urethra infections can impact male reproductive health (Hamed, 2018).

Stress can impact adolescent and adult women's menstruation. Stress can cause absent or irregular menstrual cycles, more painful periods, and cycle duration variations. Continuously, women accomplish personal, family, professional, and financial obligations. Stress, distraction, weariness, etc. can decrease sexual desire, especially for women having early childhood or sick family members, having chronic medical problems, feeling unhappy, experiencing relationship problems, etc. Stress affects a woman's fertility. Stress can affect a woman's fertility, pregnancy, and postpartum adjustment. Pregnancy and postpartum depression are common. Stress during this time causes melancholy and anxiety. Maternal stress can harm prenatal and toddler development and hinder postpartum bonding. Premenstrual symptoms can be distressing, and stress might worsen them. Cramps, fluid retention, bloating, irritability, and mood changes are the symptoms. Hormone levels fluctuate as menopause approaches. This causes anxiety, mood fluctuations, and misery. Menopause can be stressful. Menopause's physical changes, notably hot flushes, can be challenging. Stress might worsen physical issues. Anxious women may have more and/or more severe hot flashes (Gu et al., 2018).

10.8 ROLE OF DIETARY NEUROTRANSMITTERS IN STRESS

Nutrients and dietary supplements help to maintain the health of the human neurological system because dietary phytochemicals are enriched with phytochemicals. These phytochemicals include precursors to neurotransmitters (NTs), such as acetylcholine (ACh), glutamate, and gamma-aminobutyric acid (GABA), as well as biogenic amines such as dopamine, serotonin (5-HT), and histamine. The increasing use of dietary methods in neuropsychiatry has made it necessary to identify dietary neurotransmitters (NTs). Naturally, food is a source of Ach, glutamate, GABA, dopamine, 5-HT, and histamine, as researched in PubMed and Scopus. Meat and dairy, fruits, plants, roots, and phytochemicals contain NTs. These biologically active molecules may exist in nature as a result of metabolic processes and environmental influences, or they may be the result of regulated or uncontrolled activity involving food technology (Table 10.1) (Briguglio et al., 2018).

TABLE 10.1 Dietary Neurotransmitters and Their Food Sources.

Dietary neurotransmitter	Foods and botanicals sources
Acetylcholine	Aubergine, bitter orange, common bean, foxglove, mistletoe, mung bean, nettle species, pea, radish, spinach, squash, and wild strawberry
Glutamate	Caviar, cheese, crackling, chips, dried cod, fermented beans, fish sauces, gravies, instant coffee powder, meats, miso, mushrooms, noodle dishes, oyster sauce, Parmesan cheese, ready-to-eat meals, salami, savory snacks, seafood, seaweeds, soups, soy sauces, spinach, stews, tomato, and tomato sauce
GABA	Adzuki bean, barley, broccoli, buckwheat, chestnut, common bean, kale, lupine, maypop, mouse-ear hawkweed, oat, pea, pokeroot, potato, rice, shiitake, soybean, spinach, St John's wort, sweet potato, tea, tomato, valerian, wheat, and wild celery
Dopamine	Aubergine, avocado, banana, common bean, apple, orange, pea, plantain, spinach, tomato, and velvet bean
Serotonin	Bananas, chicory, Chinese cabbage, coffee powders, green coffee bean, green onion, hazelnut, kiwi, lettuce, nettle, *Griffonia simplicifolia*, paprika, passion fruit, pawpaw, pepper, pineapple, plantain, plum, pomegranate, potato, spinach, strawberry, tomato, velvet bean, and wild rice
Histamine	Anchovy, beer, billfish, Champagne and Sherry, dandelion, fermented sausages, ham and other cured dry meat products, herring, ketchup, aged cheeses, nettle, red, white, and dessert wines, sardine, sauerkraut, Scomberesocidae (e.g., sauries), Scombridae (e.g., tuna, mackerel, and bonitos), soybean food products (e.g., soy, tempeh, soy sauce, soybean milk, doenjang, doufu, and nattō), sweet or sour cream, UHT, pasteurized and fresh milk, and yogurt

Source: Briguglio et al., 2018; Zhang et al., 2022.

10.9 FUNCTIONAL AND NUTRACEUTICAL FOODS AND BRAIN HEALTH

10.9.1 FRUITS

For cognitive wellness, fruits and vegetables were consumed. Wang et al. (2022) published research on the therapeutic benefits of fruits. Consuming citrus fruits and blueberries, which are high in vitamin C and polyphenols, has been linked to improved mental function (Briguglio et al., 2018). In the sections that follow, we'll talk in more depth about some of the fruits in the list (Table 10.2).

TABLE 10.2 Various Phytoconstituents Present in Fruits that Function as Anti-Stress Agents.

Fruits	Phytochemical compounds
Strawberries	Kaempferol, fisetin, matairesinol, secoisolariciresinol, gallic acid, ellagic acid, and chlorogenic acid
Blackberries	Ellagic acid
Blueberries	Chlorogenic acid, secoisolariciresinol, and pterostilbene
Raspberries	Ellagic acid, quercetin, gallic acid, cyanidins, pelargonidins, catechins, kaempferol, and salicylic acid
Plum	Lutein and cyaniding
Prunes	Lutein and ursolic acid
Cherries	Limonene
Oranges	Rutin and lutein
Red grapes	Proanthocyanidins
Pomegranates	Ellagitannins, delphinidin, cyanidin, pelargonidin glycosides, catechins, gallocatechins, and prodelphinidins
Green and chamomile tea	Theanine and epigallocatechin-3-gallate (EGCG)

Source: Keservani et al., 2016.

10.9.2 BERRIES

Berries are high in antioxidants, which have numerous health benefits. Berries such as raspberries, strawberries, and even blackberries are good sources of vitamin C, which can help with stress management. Blackberries are abundant in fiber and vitamins C and K. Blackberries contain soluble fiber. One cup (144 g) of blackberries has half the daily vitamin C and fiber recommendations. Red and blackberries' high polyphenol and anthocyanin contents have health benefits (also known as phytochemicals). Blueberries, strawberries, blackberries, and other berry fruits can help prevent age-related memory loss. The berries have antioxidant and anti-inflammatory neuroactive substances. Berries provide the most antioxidants (polyphenols, carotenoids, and vitamin C) (Briguglio et al., 2018). Berry species, cultivars, and growth circumstances affect total polyphenol concentration. Black currant, raspberry, and strawberry are high in polyphenols. Natural polyphenols in berries help improve memory, learning, and cognition. According to preclinical studies, flavonoids may counteract age-related impairments in memory and learning. Beneficial effects include avoiding ischemia and neurodegenerative illnesses; lowering neuronal apoptosis; and increasing memory, learning, and cognitive skills (Higbee et al., 2022).

10.9.3 BLUEBERRIES

Blueberries are *Vaccinium* perennials with indigo berries (gooseberries, bilberries, and cranberries are all members of the genus *Vaccinium*). Blueberries are 84% water, 9.7% carbohydrates, 0.6% protein, and 0.4% fat. Blueberries give 192 kJ per 100 g. Blueberries have 3–3.5% dietary fiber. 100 g of blueberries provides 10 mg of ascorbic acid, or 1/3 of the daily recommended consumption (Keservani et al., 2016). Blueberry anthocyanins and cocoa flavanols boost memory, especially in the elderly, according to recent studies. Long-term (3 months) blueberry juice supplementation improved working memory and reduced depressive symptoms. Rich in flavonoids, fruit liquids, especially blueberry juice, increased short-term cognitive action in geriatric trials. Anthocyanidins in berries can penetrate the blood-brain barrier and concentrate on learning and memory (Tran and Tran, 2021).

10.9.4 STRAWBERRIES

A strawberry is the edible fruit of numerous plant species in the *Rubus* genus of the rose family, the majority of which are in the subgenus *Idaeobatus*. *R. idaeus* and *R. strigosus* hybrids are commercially grown for red raspberry. Purple raspberries are a horticultural hybrid of red and black raspberries that occur wild in Vermont. Prince Edward County, Ontario, is known for blue raspberry farming. Red raspberries were crossed with the loganberry, another *Rubus* species. Boysenberry and tayberry are hybrids. Red raspberries and Asiatic *Rubus* have also been hybridized. Quercetin, gallic acid, catechins, kaempferol, and salicylic acid are all found in blueberries. Yellow fruits lack anthocyanins. Red raspberries have anthocyanins covering their carotenoids (Keservani et al., 2016).

Strawberries' neuroprotective efficacy was investigated in vitro on PC12 cells treated with H_2O_2 due to their high phytochemical and antioxidant content. Their preventive effects and antioxidant capacity were compared to those of bananas and oranges, the most popular US fruits. Inhibition of oxidative stress-induced neurotoxicity in the MTT cell viability experiment, because oxidative stress increases neuronal cell membrane disintegration, LDH and trypan blue exclusion experiments were also performed. Strawberries had the most cell protection; strawberry > banana > orange in three trials for neural cell protection. Strawberry anthocyanins seemed to be the leading factor in their protective effects (Keservani et al., 2016).

10.9.5 ORANGES

Oranges account for 75% of all cultivated citrus fruits. Iran grows a lot of "Queen" oranges (*Citrus sinensis* (L.) Osb). Mid-season, red, high dissolved solids, flavored, seedless, and bears fruit on the tree vigorously. The tree is hardy, productive, and resistant to cold. 100 g of orange pulp provides roughly 64% of the daily vitamin C requirement. Plentiful quantities of extra-essential nutrients like carotenoids (lutein, beta-carotene, and beta-cryptoxanthin), flavonoids (naringenin), and volatile organic compounds (alcohols, aldehydes, esters, terpenes, and ketones) are among the phytochemicals found in an orange. It is crucial to get a better understanding of the role that flavanone-rich foods and beverages play in the progression of cognitive decline and aging. Folate (folic acid) is found in spinach, orange juice, and yeast. Following vitamin B absorption in the intestine, the liver produces various types of folate. A lack of dietary folate causes many physiological anomalies throughout development and maturation. Folate deficiency is linked to several neurological problems, such as depression and memory loss.

10.9.6 PLUMS

The plum belongs to the subgenus *Prunus*. The fruit contains a furrow and a pit. Plums are rich in flavonoids, notably anthocyanins, and may be an antioxidant source. Old rats with dementia benefit from plum juice. Plums maintained spatial learning against radiation-induced oxidative damage. Plum protects against radiation-induced metabolic problems and improves spatial learning. Plum-exposed mice were faster to reach the colored platform in the water tank (a proxy for spatial learning and memory) (Keservani et al., 2016). Kao-Ting et al. (2013) examined the effects of 2-month plum consumption on cognitive function and brain neurodegeneration-related protein in diabetic rats. The plum-supplemented diet improved spatial memory and learning using the Morris water maze. Alzheimer's-related beta-amyloid was also reduced.

10.9.7 PRUNES

Prunes are dried plums (*Prunus domestica* or European plum). Except for types developed for drying, the word is obsolete for fresh fruit. Prunes are a nutritious food since they include significant amounts of carbohydrates, vitamins, and minerals. Prunes and their products have therapeutic value. Dietary fiber and carbohydrates are important nutrients in prunes. Vitamin A, vitamin B-complex, and vitamin K are among the important elements in prunes. The soluble portion (80%) is made up of pectin, hemicellulose, cellulose, and lignin. Drying increases total dietary fibers. Anxiolytic effects of chlorogenic acid (20 mg/kg) have been shown in anxiety-prone mice, possibly via benzodiazepine receptor activation. The function of oxidative stress in anxiety etiology has recently been discovered. Prunes' chlorogenic acid and antioxidant contents are beneficial for anxiety ailments (Keservani et al., 2016).

10.9.8 RED GRAPES

Grape phytochemicals, including resveratrol (a polyphenol), have been shown to inhibit degenerative neurological disease, viral infections, cancer, heart disease, and Alzheimer's disease. Resveratrol's antioxidant action protects the genome. In clinical trial studies, resveratrol is transcriptionally linked to calorie reduction in the heart, skeletal muscle, and brain. The grape is one of the fruits that is consumed the most frequently. It has several biological functions due to its high polyphenol content, which is found in its seeds (60–70%) and skin (30%). In vitro, grape seed polyphenols may protect DNA from oxidative damage (Keservani et al., 2016). In clinical trials, proanthocyanidins greatly enhanced spatial memory, prevented the formation of amyloid precursor protein and tau protein pathology, and decreased presenilin-1 mRNA expression levels, thereby reducing oxidative stress. A biosynthetic brain-targeted proanthocyanidin metabolite called 3′-O-Me-EC-Gluc at a physiologically appropriate concentration can increase basal synaptic transmission and lipid transfer protein by activating cAMP response element-binding protein signaling. This is important for memory and learning in Alzheimer's disease, which is caused by a buildup of plaques in the brain (Unusan, 2020).

10.9.9 POMEGRANATES

The best pomegranates were cultivated in Carthage, which was given the genus *Punica* (the Roman name). Pomegranates are 5–8 m (16–26 ft) deciduous shrubs or trees. Pomegranate seeds contain dietary fiber (20% dry volume (DV)). Rejecting seeds wastes fiber and micronutrients. The pomegranate seed oil contains 65.3% punicic acid, 4.8% palmitic acid, 2.3% stearic acid, 6.3% oleic acid, and 6.6% linoleic acid. Pomegranate juice contains ellagitannins, which are formed when ellagic and/or gallic acids bond with a carbohydrate (Keservani et al., 2016). Pomegranate polyphenols showed neuroprotective properties in an Alzheimer's disease animal model. These results suggest that pomegranate juice is neuroprotective as it reduces soluble amyloid-beta deposition and hippocampus amyloid buildup in transgenic Alzheimer's-like mice. The mice also learned more quickly and swam faster than control animals (Ticinesi et al., 2022).

10.10 OTHER FUNCTIONAL FOODS FOR COGNITIVE AND BRAIN HEALTH

10.10.1 BEANS

Beans are high in protein and fiber, both of which aid in keeping blood sugar levels constant and consistent. Beans are high in folate and assist in reducing blood sugar spikes and falls, which can have an impact on our mood. Folate helps produce blood cells, DNA, and RNA and metabolize proteins (Briguglio et al., 2018; Sun et al., 2022). Garbanzo beans (commonly known as chickpeas) are extremely high in folate, providing more than 100% of the daily required dose in just a half cup. Pinto beans are another great choice. A half-cup serving gives you 37% of the folate you need for the day (Sulekha, 2022).

10.10.2 SEEDS

Flax (*Linum usitatissimum*, Linaceae family) is grown in more than 50 countries, with Canada leading the way. Flaxseed is now widely used in diet and disease research due to its health benefits and disease prevention properties. The main constituent of flaxseed (36–40%) is oil, while linolenic acid (LNA) (57%) is the main constituent of flaxseed oil. Flaxseed contains 30% fiber and 20% protein, and it is high in phenolic compounds known as lignans, which are responsible for its antioxidant activity. Furthermore, flaxseed has been linked to increased nutritional value by increasing omega-3 fatty acid concentrations in a variety of animals and foods, including fish, ruminants, and dairy goats. Because of their reported benefits in cardiovascular disease, cancer, neurological, and hormonal disorders, as well as their antioxidant activities, chia, perilla, and flaxseeds have grown in popularity as functional foods. Chia (*Salvia hispanica* L., Labiatae) is a plant native to Mexico and Guatemala. Some seeds contain more protein (19–23%) than traditional crops such as wheat, corn, rice, oats, barley, and amaranth. The residual meal from the extraction of the chia seed oil is high in dietary fiber and phenolic compounds with antioxidant properties. Chia seeds contain 25–38% oil and the highest known percentage of alpha-linolenic fatty acid (LNA, 18:3n-3), at around 60% (Didinger et al., 2022).

10.10.3 PROBIOTICS

Probiotics help improve gut health. They may also indirectly improve the functioning of the brain. The connection between the gut and the brain is referred to as the gut-brain axis, and it has been demonstrated by research. Both the enteric nervous system, which is located in the digestive tract, and the central nervous system are connected by biochemical signaling. The vagus nerve, which is the longest nerve in the body, acts as the principal information connection between the brain and the gastrointestinal tract. Because it produces many of the same neurotransmitters that the brain does, including serotonin, dopamine, and gamma-aminobutyric acid, the stomach has been referred to as a "second brain." These neurotransmitters all play an important part in the regulation of mood. It is believed that the digestive tract is responsible for the production of 90% of serotonin. Kimchi, kombucha, miso, sauerkraut, tofu, tempeh, and yogurt are some examples of foods that contain probiotics (Sun et al., 2022).

10.10.4 NOOTROPIC AND ADAPTOGENIC (ANTI-STRESS ACTIVITY) HERBS

An adaptogen is a herb that aids the body in adapting to stress. Adaptogens lower cortisol levels, reducing stress, weariness, and restlessness. These supplements are thought to boost brainpower. The most widely used and researched adaptogen appears to be *Withania somnifera*, followed by

Eleutherococcus senticosus and *Panax ginseng*. The adaptogen *Schisandra chinensis* is widely used in traditional Chinese medicine (TCM). Some herbs that are being studied for their adaptogenic effects are *Centella asiatica*, *Glycyrrhiza glabra*, *Bacopa monniera*, and *Rhodiola rosea* (Satapathy et al., 2022).

10.10.5 RED WINE AND RESVERATROL

Resveratrol is a phytonutrient found in the skin and seeds of grapes and berries. While resveratrol has been shown to have antidepressant properties, its link to phosphodiesterase 4, an enzyme influenced by the stress hormone cortisol, is unclear. Resveratrol also has neuroprotective properties due to its antioxidant and NO-promoting properties in gerbils. Wang et al. (2022) revealed that resveratrol diminished cerebral microglial activation and delayed neuronal cell death (Vejarano et al., 2022). In previous clinical trials, resveratrol was found to raise baseline levels of adenosine and inosine, prevent hypoxanthine and xanthine elevations, lower xanthine oxidase activity, and lower levels of an oxidative biomarker called 8-isoprostane. According to the study, resveratrol's cerebroprotective effect is mediated by its antioxidative and anti-inflammatory properties. In brain I/R injury, resveratrol therapy reduced oxidative stress and inflammatory markers such as isoprostane, TNF-, IL-6, MPO, and ICAM-1. Antioxidant and anti-inflammatory markers such as superoxide dismutase, catalase, and IL-10 were increased. Resveratrol inhibited astroglial and microglial activation by inhibiting NF-B and JNK activation and decreasing iNOS and COX-2 production. According to a recent study, intracortical resveratrol reduces rat cortex infarct volume. Infusions of resveratrol, estrogen receptor (ER), and ER antagonists inhibited this neuroprotective effect (Vejarano et al., 2022; Li et al., 2022).

10.11 MEGADOSAGES STRESS THERAPY

Adequate amounts of vitamins and minerals are essential for several physical functions that have direct (e.g., neurotransmitter synthesis) and indirect (e.g., energy metabolism and cerebral blood supply) impacts on brain function (Aller, 2005). Vitamin consumption and cognitive performance are unsurprising. The megavitamin treatment uses vitamin doses several times the recommended dietary allowance (RDA) to prevent or treat disease.

Megavitamin treatment is utilized by producing good-quality medicine professionals (Lesperance et al., 2022). Vitamins are important in preventing and treating illnesses related to dietary vitamin deficiencies. However, medical research concludes that promoters of megavitamin therapy make unproven promises of disease treatment and advise taking them for a short period. Thiamine, which is a type of vitamin B1, is a cofactor that is needed to make the memory and learning neurotransmitters, GABA and acetylcholine. Additionally, it enhances the immune system, aids in blood sugar regulation, and increases the body's ability to resist stressful situations. Since vitamin B3 (niacin) is required for the generation of stress hormones, the body's supply diminishes during times of stress. Niacin also acts as an anti-inflammatory. When brain cells are inflamed, they can't make energy, which can cause stress, anxiety, brain fog, mental fatigue, and depression. Stress is the main cause of inflammation that lasts for a long time all over the body, and this is not a coincidence. Vitamin B5 (pantothenic acid) is required for the adrenal glands to produce stress hormones. Thus, stressful conditions deplete pantothenic acid's availability for its other functions, including the conversion of food to energy and the maintenance of a healthy neurological system. Five vitamins are often used to help with anxiety and stress. These vitamins include B-complex, vitamin E, vitamin C, GABA, and 5-HTTP (Kennedy, 2016).

10.12 CONCLUSION

Diets impact the brain, according to previous studies. A poor diet might make mood disorders like anxiety and depression worse, and a diet enriched in vegetables, fruits, and essential oils, such as the Mediterranean diet, may reduce anxiety and depression. Food can affect hormone production and secretion through neural responses and the gastrointestinal tract. The fundamental purpose of food is to provide energy and healing, and its secondary effect is to stimulate metabolites and hormones to circulate in the body. Having healthier fruits and vegetables helps improve their brain functions well. Phytochemicals can reduce disease's devastating effects by reducing oxidative stress and other processes. Dietary variables affect neuronal processing and activity, which explains how nutrition maintains brain health and mental activity. More research is necessary to confirm how phytoconstituents improve depression. Previous research on dietary components and phytochemicals' beneficial properties nowadays manufactures and markets nutraceuticals as dietary supplements containing high amounts of nutrients known as megadoses. Nutraceutical manufacturers promote megadose therapy for prevention and treatment. It is imperative that the efficacy of medications and the molecular underpinnings of their curative abilities be determined through meticulous investigation. This can be done with evidence-based medicines that can include the molecular basis of herbs' pharmacodynamics and pharmacokinetics.

CONFLICTS OF INTEREST

The authors declare that there is no conflict of interest regarding the publication of this chapter.

ACKNOWLEDGMENTS

We would like to thank Dr. Pratibha Arya for her assistance in the submission of this chapter compilation.

KEYWORDS

- **stress**
- **neurotransmitters**
- **antioxidants**
- **fruits**
- **vegetables**
- **green tea**
- **red wine**

REFERENCES

Briguglio, M.; Dell'Osso, B.; Panzica, G.; Malgaroli, A.; Banfi, G.; Zanaboni Dina, C.; Galentino, R.; Porta, M. Dietary Neurotransmitters: A Narrative Review on Current Knowledge. *Nutrients* **2018,** *10*, 591.

Daiber, A.; Kröller-Schön, S.; Frenis, K.; Oelze, M.; Kalinovic, S.; Vujacic-Mirski, K.; Kuntic, M.; Bayo Jimenez, M.T.; Helmstädter, J.; Steven, S.; et al. Environmental Noise Induces the

Release of Stress Hormones and Inflammatory Signaling Molecules Leading to Oxidative Stress and Vascular Dysfunction—Signatures of the Internal Exposome. *BioFactors* **2019,** *45* (4), 495–506.

Daskalakis, N. P.; Meijer, O. C.; de Kloet, E. R. Mineralocorticoid Receptor and Glucocorticoid Receptor Work Alone and Together in Cell-Type-Specific Manner: Implications for Resilience Prediction and Targeted Therapy. *Neurobiol. Stress* **2022,** *18*, 100455.

de Kloet, E. R. Brain Mineralocorticoid and Glucocorticoid Receptor Balance in Neuroendocrine Regulation and Stress-Related Psychiatric Etiopathologies. *Curr. Opin. Endocr. Metab. Res.* **2022,** *24*, 100352.

Didinger, C.; Foster, M. T.; Bunning, M.; Thompson, H. J. Nutrition and Human Health Benefits of Dry Beans and Other Pulses. In *Dry Beans and Pulses*; Wiley, 2022; pp. 481–504.

Fan, X.; Zhao, Z.; Huang, Z.; Wu, M.; Wang, D.; Xiao, J. Mineralocorticoid Receptor Agonist Aldosterone Rescues Hippocampal Neural Stem Cell Proliferation Defects and Improves Postoperative Cognitive Function in Aged Mice. *World J. Biol. Psychiatry.* **2023,** *24*, 149–161.

Forresi, B.; Michelini, G.; Sapuppo, W.; Costa, G.; Castellini, G.; Livellara, S.; Gregori Grgič, R. Anger, Personality Traits and Psychopathological Symptoms in Subjects Exposed to Negative Interpersonal Actions in Workplaces: An Observational Study in a Large Sample Attending a Center for Occupational Stress. *Int. Arch. Occup. Environ. Health* **2022,** *95*, 1763–1773.

Gu, S.; Jing, L.; Li, Y.; Huang, J. H.; Wang, F. Stress Induced Hormone and Neuromodulator Changes in Menopausal Depressive Rats. *Front. Psychiatry* **2018,** *9*, 253.

Hamed, S. A. Sexual Dysfunctions Induced by Pregabalin. *Clin. Neuropharmacol.* **2018,** *41*, 116–122.

Higbee, J.; Solverson, P.; Zhu, M.; and Carbonero, F. The Emerging Role of Dark Berry Polyphenols in Human Health and Nutrition. *Food Front.* **2022,** *3*, 3–27.

Jürg, H. Vitamins and Brain Function. In *Nutritional Neuroscience*; Lieberman H. R., Kanarek, R. B., Prasad, C., Eds.; CRC Press: Boca Raton, FL, 2005.

Kalmakis, K. A.; Chiodo, L. M.; Kent, N.; Meyer, J. S. Adverse Childhood Experiences, Post-Traumatic Stress Disorder Symptoms, and Self-Reported Stress Among Traditional and Nontraditional College Students. *J. Am. College Health* **2020,** *68*, 411–418.

Kennedy, D. B Vitamins and the Brain: Mechanisms, Dose and Efficacy—A Review. *Nutrients* **2016,** *8*, 68.

Keservani, R. K.; Sharma, A. K.; Kesharwani, R. K. Medicinal Effect of Nutraceutical Fruits for the Cognition and Brain Health. *Scientifica* **2016,** *2016*, 1–10.

Khan, K. S.; Mamun, M. A.; Griffiths, M. D.; Ullah, I. The Mental Health Impact of the COVID-19 Pandemic Across Different Cohorts. *Int. J. Ment. Health Addict.* **2022,** *20*, 380–386.

Kim, E. J.; Pellman, B.; Kim, J. J. Stress Effects on the Hippocampus: A Critical Review. *Learn. Memory* **2015,** *22*, 411–416.

Lefebvre, C.; Fortin, C.; Guay, S. Quality of Life After Violent Crime: The Impact of Acute Stress Disorder, Posttraumatic Stress Disorder, and Other Consequences. *J. Trauma. Stress* **2021,** *34*, 526–537.

Lesperance, M. L.; Olivotto, I. A.; Forde, N.; Zhao, Y.; Speers, C.; Foster, H.; Tsao, M.; MacPherson, N.; Hoffer, A. Mega-Dose Vitamins and Minerals in the Treatment of

Non-Metastatic Breast Cancer: An Historical Cohort Study. *Breast Cancer Res. Treat.* **2002,** *76*, 137–143.

Li, R.; Li, E.; Kamili, G.; Ou, S.; Yang, D. Effect of Resveratrol on Superovulation in Mice. *Biomed. Pharmacother.* **2022,** *146*, 112565.

Loman, L.; Schuttelaar, M. L. A. Hand Eczema and Lifestyle Factors in the Dutch General Population: Evidence for Smoking, Chronic Stress, and Obesity. *Contact Dermatitis* **2022,** *86*, 80–88.

Lupien, S. J.; Leclaire, S.; Majeur, D.; Raymond, C.; Jean Baptiste, F.; Giguère, C. E. 'Doctor, I am so Stressed Out!' A Descriptive Study of Biological, Psychological, and Socioemotional Markers of Stress in Individuals Who Self-Identify as Being 'Very Stressed Out' or 'Zen'. *Neurobiol. Stress* **2022,** *18*, 100454.

Marsh, S. E.; Walker, A. J.; Kamath, T.; Dissing-Olesen, L.; Hammond, T. R.; de Soysa, T. Y.; Young, A. M. H.; Murphy, S.; Abdulraouf, A.; Nadaf, N.; et al. Dissection of Artifactual and Confounding Glial Signatures by Single-Cell Sequencing of Mouse and Human Brain. *Nat. Neurosci.* **2022,** *25*, 306–316.

Roustazade, R.; Radahmadi, M.; Yazdani, Y. Therapeutic Effects of Saffron Extract on Different Memory Types, Anxiety, and Hippocampal BDNF and TNF-α Gene Expressions in Sub-Chronically Stressed Rats. *Nutr. Neurosci.* **2022,** *25*, 192–206.

Satapathy, D. K.; Pattnaik, G.; Tripathy, S. Rational of Medicinal Ghrita on Treatment of CNS Disorders. *Syst. Rev. Pharm.* **2022,** *13*, 79–82.

Seo, W. S. An Update on the Cause and Treatment of Sleep Disturbance in Children and Adolescents with Autism Spectrum Disorder. *Yeungnam Univ. J. Med.* **2021,** *38*, 275–281.

Shahrajabian, M. H.; Sun, W.; Soleymani, A.; Cheng, Q. Traditional Herbal Medicines to Overcome Stress, Anxiety and Improve Mental Health in Outbreaks of Human Coronaviruses. *Phytother. Res.* **2021,** *35*, 1237–1247.

Sulekha, S. M. P. Traditional Siddha Approach to Treatment of Cognitive Impairment in Menopause. *Curr. Pharmacol. Rep.* **2022,** *8*, 312–320.

Sun, Y.; Li, L.; Xie, R.; Wang, B.; Jiang, K.; Cao, H. Stress Triggers Flare of Inflammatory Bowel Disease in Children and Adults. *Front. Pediatr.* **2019**, *7*, 432.

Sun, H.; Zhao, F.; Liu, Y.; Ma, T.; Jin, H.; Quan, K.; Leng, B.; Zhao, J.; Yuan, X.; Li, Z.; et al. Probiotics Synergized with Conventional Regimen in Managing Parkinson's Disease. *NPJ Parkinson's Dis.* **2022,** *8*, 62.

Ticinesi, A.; Mancabelli, L.; Carnevali, L.; Nouvenne, A.; Meschi, T.; Del Rio, D.; Ventura, M.; Sgoifo, A.; Angelino, D. Interaction Between Diet and Microbiota in the Pathophysiology of Alzheimer's Disease: Focus on Polyphenols and Dietary Fibers. *J. Alzheimer's Dis.* **2022,** *86*, 961–982.

Tran, P. H. L.; Tran, T. T. D. Blueberry Supplementation in Neuronal Health and Protective Technologies for Efficient Delivery of Blueberry Anthocyanins. *Biomolecules* **2021,** *11*, 102.

Unusan, N. Proanthocyanidins in Grape Seeds: An Updated Review of their Health Benefits and Potential uses in the Food Industry. *J. Funct. Foods* **2020,** *67*, 103861.

Vejarano, R.; Luján-Corro, M. Red Wine and Health: Approaches to Improve the Phenolic Content During Winemaking. *Front. Nutr.* **2022,** 9, 890066.

Violanti, J. M.; Ma, C. C.; Mnatsakanova, A.; Fekedulegn, D.; Hartley, T. A.; Gu, J. K.; Andrew, M. E. Associations Between Police Work Stressors and Posttraumatic Stress Disorder Symptoms: Examining the Moderating Effects of Coping. *J. Police Crim. Psychol.* **2018,** *33*, 271–282.

Wang, Y.; Haskell-Ramsay, C.; Gallegos, J. L.; Lodge, J. K. Effects of Chronic Consumption of Specific Fruit (Berries, Cherries and Citrus) on Cognitive Health: A Systematic Review and Meta-Analysis of Randomised Controlled Trials. *Euro. J. Clin. Nutr.* **2023,** *77*, 7–22.
Wiegman, C. H.; Li, F.; Ryffel, B.; Togbe, D.; Chung, K. F. Oxidative Stress in Ozone-Induced Chronic Lung Inflammation and Emphysema: A Facet of Chronic Obstructive Pulmonary Disease. *Front. Immunol.* **2020,** *11*, 1957.
Yang, L.; Zhao, Y.; Wang, Y.; Liu, L.; Zhang, X.; Li, B.; Cui, R. The Effects of Psychological Stress on Depression. *Curr. Neuropharmacol.* **2015,** *13*, 494–504.
Yaribeygi, H.; Panahi, Y.; Sahraei, H.; Johnston, T. P.; Sahebkar, A. The Impact of Stress on Body Function: A Review. *EXCLI J.* **2017,** *16*, 1057–1072.
Zhang, X.; Yoshihara, K.; Miyata, N.; Hata, T.; Altaisaikhan, A.; Takakura, S.; Asano, Y.; Izuno, S.; Sudo, N. Dietary Tryptophan, Tyrosine, and Phenylalanine Depletion Induce Reduced Food Intake and Behavioral Alterations in Mice. *Physiol. Behav.* **2022,** *244*, 113653.
Zydlik, Z.; Cieśliński, S.; Chung Mai, V.; Ebru Kafkas, N.; Morkunas, I. Soil Preparation, Running Highbush Blueberry (Vaccinium corymbosum L.) Plantation and Biological Properties of Fruits. In *Modern Fruit Industry*; IntechOpen, 2019.

CHAPTER 11

AN UPDATE ON THE ROLE OF ANTIOXIDANTS IN HEALTH AND DISEASE PREVENTION

MRUGENDRA BHOJRAJ POTDAR[1], KIRAN PATIL[1],
MD. RAGEEB MD. USMAN[2], and RAJU RATAN WADEKAR[3]

[1]*Department of Pharmaceutics, Shri Vile Parle Kelavani Mandal's Institute of Pharmacy, Dhule, Maharashtra, India*

[2]*Smt. Sharadchandrika Suresh Patil College of Pharmacy, Chopda, Maharashtra, India*

[3]*Department of Pharmacognosy, Shri Vile Parle Kelavani Mandal's Institute of Pharmacy, Dhule, Maharashtra, India*

ABSTRACT

The incidence of allergies and asthma has risen significantly during the past few decades. Although the origins of this phenomenon are still a mystery, many people believe that shifting dietary and behavioral patterns are to blame. One of these is an overly clean atmosphere, which can make people more susceptible to allergic reactions. There is also an increasing use of preservatives and colorants in dietary supplements. Oxidative substances like vitamins C and E, as well as food preservatives and colorants, decrease. The immune activation cascade in newly isolated human peripheral blood mononuclear cells in vitro, antioxidant chemicals, and proinflammatory signaling cascades, including nuclear factor-B, may be involved in the observed results. Therefore, maintaining and restoring oxidative status through natural nutrition strategies are

Antioxidants as Nutraceuticals. Nayan A. Gujarathi, Raj K. Keservani, Rajesh K. Kesharwani, Bhushan R. Rane, Yogeeta Sameer Goyal (Eds.)

critical for normal physiological processes in animals. Oxidative stress inhibits animals' health, performance, and production. Antioxidants found in plants, referred to as phytochemicals, are among the most promising new ingredients for animal feed. In nature, carotenoids are a common type of isoprenoid pigment. Singlet oxygen is effectively quenched, and other reactive oxygen species are scavenged by them. During the process of oxygenation, carotenoids can act as chemical quenchers, but this action is irreversible. A lot of the molecular mechanisms that underlie these reactions are still not fully understood. This is especially true for carotenoids, which are present in the blood and tissues of both humans and animals but aren't synthesized by either. Carotenoids thus play a role in numerous biochemical processes. "Oxidative stress" is a significant element in the pathogenic processes associated with many chronic diseases, and a deficiency in antioxidant-reactive oxygen species balance can lead to this stress. This chapter deals with the potential role of antioxidants for health benefits as well as their potential therapeutic benefits in a disease condition.

11.1 INTRODUCTION

Antioxidant properties can protect cells from free radicals, which are unstable molecules that can cause damage. Antioxidants interact with free radicals and stabilize them, potentially mitigating some of the damage they cause. The damage caused by free radicals has the potential to cause serious harm. Antioxidants include beta-carotene, lycopene, vitamins C, E, and A, as well as other compounds. An antioxidant is a chemical that can slow or halt other molecules from oxidizing (Hamid et al., 2010). A chemical reaction in which electrons can flow from a material to an oxidizer is known as oxidation. Oxidation processes produce free radicals, which begin chemical changes that damage cells (Tekwani, 2008). Antioxidants break the chain by reducing free radical mediators and inhibiting the oxidation process by becoming oxidized themselves. As a result, reducing agents such as thiols, ascorbic acid, and polyphenols are commonly used (Bagchi and Puri, 1998). Plants and animals have extensive antioxidant systems, which include glutathione, vitamin C, and vitamin E, as well as enzymes like catalase, superoxide dismutase, and many peroxidases (Pham-Huy et al., 2008). Lack of antioxidants or suppression of antioxidant enzymes creates oxidative stress, which can harm or kill cells (Lobo et al., 2010).

Antioxidants are being explored intensively in pharmacology, notably as medications for brain and neurodegenerative diseases, because oxidative stress may play a role in a range of human disorders (Chakraborty et al., 2009; Balakrishnan et al., 2014).

Antioxidants are also extensively used as ingredients in dietary supplements to help people stay healthy and avoid diseases like cancer and coronary heart disease (Wu and Cederbaum, 2003). Although past research stated that antioxidant supplements could improve health, subsequent large clinical trials found no impact and instead suggested that excessive intake could be harmful (Abd El, 2012). Other industrial uses for natural antioxidants include preservatives in food and cosmetics and the prevention of the deterioration of rubber and fuel, in addition to these medical ones (Somogyi et al., 2007). It has long been understood by chemical scientists that free radicals are a source of oxidation that can be mitigated or even prevented by the application of various antioxidants (Thomas, 1995). Liquid lubricating oils must not dry out like paints and must maintain their stability. As a result, these oils typically include a tiny amount of antioxidants, such as phenols or amines (David et al., 2016). Even though free radicals commonly generate plastics, they may also break them down; thus, antioxidants like phenols or naphthol must be used to guard against this. Carbon black, which absorbs ultraviolet light and induces radical formation in low-density polythene, also serves to protect it (Gomes et al., 2012).

11.1.1 SOURCES AND ORIGIN OF ANTIOXIDANTS

In addition to fruits and vegetables, antioxidants can be found in a wide range of other foods, such as nuts, cereals, and some meat, chicken, and fish (Aversa et al., 2016). Plants rich in antioxidant flavonoids, also known as nature's tender drugs, possess a wide spectrum of chemotherapeutical and pharmacological activities that include anti-neoplastic, antibiotic, antiviral, antiulcer, hepatoprotective, anti-inflammatory, immunomodulatory, and antithrombotic activities. Table 11.1 describes certain flavonoid-rich plants that are traditionally important and are used for the treatment of inflammation and inflammation-associated disorders. Further, it also indicated some active phytochemicals or phytoconstituents of the flavonoids group and their likely pharmacological activities along with therapeutic implications.

TABLE 11.1 The Various Plant Species Containing Flavonoids with Significant Anti-Inflammatory Activities.

Traditional flavonoids herbs/plant originated (country)	Plant species	Reported phytochemicals	Pharmacological activity and mechanism(s) of action
Latin America and Italy	*Griendella robust* Nuff; *Cistus laurifolius*	Quercetin-3 methyl ester, 3-O-methyl quercetin, 3,7-O-dimethyl quercetin, and 3,7-O-dimethyl kaempferol	Anti-inflammatory activity (inhibition of human neutrophil elastase activity, potent antioxidant activity).
Brazil, Argentina, and Bolivia	*Eupatorium arnottianum*	Nepetin, jaceosidin, and hispidulin	Anti-inflammatory activity inhibits nuclear kappa-δB (NF-δB) induction, which is necessary for the expression of intracellular proinflammatory mediators.
Latin America and Cuba	*Boldoa purpurascens*	Flavonoid glycosides (4,5-dihydroxy-6,7 methylene dioxy lavonol3-o-α-L-rhamnopyranosyl-(1-2) β-D-xylopyranoside)	Through the suppression of inflammatory mediator release, it is effective in both acute and chronic inflammation.
Brazil, Peru, and Colombia	*Cayaponia tayuya* Well	Vincenin-2, acacetin, apigenin, demethylnobiletin, nobiletin, swertisin, and spinosin	Anti-inflammatory activity mainly through the inhibition of COX and NOS induction.
China	*Sophora flavescens* (Leguminosae)	Kurarinone and sophoraflavanone G	Useful in inflammatory disorders, ulcers and skin burns, arthritis, passive and cutaneous anaphylaxis. The major active compounds shown to inhibit Cox-I, Cox-2, 5-lipoxygenase and 12-Lox.
Vietnam, Korea, and China	*Citrus aurantium* (Rutaceae)	Nobiletin, naringin, and hesperidin	Inflammatory conditions are beneficial. Blocking nuclear factor kappa 8 (NF-κ8) and nitrogen-activated protein kinase signaling in lipopolysaccharides (LPS) primed RAW 264.7 macrophages cell line inhibits proinflammatory mediators and cytokines. In LPS-induced macrophages, these flavonoids decrease COX-2 and iNOS mRNA and protein expression.

Sweet potatoes, carrots, cantaloupe, squash, apricots, pumpkins, and mangoes all contain beta-carotene, which is a type of vitamin A. Beta-carotene can be found in a variety of green leafy foods, such as collard greens, spinach, and kale (Sundaram Sanjay and Shukla, 2021).

Green leafy foods, including collard greens, spinach, and kale, are high in lutein, a carotenoid renowned for its connection to good vision (Sakhi, 2008). Lycopene, a potent antioxidant, is found in a wide variety of fruits and vegetables, such as tomatoes, guavas, papayas, apricots, pink grapefruits, and blood oranges, to name a few. An estimated 85% of the lycopene Americans consume originates from tomatoes and tomato-based foods (Engwa, 2018).

Selenium is not only a mineral but also an antioxidant (Valko et al., 2007; Buřičová and Reblova, 2008). Selenium is mostly found in plant foods like rice and wheat, which are common staples in many cultures' diets. The amount of selenium in food depends on the soil selenium content, which varies by region. Those animals that eat grain or plants cultivated in selenium-rich soil have higher levels of selenium in their muscles. Selenium is commonly found in meats and breads in the American diet (Valenzuela et al., 2003).

Selenium is also found in considerable amounts in Brazil nuts. 3-hydroxyretinol (vitamin A3) and retinol (vitamin A1) are the most common forms of vitamin A. Milk, eggs, and mozzarella cheese are some of the best sources of vitamin A (Ruiz-Rodríguez et al., 2014). The liver is also a good source of vitamin A. Ascorbic acid, another name for vitamin C, can be found in high concentrations in a wide variety of foods, including fruits, vegetables, grains, red meat, chicken, and fish (Beara et al., 2009; Stolarzewicz et al., 2013). In addition to almonds, which contain high levels of vitamin E (also known as alpha-tocopherol), other foods that contain alpha-tocopherol include mangoes, nuts, broccoli, and a variety of vegetable oils (Schmidt and Pokorný, 2005).

11.2 CLASSIFICATION OF ANTIOXIDANTS

11.2.1 ENDOGENOUS ANTIOXIDANTS

Antioxidants have a variety of roles in the body's defensive system, which includes both intracellular and extracellular antioxidants. H_2O_2 is converted to O_2 and H_2O by catalase, while the superoxide radical is converted to H_2O_2 and O_2 by SOD. Many different kinds of antioxidant enzymes can be found. There are membrane, cytosolic, and plasma forms of glutathione peroxidase, and SOD exists in all three forms. For cell viability, these antioxidants must be carefully managed. Most superoxides and peroxides are removed from cells by enzymes such as SOD, GPX, and catalase (CAT) before they can combine with metal ions to produce more reactive free radicals. Water- or lipid-soluble antioxidants that disrupt peroxidative chain reactions started by free radicals that eluded antioxidant defenses put an end to the chain reaction (Shah et al., 2014).

11.2.2 EXOGENOUS ANTIOXIDANTS

By delivering key nutrients such as vitamin E, C, and beta-carotene, flavonoids, and essential minerals that create important antioxidant enzymes, diet plays a vital role in the formation of the antioxidant defense system. Zinc and selenium are found in SOD and glutathione peroxidase, respectively. The substrates that are subject to oxidation are affected by diet, which plays a significant role in the oxidation process. The oxidation of lipids is the best example. As the number of double bonds in a polyunsaturated fatty acid (PUFA) grows, it becomes more vulnerable to free radical attack (Rizzo et al., 2010). To avoid oxidation of a nearby fatty acid, antioxidants present at the attack site are preferentially oxidized by the attacking radical. A person's diet is the primary factor in determining the fatty acid composition of their membrane and lipoproteins. Examples include arachidonic acid (20:4) from meat intake, eicosapentaenoic acid (20:5) from eating fish, and docosahexaenoic acid (20:6) from fish consumption (10:1), (22:6). A vegetarian diet has less total fat and polyunsaturated fatty acids on average than a diet that contains animal products. This could explain why vegetarianism has been linked to a number of health advantages. Olive oil's protective effects on LDL oxidation may be ascribed to the oil's higher concentration of monounsaturated fatty acids than polyunsaturated fatty acids, in addition to the presence of antioxidants such as flavonoids and other phenolic compounds found in olives (Guerra-Araiza et al., 2013).

Antioxidants can also be categorized as:

1. Primary or natural antioxidants.
2. Secondary or synthetic antioxidants.

11.2.2.1 PRIMARY OR NATURAL ANTIOXIDANTS

Lipid radicals are chain-breaking antioxidants that turn them into more stable molecules by reacting with them. Some of the most common antioxidants in this category are phenolic in structure (Žebeljan et al., 2021).

In addition to antioxidant enzymes, these minerals act as cofactors. Many macromolecules, such as carbohydrates, will be affected if they are not present in sufficient amounts. Minerals such as manganese and selenium are examples (Agati et al., 2020).

Most bodily metabolic processes necessitate the intake of antioxidant vitamins. Vitamin C, vitamin E, and vitamin B are a few examples.

There are three types of phytochemicals: (1) vitamins and minerals; (2) phenolic compounds; and (3) phytochemicals. These are some examples: Vegetables, fruits, seeds, leaves, flowers, and bark are all colored by phenolic chemicals known as flavonoids. Catechins, which are found in green and black tea and sesamol, are the most potent antioxidants. Carotenoids, the pigments found in various fruits and vegetables, are fat-soluble. Beta-carotene, which is found in carrots, can be converted to vitamin A if the body is deficient. Zeaxanthin, found in spinach, is also found in high concentrations in tomatoes and other dark greens. Herbs and spices include diterpene, rosmariquinone, thymol, nutmeg, and cloves, as well as black pepper, ginger, garlic, and curcumin (Díaz et al., 2014).

11.2.2.2 SECONDARY OR SYNTHETIC ANTIOXIDANTS

These are phenolic compounds that capture free radicals and inhibit chain reactions, and they include:

I. Butylated hydroxyl anisole (BHA).
II. Butylated hydroxy toluene (BHT).
III. Propyl gallate (PG) and metal chelating agent (EDTA).
IV. Tertiary butyl hydroquinone (TBHQ).
V. Nordihydroguaiaretic acid (NDGA).

11.3 TYPES OF ANTIOXIDANTS

11.3.1 ASCORBIC ACID

Vitamin C is a monosaccharide antioxidant found in both animals and plants. Ascorbic acid is categorized as a vitamin since one of the enzymes required for its synthesis has been lost over time in humans. The majority of other animals can synthesize this molecule and do not require it in their diet. Two enzymes, protein disulfide isomerase and glutaredoxins, can assist cells in keeping glutathione in its reduced form. Reduced ascorbic acid can help to neutralize reactive oxygen species like hydrogen peroxide (Bhattacharya, 2015).

11.3.2 GLUTATHIONE

Most aerobic living forms produce glutathione, a cysteine-containing peptide. Amino acids that make up the protein are produced in the cells rather than ingested in the diet. Glutathione's cysteine moiety has a thiol group that may be reduced and oxidized reversibly, making it an antioxidant. Ascorbate in the glutathione-ascorbate cycle, glutathione peroxidases, and glutaredoxins are all reduced by the enzyme glutathione reductase, which in turn reduces other metabolites and enzyme systems. It also reacts directly with oxidants. There's no doubt that glutathione is an important antioxidant in the body because of its large concentration and its central role in keeping cells in balance. Mycothiol and trypanothione are substitutes for glutathione in some organisms, such as actinomycetes and kinetoplastids (Heidari et al., 2021).

11.3.3 MELATONIN

Melatonin is a potent antioxidant that can quickly pass through cell membranes and the blood-brain barrier, making it ideal for treating insomnia. Antioxidants such as vitamin C and beta-carotene, which are well-known for their redox cycling properties, do not include the antioxidant melatonin on their list. Redox cycling may allow other antioxidants (such as vitamin C) to become prooxidants and encourage free radical production. There are various stable compounds formed when free radicals react with oxidized melatonin; therefore, it can't be returned to its original state. Terminal (or suicidal) antioxidants have so been referred to (Sharafati-Chaleshtori et al., 2017).

11.3.4 TOCOPHEROLS AND TOCOTRIENOLS (VITAMIN E)

Tocopherols and tocotrienols, which are fat-soluble vitamins with anti-oxidant characteristics, are known as vitamin E. Most research has been done on alpha-tocopherol due to its high bioavailability and preference for absorption and metabolism by the body. The most important lipid-soluble antioxidant, α-tocopherol, is said to react with lipid radicals produced in the lipid peroxidation chain reaction to protect membranes from oxidation (Kamal-Eldin and Appelqvist, 1996); it stops the process by removing the free radical intermediates. Other antioxidants, such as ascorbate and retinol, which can be found in a variety of foods, can decrease these radicals back to their active state (Shahidi and Zhong, 2015). Water-soluble antioxidants are inadequate at protecting glutathione peroxidase (GPX4)-depleted cells from cell death. GPX4 is the only enzyme known to successfully reduce lipid hydroperoxides in biological membranes (Shahidi and Zhong, 2015).

11.4 TECHNIQUES FOR MEASUREMENT OF ANTIOXIDANT ACTIVITY

Antioxidant activity can be measured in a variety of samples using one of three methods.

11.4.1 CHEMICAL ASSAYS FOR ANTIOXIDANT ACTIVITY

Antioxidant activity in products can be evaluated using a wide variety of chemical assays (herbal, nutraceuticals, and food items). Listed below are some of the best-known and most often used approaches (Shahidi and Zhong, 2015).

11.4.2 OXYGEN RADICAL ABSORPTION CAPACITY

An azo-compound, such as 2,2′-azobis (2-amidinopropane) dihydrochloride (AAPH), is used as a radical generator in the oxygen radical absorption capacity (ORAC) method. The thermal breakdown of AAPH inhibits peroxyl radical-induced oxidation, as measured by this assay. Fluorescein's fluorescence fades with time because of the free radicals produced by the heat breakdown of AAPH. Fluorescein decay is inhibited by either a single antioxidant or a complex mixture of antioxidants, resulting in a more stable fluorescence signal. Fluorescence degradation is an indicator of the antioxidant's ability (Bisby et al., 2008).

11.4.3 DETERMINATION OF TOTAL PHENOLIC CONTENT (TPC)

Folin–Ciocalteu (FC) reagent with a spectrophotometer set at 725 nm measures the total phenolic content of the extracts. Phenolic functional groups are used because of their potential to reduce compounds. The phenolate ion undergoes oxidation and reduction reactions when the pH is low. In this case, the color of the FC reagent (Folin–phosphomolybdenum complex) will change to blue. When the extract includes more phenolic chemicals, the reduction of complex will be more pronounced. Because of this, the color and absorbance are darker, indicating that the antioxidant activity is higher (Lu et al., 2011).

11.4.4 DPPH ASSAY (1,1-DIPHENYL-2-PICRYLHYDRAZYL)

By dissolving DPPH in methanol, one obtains the free radical DPPH, which can be stored in darkness at 20°C until needed. The color of the solution changes from violet to yellow when DPPH reacts with the antioxidants in the sample, and the absorbance at 515 nm of the resulting solution is measured spectrophotometrically (Nanjo et al., 1996).

11.4.5 TROLOX EQUIVALENT ANTIOXIDANT CAPACITY

To get a blue color, ABTS+ is formed when potassium persulfate combines with the chemical. In the presence of foodborne phenolic compounds such as thiols or vitamin C, the free radical ABTS+ is scavenged by these compounds and converted into its neutral colorless form. Light at 734 nm is absorbed by ABTS+ (van den Berg et al., 1999).

11.4.6 FERRIC-REDUCING ANTIOXIDANT POWER

Low-pH reactions between TPTZ and ferric chloride result in the creation of an iron triazine complex when ferric chloride is transformed to iron. The absorbance shift at 593 nm in reaction mixtures with those containing ferrous ions at known concentrations is used to calculate FRAP values (Benzie and Szeto, 1999).

11.4.7 DETERMINATION OF TOTAL REDUCING POWER (TRP)

The ability to convert potassium ferricyanide (Fe3+) to potassium ferricyanide (Fe2+) can be evaluated spectrophotometrically if the sample contains appropriate amounts of antioxidant chemicals. The antioxidant chemicals react with ferric chloride to generate ferric ferrous complex, which absorbs light at 700 nm (Christodouleas et al., 2014).

11.4.8 BIOCHEMICAL ASSAYS FOR ANTIOXIDANT ACTIVITY ASSESSMENT

In addition to in vitro and in vivo models, antioxidant activity can also be assessed in biological systems. These include the measurement of ROS adducts and end products, such as lipids, proteins, DNA, and other compounds, as well as other oxidative stress markers. TBARS, SOD, CAT, GPx, GSH, and the ferrous oxidation-xylenol orange (FOX) assay are a few of the methods available (Kulkarni et al., 2019). Blood, urine, breath, and tissues can all be used for these tests. The following are a few examples:

11.4.9 TBARS

Lipid peroxidation can be measured using TBARS. Thiobarbituric acid (TBA) and malondialdehyde (MDA) react to form TBARS, a reaction product that is detected by spectrophotometry at 532 nm after lipid hydroperoxide's decomposition in the sample (Puntel et al., 2005).

11.4.10 PROTEIN CARBONYL

The oxidative cleavage of proteins produces protein carbonyl content. 2,4-dinitrophenylhydrazine (DNPH) and protein carbonyl create a Schiff base, resulting in the equivalent hydrazone in this case. An absorbance of 360–380 nm is used to measure the amount of protein hydrazone generated (Dalle-Donne et al., 2003).

11.4.11 FOX

In order to evaluate how much hydroperoxide a lipid has in it, we can look at its ability to convert $Fe2+$ to $Fe3+$. The xylenol orange reagent (bluish-purple color) and $Fe3+$ generated a combination that was visible at 560 nm (Meade et al., 1999).

11.4.12 SOD

NADH, an adenine dinucleotide, is the substrate of choice. At 560 nm, the spectrophotometer measures the chromogen's color intensity (purple) in the butanol layer against butanol (blank) (Menvielle-Bourg, 2005).

11.4.13 ROS

In this test, 2′,7′-dichlorofluorescein diacetate (DCFDA) is used to evaluate ROS levels. The very fluorescent dichlorofluorescein (DCF) undergoes cellular oxidation by ROS and is converted into DCF (Snezhkina et al., 2019).

11.5 CHARACTERISTICS OF ANTIOXIDANTS

Many monohydroxy or polyhydroxy phenol molecules with different ring substitutions are currently the most common food-based antioxidants. The activation energy of these molecules to give hydrogen is minimal. It's because of this that the antioxidant radical doesn't start another free radical as it's stabilized. Antioxidants and metal chelating agents donate hydrogen to the chain reaction, delaying or preventing its commencement. There is no quick oxidation of the antioxidant free radical as a result of its high stability. By forming a stable complex compound, antioxidant free radicals and lipid free radicals can reduce some of the damage that the radicals do to the body (Logan et al., 1998).

11.6 ANTIOXIDANTS SYSTEM IN OUR BODY

Many antioxidant systems have been established by the body to deal with ROI generation. There are enzymatic systems and nonenzymatic systems in these systems. In addition to superoxide dismutase (SOD), which catalyzes the conversion of oxygen and oxygen dioxide (O_2), other enzymatic antioxidants include glutathione peroxidase, which converts hydrogen peroxide (H_2O_2) to water. Another class of antioxidants is composed of vitamins that are not enzymes, such as lipid-soluble vitamin E, provitamin A, and water-soluble vitamin C (Aslani and Ghobadi, 2016). Vitamin E has been referred to as the human body's most powerful antioxidant. One of its functions is to prevent lipid peroxidation from occurring, as well as to modulate the internal signaling pathways that are dependent on ROI. Adding a little vitamin E to your diet can help you stay cool. Alpha-tocopherol and beta-tocotrienol were tested for their antioxidant effects since they contain 45% tocopherol and 55% tocotrienol. Tocopherol and tocotrienol were shown to accumulate in the hearts and livers of vitamin E-deprived rats more slowly than tocopherol. In vitro, two-thirds of the rate of lipid peroxidation in cardiac homogenate from rats fed tocotrienol was created. As a result, palm oil vitamin E may be more effective than –tocopherol alone in preventing heart damage caused by ischemia and reperfusion. Because alpha-tocopherol or beta-tocotrienol supplementation protects skeletal muscles from exercise-induced increases in protein oxidation, palm oil vitamin E protects biological systems from both lipid and protein oxidation. Lipid peroxidation in biological membranes caused by free radicals has been linked to the onset of a variety of diseases. Despite its low concentration, vitamin E is extremely helpful in preventing heart disease, cancer, cataracts, neuropathies, and myopathies. Berry consumption has been linked to a number of health benefits, including the prevention of stroke, degenerative illnesses associated with aging, and cancer. According to some of these research, berry phytochemicals with strong antioxidative potential may contribute to or enhance the intrinsic antioxidant capacity of live cells or organisms by induction (Sen et al., 2010).

11.7 EFFECTS OF ANTIOXIDANTS

A "free radical" is the enemy of a healthy cell. The outer membranes of healthy cells are constantly targeted by free radicals, which eventually lead to cellular degeneration and death. According to current research, free radicals are responsible for most diseases, infections, stress, and aging. Free radicals can potentially harm athletic performance by lowering aerobic capacity and slowing or stopping muscle growth. Furthermore, free radicals have been found to cause mutations in the genetic material of the cell, that is, RNA and DNA. Most molecules in the human body have a paired group (two electrons) in their outer shell (De la Fuente, 2002). A free radical is a molecule that has only one unpaired electron in its outer shell. Oxygen in the bloodstream combines with a wide range of chemicals, including those found in polluted air, primary and second-hand cigarette smoke, and known damage is accelerated by the normal radiation found in sunlight and increasing exercise, especially running and other aerobic activities. Free radicals occur naturally. To put it simply, aerobic activity can raise oxygen consumption 10–20-folds. Free radical generation increases as a result of increased blood oxygenation. Free radicals continue to damage muscle even after you've stopped working out. It is possible to counteract free radical damage by including antioxidants in your diet or using antioxidant supplements. Dietary antioxidant complexes have an advantage over supplements since they contain a wide variety of antioxidants that target and eliminate free radicals in a wide range of cells. It is only the outside fatty layers of the cell that are protected by a single antioxidant, such as vitamin E. It will not be able to maintain DNA stability, which is one of the key impacts of vitamin C, for example. Antioxidant synergy refers to the way different antioxidants spread throughout the body to protect cells in various locations. Free radicals in the bloodstream are neutralized by certain antioxidants when they come into contact with them at their suitable action sites. Increased antioxidant levels, as a result of increased supplementation with antioxidants from more diverse sources, result in less cellular damage as well as better health. As a matter of fact, antioxidant supplementation has been shown to reduce athletic training-related injuries significantly. Polyunsaturated lipids, which lipid peroxidation targets, are particularly abundant in the brain, making it particularly prone to oxidative harm. This has led to the widespread use of antioxidants in the treatment of a variety of brain injuries. Sodium thiopental and propofol, which mimic superoxide dismutase, are used to treat reperfusion injury and traumatic brain injury in stroke patients (Kaneto et al., 1999).

11.8 MEDICINAL APPLICATIONS OF ANTIOXIDANTS

11.8.1 LANTHANIDES AS ANTICANCER AGENTS

New therapeutic and diagnostic metal complexes are influencing medical practice as a result of the rapid development of inorganic chemistry in medicine. Improved molecules designed to decrease harmful effects and better understand their mechanisms of action require advancements in biocoordination chemistry. The treatment of cancer involves the use of many metal-based medicines (Chan et al., 2014).

11.8.2 LYCOPENE AS A POTENTIAL ANTICANCER AGENT

Most common chronic diseases can be controlled using a low-cost approach to dietary chemoprevention, including cancer. Tomatoes and tomato-based products, in particular, have been found to provide a wide range of health advantages. According to an epidemiological study, tomatoes have been demonstrated to reduce the prevalence of ROS-related illnesses, such as cardiovascular disease and cancer, by boosting the antioxidant carotenoid known to be a more lasting and potent singlet oxygen-quenching agent than other carotenoids. In addition to its antioxidant capabilities, lycopene possesses a wide spectrum of biological effects, including cardioprotective, anti-inflammatory, antimutagenic, and anticarcinogenic properties (De la Fuente, 2002).

11.8.3 SELENIUM DERIVATIVES AS CANCER-PREVENTIVE AGENTS

Recently, laboratory research, clinical trials, and epidemiological data have confirmed selenium's involvement in cancer prevention. This has resulted in the use of selenium supplementation for therapeutic purposes, such as cancer chemoprevention and heart failure treatment, rather than merely to make up for nutritional deficiency (Bhuvaneswari and Nagini, 2005).

11.8.4 ANTICANCER ACTIVITY OF BERBERIN AND COPTIS

To sustain their proliferative abilities and high metabolic rate, cancer cells require high quantities of reactive oxygen species (ROS) during carcinogenesis (Bystrom et al., 2014). ROS also have a role in the activation of transcription factors such as AP-I, NF-κB, and cAMP, which are critical for cancer cell growth. Furthermore, by causing DNA damage and mutations, oxidative stress contributes to genomic instability. Berberine's antioxidant effect has been extensively documented, and multiple investigations have indicated that berberine increases caspase-dependent cell death in tumors via inducing ROS generation (e.g., in human glioblastoma T98G cells). Berberine also induced caspase-dependent apoptosis and mitochondrial malfunction via activating the ER-stress pathway, which was activated by ROS. Similarly, berberine also increases ROS secretion due to xanthine oxidase, leading to damage of mitochondrial membrane potential and cellular apoptosis. But such effects could not be demonstrated in normal epithelial cells; therefore, this effect has been considered as its specific effect on cancer cells (Casey et al., 2015).

Such selective activity has also been discovered in an in vitro colon cancer model. In a mouse model of Den and CCl4-induced hepatocarcinogenesis, berberine's anticancer effectiveness was also demonstrated in vivo. The inhibitory effect on hepatocarcinoma has been attributed to the reduction of ROS production and the prevention of AKT-mediated cell proliferation, as well as p53 degradation via the Nrf2/HO-1 signaling cascade. Berberine also inhibited JNK and protein phosphatase-2 expression, which resulted in BC12 dephosphorylation and Bax accumulation, resulting in apoptosis induction. Such a dual action is likely to protect normal cells against the development of carcinoma while simultaneously slowing the advancement of cancer cells (Wang et al., 2015).

Coptis and berberine also possess anti-inflammatory properties. Inflammation is regarded as the activation of inflammatory molecules involved in signaling pathways that mediate inflammation, and berberine has been demonstrated to participate in the regulation of anti-inflammatory activity and thus produce significant anti-inflammatory effects. Berberine and Coptis anti-inflammatory effects are also believed to be substantially mediated by a key pathway including nuclear factor-kappa B (NF-κB), mitogen-activated protein kinase, and adenosine monophosphate-activated protein kinase. Immune malfunction, tissue degradation, and even cell death will occur if the NF-κB component is impaired. The inhibitors of kB (IKB) work with the NF-κB subunits to regulate gene expression in various tissues, and IKK regulates IkB phosphorylation. As a result, these biomolecules are likely targets for NF-κB therapeutics (Ehteshamfar et al., 2020).

In an endotoxemic mouse model, berberine was found to be protective. Endotoxemia is an inflammatory condition caused by endotoxin, which causes a disruption in the immune system. Berberine's anti-inflammatory properties are mostly attributable to a decrease in proinflammatory cytokine release (Rook et al., 2006). Berberine, which inhibits nuclear translocation of the NF-κB p65 subunit and the myosin light chain kinase pathway, caused tight junction disruption in intestinal epithelial cells (Zhou et al., 2017). Berberine also reduced IFN/TNF-associated ER stress and apoptosis in an epithelial cell model (in vitro), suggesting its protective effect in inflammatory bowel disease. Berberine has been traditionally used by the Chinese in antidiarrhea-associated inflammatory bowel disease. Berberine also showed a protective effect against visceral hypersensitivity (the principal symptom of irritable bowel syndrome), and NO release by berberine may be a major contributing factor for such a pharmacological effect (Farzaei et al., 2016). Alzheimer's disease's occurrence has largely been attributed to neuron inflammation induced by the amyloid-beta peptide. By deactivating the NF-κB factor, berberine inhibits peptides and completely blocks inducible nitric oxide synthase (iNOS) and COX-2 expression in microglia. Rho GTPase belongs to families of small G-proteins, and earlier research findings have demonstrated their involvement in the mediation of NF-κB activity in various inflammatory-related diseases (Travaglione et al., 2008). It was observed that, as a potent inhibitor of the Rho GTPase family proteins RhoA Rac and cdc42, berberine produces greater inhibition of the GTPase activity in cancer. It is presumed that the inhibition of cancer cell migration by Coptis and berberine is directly related to this property as well as the inflammation-associated NF-κB pathway (Lan et al., 2022).

11.8.5 BETULINIC ACID

Betulinic acid is a pentacyclic triterpene that is chemically related to betulin. Betulin is found in the outer bark of *Betulla alba*, a white birch tree (Hordyjewska et al., 2019). Antiviral, antineoplastic, and antiplasmodial properties are all produced by betulinic acid. On cultured human melanoma, neuroblastoma, malignant brain tumor, leukemia cells, lung carcinomas, ovarian, and cervical carcinomas, betulinic acid has a specific antitumor action with no unfavorable or side effects (Hordyjewska et al., 2019). Its anti-neuroectodermal activity has also been proven, and it is mostly related to the activation of apoptosis by direct mitochondrial changes. In vitro, betulinic acid had a synergistic cytotoxic effect on the proliferation and metastasis of melanoma cells (B16F10) when combined with the anticancer medication vincristine. This effect is ascribed to cell cycle arrest at several sites, which resulted in melanoma cell apoptosis. Because of its low toxicity to normal cells, betulinic acid has a high therapeutic index, indicating that it is a prospective anticancer drug that should be pursued. Only a greater knowledge of the underlying mechanism of cytotoxicity can unlock its potential clinical applicability (Zhang et al., 2015).

11.8.6 PODOPHYLLOTOXIN

Podophyllotoxin, a promising second-generation anticancer drug obtained from the resin of *Podophyllum hexandrum* and *Podophyllum pettatum* (Berberidaceae), was reported to be highly toxic, and derivatives have been used recently in clinical medicine, which are comparatively less toxic. Etoposide phosphate acts by inhibiting topoisomerase II and breaking the DNA strands. It is administered orally or intravenously, either alone or along with other drugs. It is effective in the treatment of lung cancer, Ewing sarcoma, testicular cancer, and lymphoma. It is also used prior to bone marrow or blood stem cell transplantation. Etopophos is a water-soluble ester of etoposide that has shown metaphase arrest in chick fibroblasts and DNA-topoisomerase II-dependent arrest in the G2 portion of the mammalian cell cycle. This is used for refractory testicular tumor and small-cell lung cancer. Teniposide is the other derivative (a substitution of the thenylidine group on the glucopyranoside ring). It is used to treat childhood acute lymphocytic leukemia (Silva et al., 2017).

11.8.7 CAPSAICIN

It's a homovanillic acid derivative that's the main pungent component in red and chili peppers made from capsicum fruit extracts. Its pretreatment was reported to protect rats exposed to sulfur dioxide and nitrogen dioxide from free radical-induced lung injury. It is also an irritant and produces neurogenic inflammation mainly due to the release of substance P and calcitonin gene-related peptide via activating transient receptor potential vanilloid-1 (Peng et al., 2022). Documented research reports state that capsaicin showed anticancer activity against a wide variety of cancers. Capsaicin has shown protective activity against benzo(a)pyrene-induced carcinogenesis in mice model. Capsaicin (10 mg/kg body weight) supplementation effectively reversed various biochemical changes such as elevation in polyamines' content, DNA and RNA levels, and induction of DNA damage during experimental lung cancer. Therefore, capsaicin could be a promising drug candidate for inhibiting lung carcinogenesis.

11.8.8 (+)-CATECHIN

(+)-Catechin reportedly inhibited HepG2 cell proliferation through a caspase-related pathway. Catechin was found to downregulate Ccl-2, stimulate the release of cytochrome into the cytosol, and upregulate Bax, caspase-3, 9, and p53 in the oncogenic cells. The chemopreventive efficacy of (+)-catechin-rich extract of *Acacia catechu* Willd (Fabaceae) heartwood against 7,12-dimethyl-benz [a] anthracene-induced hepatocarcinoma in Bulb/c mice has been reported in Figure 11.1 (Isemura, 2019).

11.8.9 (–)-EPICATECHIN

(−)-Epicatechin has been shown to potentiate etoposide-induced antileukemic effects in rats with myeloid leukemia. Epicatechin exhibited a promising protective effect against radiation-induced injury during cancer therapy. This is largely due to the stimulation of mitochondrial activity and the selective sensitization of cancer cells to radiation. This is also beneficial in protecting normal cells against cancer radiotherapy (Gaobotse et al., 2023). Epigallocatechin-3-O-gallate exhibits an antiproliferative effect on Caco-2 colon cancer cells. The chemopreventive actions of quercetin and epigallocatechin-3-O-gallate have been considered due to in general induction apoptosis. This

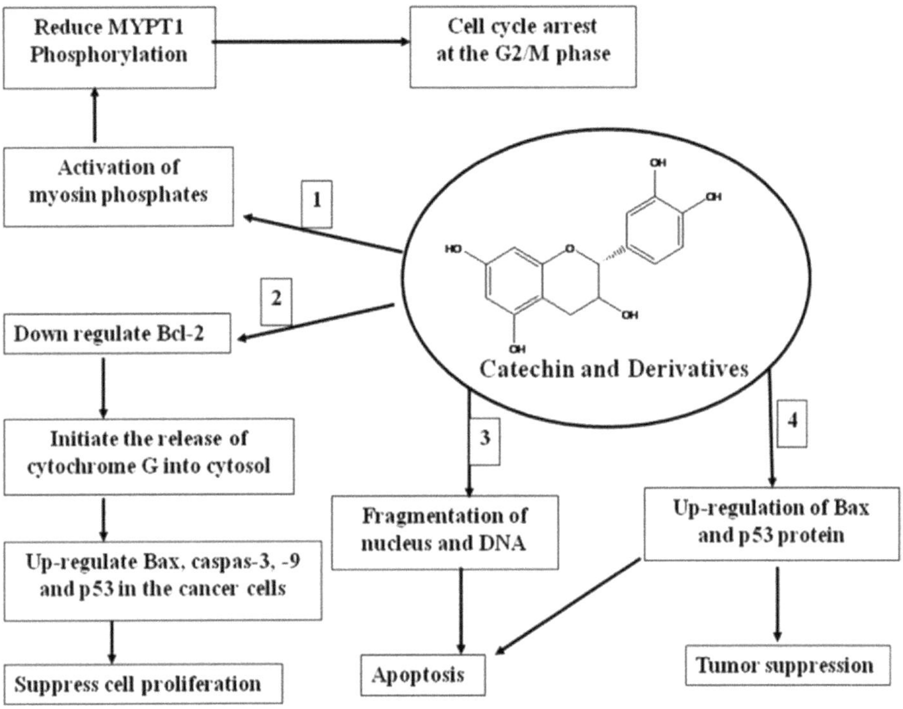

FIGURE 11.1 Mechanism of catechin and derivatives as anticancer agents (1 = epigallocatechin-3-O-gallate; 2 = (+)-catechin; 3, 4 = (−)-epicatechin).

compound also inhibits the proliferation of mammary and epidermal cancer cells. This compound induces the downregulation of Erb B1 and Erb B2 in these cells. Gallic acid has been reported to be cytotoxic for human prostate cancer LNCap cells, which was enhanced when combined with flutamide. Autooxidation of gallic acids leads to the formation of reactive oxygen species (ROS) and is responsible for gallic acid-induced death in LNCaP cells (Zhang et al., 2020). Figure 11.2 demonstrates the mechanism of action of catechin for its anticancer activity and the mechanism of gallic acid as an anticancer compound.

11.8.10 QUERCETIN

Quercetin has been reported to possess antimelanoma activity. Quercetin treatment inhibited proliferation of melanoma cells, induction of cell apoptosis, and decreased migration and invasion properties. The possible

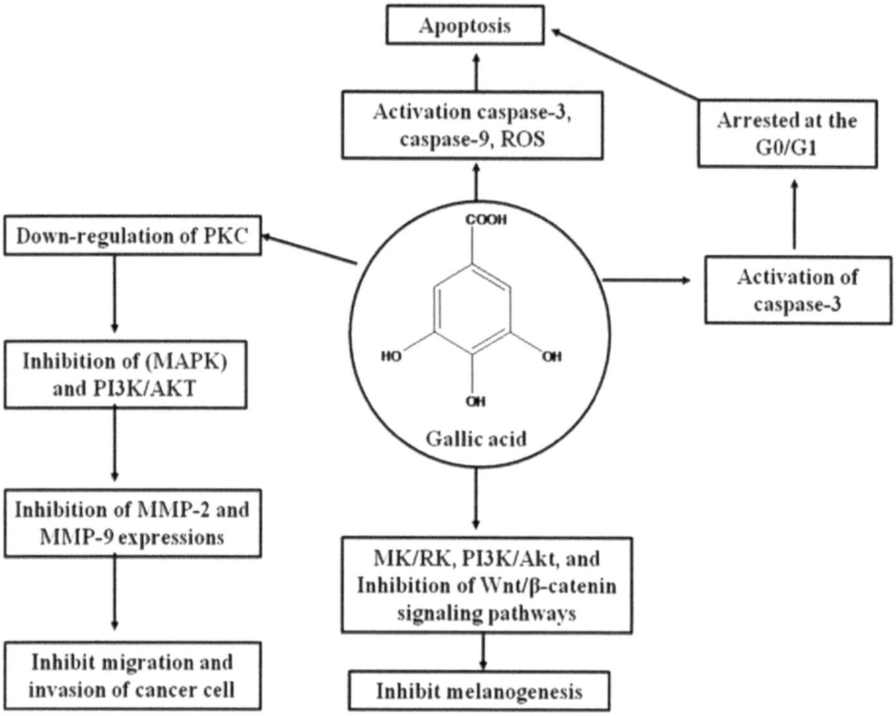

FIGURE 11.2 Mechanism of gallic acid as anticancer agent.

mechanisms involved are: (1) inhibition of the activation of STAT-3 signaling by interfering with STAT-3 transcription activity; (2) downregulation of STAT-3 targeted genes Mcl-1 (induced myeloid leukemia cell differentiation protein), MMp-2, MMP-9, and vascular endothelial growth factor, which participate in cell growth, migration, and invasion. In addition, quercetin is known to suppress A-375 tumor growth and STAT-3 activities in xenografted mice model. These findings indicate that inhibition of melanoma by quercetin may be due to interference in STAT-3 signaling (Cao et al., 2014).

A rat model of prostate cancer (induced by the administration of testosterone and N-methyl-N-nitrosourea) showed enhanced lipid peroxidation, increased hydrogen peroxide, and reduced glutathione levels. These biochemical changes were significantly inhibited with the administration of quercetin (Lindshield et al., 2010).

Quercetin also delayed the formation of tumors and decreased tumor multiplicity in a skin cancer mice model. In addition, quercetin inhibited inhibitory growth factor-1 (IGF-1)-driven phosphorylation of the IGF-1 receptor insulin receptor substrate, AKt, and S6k in the MT1/2 cutaneous papilloma cell line. These data suggest that quercetin can prevent skin cancer by inhibiting IGF-1 signaling.

Quercetin considerably increased the apoptic action (shown in Fig. 11.3) of tumor necrosis factor-related apoptosis-inducing ligand (TRAIL) in human ovarian carcinoma cells via the CCAAT enhancer-binding protein homologous protein (CHOP)-death receptor 5 (DRS) pathway mediated by reactive oxygen species (ROS). Activation of JNK and upregulation of CHOP were key factors in DR5 stimulation. In addition, activation of apoptosis, stimulation of caspase-3, CHOP, and DRS were all implicated with quercetin-mediated augmentation of TRAIL-mediated suppression of tumor development in human SKOV-3 (Imran et al., 2019).

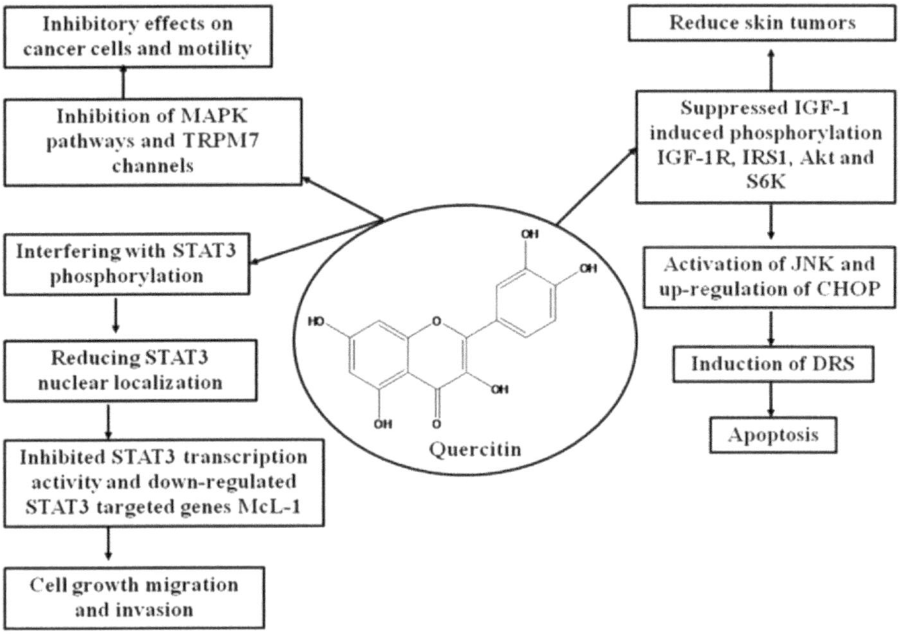

FIGURE 11.3 Mechanism of quercetin as anticancer agent.

11.9 MARINE-DERIVED ANTICANCER MOLECULES

Cancer is among the most challenging diseases humans have ever encountered. Malignant neoplasia is a phrase used to describe a group of diseases distinguished by uncontrolled cell growth and tumor formation. Each year,

14.1 million new cancer cases are identified, 8.2 million people die from cancer, and 32.6 million people live with cancer, according to verifiable data. These are estimates of all cancers' incidences, fatality, and prevalence in 2012 (excluding nonmelanoma skin cancer). Despite the fact that marine compounds are underrepresented in today's pharmacopoeia, the marine environment, which accounts for 95% of the biosphere, is likely to become a significant source of novel compounds in the future. However, the discovery of marine floral compounds as bioactive molecules is still in its early stages due to a lack of a similar ethnomedical background in comparison to terrestrial environments, as well as the relative technological obstacles in obtaining marine flower samples. Pharmaceutical companies and academic organizations have invested heavily in the isolation and discovery of novel marine-derived, natural chemicals, notably from marine creatures, over the last few decades. Marine floras, on the other hand, are largely unknown, and these research efforts are being assessed as a foundation for future research in this area. Bacteria, actinobacteria, cyanobacteria, and fungus, as well as microalgae, macroalgae (seaweeds), and flowering plants, make up the marine flora (mangroves and other halophytes). Microflora and microalgae account for more than 90% of marine biomass in the ocean, which spans more than 71% of the earth's surface. This large maritime floral resource will offer a myriad of drug development opportunities. It's becoming clear that the ocean has a varied variety of natural products and unique chemical substances with distinct biological activities that could aid in the development of novel medications with improved efficacy, selectivity, and selectivity for the treatment of human diseases. Some aquatic organisms have been found to be dependable medication suppliers. Sponge, soft corals, sea fans, sea hares, bryozoans, and tunicates are examples of invertebrates. Seaweed dietary fibers have antioxidant, antimutagenic, anticoagulant, and anticancer effects, to name a few (Brush et al., 2020).

Although they haven't been properly researched, marine flora could be a source of anticancer compounds. Marine algae contribute 65.63% of the anticancer chemicals discovered so far, mangroves 28.12%, and bacteria 6.25%. Because of their varied chemical ecology, marine animals, particularly marine flora, have considerable promise for developing effective, less expensive, and safer anticancer medicines, which warrant more exploration. Many marine compounds include conopeptides, didemins, largazole, peptides, prenylated quinolines and hydroquinones, arsenolipids, bryostatins, multisulfide-containing metabolites, fascaplysin, tunichromes, glycosides from sponges, sea anemone toxins, myealamides, and related compounds and polyhydroxysteroids. These are sesquiterpenoids, cembrane, diterpenes, and diketopiperazine. The marine sources are cyanobacteria, microalgae, actinomycetes, gorgonians, ascidians, sea cucumbers, sponges, seaweeds and their entophytic fungi, the marine flora, and fauna in different arenas.

11.10 MECHANISM(S) OF ANTICANCER ACTIVITY OF MARINE-DERIVED PRODUCTS

Among the most significant processes in the progression of cancer is DNA damage. A mutagenic DNA damage marker will aid in the estimation of cancer risk in varied populations as well as the monitoring of chemoprevention effects. Much of this harm is caused by oxidation. Each day, a typical human cell is exposed to approximately 10.000 oxidative "hits" to its DNA. The majority of the damage is repaired by DNA repair enzymes. With age, oxidative DNA damage increases, as does the chance of cancer.

In the human system, several mechanisms protect against free radicals and other reactive oxygen species (ROS). Because they operate on distinct oxidants or in various cellular compartments, different defenses complement one another. Vitamin E, unlike other vitamins, has not been found to be linked to the function of any enzyme system. It has a well-established role as an antioxidant and scavenger of free radicals, making it an efficient guardian of lipid and phospholipid membrane integrity. Vitamin E interacts closely with other dietary systemic antioxidants, including vitamin C and glutathione, as an antioxidant. Vitamin E appears to have a variety of different effects, including control of gene expression and inflammatory responses, according to growing research.

11.11 MOLECULES ISOLATED FROM MARINE ORIGIN

11.11.1 PSAMMAPLIN-A

Psammaplin-A is isolated from Verongid sponge, chemically a symmetrical bromotyrosine disulfide possessing oxime moieties and eliciting very potent cytotoxicity via inhibiting human topoisomerase II and suppressing aminopeptidase N angiogenesis (in vitro) (Shin et al., 2004). The analogues of psammaplin-A, NVP-LAQ824, and indolic cinnamyl hydroxamate have clinical trials for leukemia (Niemann et al., 2015).

11.11.2 DIDEMNIN B

Didemnin B is a cyclic antiproliferative depsipeptidase isolated from Caribbean tunicate. Trididemnum depsipeptidase, after preclinical evaluation, was taken up for clinical trials in humans. The major site of action of this compound is the inhibition of DNA, RNA, and proteins. It is suggested that didemin B modulates the activity of the FK-506 binding protein as a part of its immunomodulatory process, thus leading to cell death via apoptosis (Altmann, 2017).

11.11.3 APLIDINE

Aplidine is a tunicate/prochloron derived from the cyclic depsipeptide didemnin B, a lead molecule for the treatment of leukemia and lymphoma, and is shown to interfere with the synthesis of DNA and protein, ultimately causing the arrest of the cell cycle. It also inhibits a rate-limiting enzyme (ornithine decarboxylase) in polyamine synthesis, a critical event in tumor growth and angiogenesis. The initial clinical trials show that aplidine is more active than didemnin B (Broggini et al., 2003).

11.11.4 DOLASTATIN

Dolastatin was isolated from *Dolabella curicularia* (sea hares) and reported to be the most potent antiproliferative against marine PS leukemia cells, a noncompetitive inhibitor of Vinca alkaloid-binding tubulin, and impaired significantly microtubule assembly and tubulin-dependent guanosine triphosphate hydrolysis (Bai et al., 1990). The other derivatives of dolastatin-15, cemadatin, and synthadatin are also under clinical trials. All these derivatives inhibited P388 leukemia growth and showed inhibitory effect on three solid tumor lines (Colon 26 adenocarcinoma, B-16 melanoma, and M507 sarcoma) and effect was greater than dolastatin (Abreu and Branco, 2003).

11.11.5 ECTEINASCID-743

Ecteinascid-743 (isolated from Caribbean tunicate, *Ecteinascidia turbinata*), chemically ecteinascid alkaloid as complex tetrahydroisoquonoles, and its dimethyl analog (ET-729) showed cytotoxicity against leukemic cells. Halichondrin B is a complex polyether isolated from the Japanese sponge *Halichondria okadai*. The likely mechanism of Halichondrin B is tubulin inhibition; it also binds noncompetitively to vinca binding sites and causes a characteristic G2M cell cycle arrest as well as disruption of the mitotic spindle. Among the different derivatives of Halichondrin B, erbulin was found to be ultrapotent (in tubulin-targeted mitotic inhibition) and hence taken up for human clinical trials. Kahalalide F is one of the families of dehydroaminobutyric containing cyclic peptides isolated from the Hawaiian mollusk (Rufencens and the green alga *Bryopsis* sp.) (Garcia-Carbonero et al., 2005).

In human cancer models of androgen-independent prostate and other solid tumors, this chemical has been shown to act on lysosomes at the cellular target (in vivo). In individuals with melanoma, colorectal cancer, and hepatocellular carcinoma, it also demonstrated promising anticancer action (De Rosa et al., 2013). Sacophytal A, a diterpenoid of the oxygenated cembrene type discovered from the Okinawan soft coral *Sarcophyton glaucum*, showed potent inhibitory effects against a variety of tumor promoters. Due to the low yield, new powerful sarcophine derivatives were created, one of which is sarcotrial, which has shown effective chemopreventive efficacy against skin cancer (Fahmy et al., 2006).

11.11.6 CURACIN A

Curacin A was isolated from *Lyngbya majuscula* and found to be a potent tubulin interactive compound (colchicines site tubulin binding) and also exhibited significant anticancer activity (Rani et al., 2021). Recently, phytochemists have identified around 5000 natural flavonoids, and very few of them have been evaluated for anticancer properties. Anthocyanins and their congeners exhibited significant anticancer and associated effects like ROS scavenging, phase II detoxification, enzyme activation, anti-inflammatory, antiproliferative, and apoptosis-inducing activities both in vitro and in vivo (Wipf et al., 2004).

11.12 SIGNIFICANCE OF ANTIOXIDANTS IN RED BLOOD CELLS

Erythrocytes have a strong attraction for red blood cells due to their aberrant hemoglobin content. HbS is known to have a strong affinity for red cell membranes, and sickle cells are particularly vulnerable to membrane peroxidation, so 20 people with sickle cell anemia who were heterozygous for the condition were studied to see how the erythrocyte antioxidant system behaved. Glutathione peroxide activity and superoxide dismutase activity in these individuals were both low, although their reduced glutathione levels were normal (Kostić et al., 1993).

11.13 THERAPEUTIC PROPERTIES OF ANTIOXIDANTS

In the treatment of Friedreich ataxia, a rare and degenerative illness that damages the nervous system, antioxidants are essential. In order for the disease to manifest in a child, an afflicted gene must be passed down from one parent to the other in an autosomal recessive form. The disease's progression can't be determined by a simple clinical examination (Al-Snafi, 2015). Neurological scales are used to assess the severity of a condition. Rheumatoid arthritis, hemorrhagic shock, cardiovascular illness, cystic fibrosis, metabolic disorders, gastrointestinal ulcer genesis, and acquired immunodeficiency are all diseases caused by excessive oxidative damage to cells. Leutinide is used as a treatment for radiation immunotherapy and photodynamic therapy (Sheu et al., 2006).

11.14 CONCLUSION

Dietary supplements that include antioxidants are popular because they aim to help people stay healthy and ward off diseases like cancer and heart disease. After a series of large clinical trials, researchers found no evidence that antioxidant supplements improved health but rather that excessive use could be harmful. Lower chronic disease risk is connected with a diet rich in fruits and vegetables as well as minimally refined grains. Because chronic degenerative illness is associated with oxidative stress, it has been hypothesized that dietary antioxidants may play a role. Antioxidants come in a wide variety of forms in all food plants. Many of these antioxidants work together in plants to reduce oxidative stress, and we predict that animals' cells may likewise require a wide variety of antioxidants to be well protected. The identification of dietary plants with high total antioxidant content can be helpful in testing this hypothesis.

KEYWORDS

- **stress**
- **neurotransmitters**
- **antioxidants**
- **fruits**
- **vegetables**
- **green tea**
- **red wine**

REFERENCES

Abd El, H. A. H. M. Lipid Peroxidation End-Products as a Key of Oxidative Stress: Effect of Antioxidant on their Production and Transfer of Free Radicals. In *Lipid Peroxidation*; IntechOpen, 2012.

Abreu, P. M.; Branco, P. S. Natural Product-Like Combinatorial Libraries. *J. Braz. Chem. Soc.* **2003,** *14*, 675–712.

Agati, G.; Brunetti, C.; Fini, A.; Gori, A.; Guidi, L.; Landi, M.; Sebastiani, F.; Tattini, M. Are Flavonoids Effective Antioxidants in Plants? Twenty Years of our Investigation. *Antioxidants* **2020,** *9*, 1098.

Alkilani, A. Z.; McCrudden, M. T.; Donnelly, R. F. Transdermal Drug Delivery: Innovative Pharmaceutical Developments Based on Disruption of the Barrier Properties of the Stratum corneum. *Pharmaceutics* **2015**, *7* (4), 438–470.

Al-Snafi, A. E. Therapeutic Properties of Medicinal Plants: A Review of Plants with Antioxidant Activity (Part 1). *Int. J. Pharmacol. Toxicol.* **2015,** *6*, 159–182.

Altmann, K. H. Drugs from the Oceans: Marine Natural Products as Leads for Drug Discovery. *Chimia* **2017,** *71*, 646.

Aslani, B. A.; Ghobadi, S. Studies on Oxidants and Antioxidants with a Brief Glance at their Relevance to the Immune System. *Life Sci.* **2016,** *146*, 163–173.

Aversa, R.; Petrescu, R. V.; Apicella, A.; Petrescu, F. I. One Can Slow Down the Aging Through Antioxidants. *Am. J. Eng. Appl. Sci.* **2016,** *9* (4), 1112–1126.

Bagchi, K.; Puri, S. Free Radicals and Antioxidants in Health and Disease: A Review. *EMHJ* **1998,** *4* (2), 350–360.

Balakrishnan, D.; Kandasamy, D.; Nithyanand, P. A Review on Antioxidant Activity of Marine Organisms. *Int. J. Chem. Tech. Res.* **2014,** *6*, 3431–3436.

Beara, I. N.; Lesjak, M. M.; Jovin, E. Đ.; Balog, K. J.; Anackov, G. T.; Orcic, D. Z.; Mimica-Dukic, N. M. Plantain (Plantago L.) Species as Novel Sources of Flavonoid Antioxidants. *J. Agric. Food Chem.* **2009,** *57*, 9268–9273.

Benzie, I. F. F.; Szeto, Y. T. Total Antioxidant Capacity of Teas by the Ferric Reducing/Antioxidant Power Assay. *J. Agric. Food Chem.* **1999,** *47*, 633–636.

Bhattacharya, S. Reactive Oxygen Species and Cellular Defense System. In *Free Radicals in Human Health and Disease*, 2015; pp 17–29.
Bhuvaneswari, V.; Nagini, S. Lycopene: A Review of its Potential as an Anticancer Agent. *Current Medicinal Chemistry-Anti-Cancer Agents*. **2005,** *5*, 627–635.
Bisby, R. H.; Brooke, R.; Navaratnam, S. Effect of Antioxidant Oxidation Potential in the Oxygen Radical Absorption Capacity (ORAC) Assay. *Food Chem*. **2008,** *108*, 1002–1007.
Broggini, M.; Marchini, S. V; Galliera, E.; Borsotti, P.; Taraboletti, G.; Erba, E.; Sironi, M.; Jimeno, J.; Faircloth, G. T.; Giavazzi, R. Aplidine, A New Anticancer Agent of Marine Origin, Inhibits Vascular Endothelial Growth Factor (VEGF) Secretion and Blocks VEGF-VEGFR-1 (flt-1) Autocrine Loop in Human Leukemia Cells MOLT-4. *Leukemia* **2003,** *17*, 52–59.
Brush, M. J.; Giani, M.; Totti, C.; Testa, J. M.; Faganeli, J.; Ogrinc, N.; Kemp, W.M.; Umani, S. F. Eutrophication, Harmful Algae, Oxygen Depletion, and Acidification. In *Coastal Ecosystems in Transition: A Comparative Analysis of the Northern Adriatic and Chesapeake Bay*, 2020; pp 75–104.
Buřičová, L.; Reblova, Z. Czech Medicinal Plants as Possible Sources of Antioxidants. *Czech J. Food Sci*. **2008,** *26*, 132–138.
Bystrom, L. M.; Guzman, M. L.; Rivella, S. Iron and Reactive Oxygen Species: Friends or Foes of Cancer Cells? *Antioxid. Redox Signal*. **2014,** *20*, 1917–1924.
Cao, H. H.; Tse, A. K. W.; Kwan, H. Y.; Yu, H.; Cheng, C. Y.; Su, T.; Fong, W. F.; Yu, Z. L. Quercetin Exerts Anti-Melanoma Activities and Inhibits STAT3 Signaling. *Biochem. Pharmacol*. **2014,** *87*, 424–434.
Casey, S. C.; Amedei, A.; Aquilano, K.; Azmi, A. S.; Benencia, F.; Bhakta, D.; Bilsland, A. E.; Boosani, C. S.; Chen, S.; Ciriolo, M. R. Cancer Prevention and Therapy Through the Modulation of the Tumor Microenvironment. In *Seminars in Cancer Biology*; Elsevier, 2015; pp S199–S223.
Chakraborty, P.; Kumar, S.; Dutta, D.; Gupta, V. Role of Antioxidants in Common Health Diseases. *Res. J. Pharm. Technol*. **2009,** *2*, 238–244.
Chan, C. F.; Tsang, M. K.; Li, H.; Lan, R.; Chadbourne, F. L.; Chan, W. L.; Law, G. L.; Cobb, S. L.; Hao, J.; Wong, W. T. Bifunctional Up-Converting Lanthanide Nanoparticles for Selective In Vitro Imaging and Inhibition of Cyclin D as Anti-Cancer Agents. *J. Mater. Chem. B* **2014,** *2*, 84–91.
Christodouleas, D. C.; Fotakis, C.; Papadopoulos, K.; Calokerinos, A. C. Evaluation of Total Reducing Power of Edible Oils. *Talanta* **2014,** *130*, 233–240.
Dalle-Donne, I.; Rossi, R.; Giustarini, D.; Milzani, A.; Colombo, R. Protein Carbonyl Groups as Biomarkers of Oxidative Stress. *Clinica Chimica Acta* **2003,** 329, 23–38.
David, A. V. A.; Arulmoli, R.; Parasuraman, S. Overviews of Biological Importance of Quercetin: A Bioactive Flavonoid. *Phcog. Rev*. **2016,** *10*, 84.
De la Fuente, M. Effects of Antioxidants on Immune System Ageing. *Euro. J. Clin. Nutr*. **2002,** *56*, S5–S8.
Díaz, G. C.; Cruz, Y. R.; Fortes, M. M.; Viegas, C. V.; Carliz, R. G.; Furtado, N. C.; Aranda, D. A. G. Primary Separation of Antioxidants (Unsaponifiables) the Wet Biomass Microalgae Chlamydomonas sp. and Production of the Biodiesel. *Natl. Sci*. **2014,** *6*, 1210.
Ehteshamfar, S.; Akhbari, M.; Afshari, J. T.; Seyedi, M.; Nikfar, B.; Shapouri-Moghaddam, A.; Ghanbarzadeh, E.; Momtazi-Borojeni, A. A. Anti-inflammatory and Immune-Modulatory Impacts of Berberine on Activation of Autoreactive T Cells in Autoimmune Inflammation. *J. Cell. Mol. Med*. **2020,** *24*, 13573–13588.

Engwa, G. A. Free Radicals and the Role of Plant Phytochemicals as Antioxidants Against Oxidative Stress-Related Diseases. *Phytochemicals* **2018,** *7*, 49–74.

Fahmy, N. M.; Mahmud, S.; Aprikian, A. G. Delay in the Surgical Treatment of Bladder Cancer and Survival: Systematic Review of the Literature. *Eur. Urol.* **2006,** *50*, 1176–1182.

Farzaei, M. H.; Bahramsoltani, R.; Abdollahi, M.; Rahimi, R. The Role of Visceral Hypersensitivity in Irritable Bowel Syndrome: Pharmacological Targets and Novel Treatments. *J. Neurogastroenterol. Motil.* **2016,** *22*, 558.

Gaobotse, G.; Venkataraman, S.; Brown, P. D.; Masisi, K.; Kwape, T. E.; Nkwe, D. O.; Rantong, G.; Makhzoum, A. The Use of African Medicinal Plants in Cancer Management. *Front. Pharmacol.* **2023,** *14*, 112–388.

Garcia-Carbonero, R.; Supko, J. G.; Maki, R. G.; Manola, J.; Ryan, D. P.; Harmon, D.; Puchalski, T. A.; Goss, G.; Seiden, M. V; Waxman, A. Ecteinascidin-743 (ET-743) for Chemotherapy-Naive Patients with Advanced Soft Tissue Sarcomas: Multicenter Phase II and Pharmacokinetic Study. *J. Clin. Oncol.* **2005,** *23*, 5484–5492.

Gomes, E. C.; Silva, A. N.; Oliveira, M. R. de Oxidants, Antioxidants, and the Beneficial Roles of Exercise-Induced Production of Reactive Species. *Oxid. Med. Cell. Longev.* **2012,** 1–12.

Guerra-Araiza, C.; Álvarez-Mejía, A. L.; Sánchez-Torres, S.; Farfan-García, E.; Mondragón-Lozano, R.; Pinto-Almazán, R.; Salgado-Ceballos, H. Effect of Natural Exogenous Antioxidants on Aging and on Neurodegenerative Diseases. *Free Radic. Res.* **2013,** *47*, 451–462.

Hamid, A. A.; Aiyelaagbe, O. O.; Usman, L. A.; Ameen, O. M.; Lawal, A. Antioxidants: Its Medicinal and Pharmacological Applications. *Afr. J. Pure Appl. Chem.* **2010,** *4*, 142–151.

Heidari, S.; Azizbeigi, K.; Bahman Pour, K. The Effect of 12 Weeks of Aerobic Exercise on Cardiac Antioxidant Enzymes in the Hypercholesterolemic Male Wistar Rats. *J. Anim. Biol.* **2021,** *13*, 57–66.

Hordyjewska, A.; Ostapiuk, A.; Horecka, A.; Kurzepa, J. Betulin and Betulinic Acid: Triterpenoids Derivatives with a Powerful Biological Potential. *Phytochem. Rev.* **2019,** *18*, 929–951.

Imran, M.; Rauf, A.; Abu-Izneid, T.; Nadeem, M.; Shariati, M. A.; Khan, I. A.; Imran, A.; Orhan, I. E.; Rizwan, M.; Atif, M. Luteolin, A Flavonoid, as an Anticancer Agent: A Review. *Biomed. Pharmacother.* **2019,** *112*, 108612.

Isemura, M. Catechin in Human Health and Disease. *Molecules* **2019,** *24*, 528.

Kamal-Eldin, A.; Appelqvist, L. The Chemistry and Antioxidant Properties of Tocopherols and Tocotrienols. *Lipids* **1996,** *31*, 671–701.

Kaneto, H.; Kajimoto, Y.; Miyagawa, J.; Matsuoka, T.; Fujitani, Y.; Umayahara, Y.; Hanafusa, T.; Matsuzawa, Y.; Yamasaki, Y.; Hori, M. Beneficial Effects of Antioxidants in Diabetes: Possible Protection of Pancreatic Beta-Cells Against Glucose Toxicity. *Diabetes* **1999,** *48*, 2398–2406.

Kostić, M. M.; Ognjanović, B.; Dimitrijević, S.; Zikić, R. V; Stajn, A.; Rosić, G. L.; Zivković, R. V. Cadmium-Induced Changes of Antioxidant and Metabolic Status in Red Blood Cells of Rats: In Vivo Effects. *Euro. J. Haematol.* **1993,** *51*, 86–92.

Kulkarni, B. D.; Hoskeri, J. H.; Vedamurthy, A. B. Neuroprotective and Anti-inflammatory Activities of Aegiceras corniculatum (L.) Blanco. *Pharmacogn. Res.* **2019,** *11* (3), 260–266.

Lan, Y.; Wang, H.; Wu, J.; Meng, X. Cytokine Storm-Calming Property of the Isoquinoline Alkaloids in Coptis chinensis Franch. *Front. Pharmacol.* **2022,** *13*, 1–17.

Lindshield, B. L.; Ford, N. A.; Canene-Adams, K.; Diamond, A. M.; Wallig, M. A.; Erdman Jr, J. W. Selenium, but not Lycopene or Vitamin E, Decreases Growth of Transplantable Dunning R3327-H Rat Prostate Tumors. *PLoS One* **2010,** *5*, e10423.

Lobo, V.; Patil, A.; Phatak, A.; Chandra, N. Free Radicals, Antioxidants and Functional Foods: Impact on Human Health. *Pharmacog. Rev.* **2010,** *4*, 118.

Logan, B. A.; Grace, S. C.; Adams III, W. W.; Demmig-Adams, B. Seasonal Differences in Xanthophyll Cycle Characteristics and Antioxidants in Mahonia repens Growing in Different Light Environments. *Oecologia* **1998,** *116*, 9–17.

Lu, X.; Wang, J.; Al-Qadiri, H. M.; Ross, C. F.; Powers, J. R.; Tang, J.; Rasco, B. A. Determination of Total Phenolic Content and Antioxidant Capacity of Onion (Allium cepa) and Shallot (Allium oschaninii) using Infrared Spectroscopy. *Food Chem.* **2011,** *129*, 637–644.

Meade, T.; Sleight, P.; Collins, R.; Armitage, J.; Parish, S.; Peto, R.; Youngman, L.; Buxton, M.; Fuller, J.; Keech, A. MRC BHF Heart Protection Study of Cholesterol-Lowering Therapy and of Antioxidant Vitamin Supplementation in a Wide Range of Patients at Increased Risk of Coronary Heart Disease Death: Early Safety and Efficacy Experience. *Euro. Heart J.* **1999,** *20*, 725-741

Menvielle-Bourg, F. J. Superoxide Dismutase (SOD), the Powerful Natural Antioxidant, Now Available Orally. *Phytothérapie* **2005,** *3*, 118–121.

Nanjo, F.; Goto, K.; Seto, R.; Suzuki, M.; Sakai, M.; Hara, Y. Scavenging Effects of Tea Catechins and their Derivatives on 1, 1-diphenyl-2-picrylhydrazyl Radical. *Free Radic. Biol. Med.* **1996,** *21*, 895–902.

Niemann, H.; Marmann, A.; Lin, W.; Proksch, P. Sponge Derived Bromotyrosines: Structural Diversity Through Natural Combinatorial Chemistry. *Natl. Prod. Commun.* **2015,** *10* (1), 219–231.

Peng, G.; Tang, X.; Gui, Y.; Yang, J.; Ye, L.; Wu, L.; Ding, Y. H.; Wang, L. Transient Receptor Potential Vanilloid Subtype 1: A Potential Therapeutic Target for Fibrotic Diseases. *Front. Physiol.* **2022,** *13*, 951980.

Pham-Huy, L. A.; He, H.; Pham-Huy, C. Free Radicals, Antioxidants in Disease and Health. *Int. J. Biomed. Sci.* **2008,** *4*, 89.

Puntel, R. L.; Nogueira, C. W.; Rocha, J. B. T. Krebs Cycle Intermediates Modulate Thiobarbituric Acid Reactive Species (TBARS) Production in Rat $_B$rain in vitro. *Neurochem. Res.* **2005,** *30*, 225–235.

Rani, D.; Garg, V.; Dutt, R. Anticancer Potential of Azole Containing Marine Natural Products: Current and Future Perspectives. *Anti-Cancer Agents Med. Chem.* **2021,** *21*, 1957–1976.

Rizzo, A. M.; Berselli, P.; Zava, S.; Montorfano, G.; Negroni, M.; Corsetto, P.; Berra, B. Endogenous Antioxidants and Radical Scavengers. In *Bio-Farms for Nutraceuticals: Functional Food and Safety Control by Biosensors*, 2010; pp 52–67.

Rook, F.; Hadingham, S. A.; Li, Y.; Bevan, M. W. Sugar and ABA Response Pathways and the Control of Gene Expression. *Plant Cell Environ.* **2006,** *29*, 426–434.

Rosa, G.; Misso, G.; Salzano, G.; Caraglia, M. Bisphosphonates and Cancer: What Opportunities from Nanotechnology? *J. Drug Deliv.* **2013,** 1–17.

Ruiz-Rodríguez, B. M.; De Ancos, B.; Sánchez-Moreno, C.; Fernández-Ruiz, V.; de Cortes Sánchez-Mata, M.; Cámara, M.; Tardío, J. Wild blackthorn (Prunus spinosa L.) and hawthorn (Crataegus monogyna Jacq.) Fruits as Valuable Sources of Antioxidants. *Fruits* **2014,** *69*, 61–73.

Sakhi, A. K. Low Molecular Weight Plasma Antioxidants in Healthy Individuals and Head and Neck Squamous Cell Carcinoma Patients, 2008.

Schmidt, S.; Pokorný, J. Potential Application of Oilseeds as Sources of Antioxidants for Food Lipids–A Review. *Czech J. Food Sci.* **2005,** *23*, 93–102.

Sen, S.; Chakraborty, R.; Sridhar, C.; Reddy, Y. S. R.; De, B. Free Radicals, Antioxidants, Diseases and Phytomedicines: Current Status and Future Prospect. *Int. J. Pharm. Sci. Rev. Res.* **2010,** *3*, 91–100.

Shah, M. A.; Bosco, S. J. D.; Mir, S. A. Plant Extracts as Natural Antioxidants in Meat and Meat Products. *Meat Sci.* **2014,** *98*, 21–33.

Shahidi, F.; Zhong, Y. Measurement of Antioxidant Activity. *J. Funct. Foods* **2015,** *18*, 757–781.

Sharafati-Chaleshtori, R.; Shirzad, H.; Rafieian-Kopaei, M.; Soltani, A. Melatonin and Human Mitochondrial Diseases. *J. Res. Med. Sci.* **2017,** *22*, 2.

Sheu, S. S.; Nauduri, D.; Anders, M. W. Targeting Antioxidants to Mitochondria: A New Therapeutic Direction. *Biochim. Biophys.* **2006,** *1762*, 256–265.

Silva, C. G.; De Almeida, V. L.; Campana, P. R. V; Rocha, M. P. Plant Cell Cultures as Producers of Secondary Metabolites: Podophyllum lignans as a Model. In *Transgenesis and Secondary Metabolism, Reference Series in Phytochemistry,* 1st Ed.; Jha, S., Ed., **2017**; pp 67–102.

Snezhkina, A. V.; Kudryavtseva, A. V.; Kardymon, O. L.; Savvateeva, M. V.; Melnikova, N. V.; Krasnov, G. S.; Dmitriev, A. A. ROS Generation and Antioxidant Defense Systems in Normal and Malignant Cells. *Oxid. Med. Cell. Longev.* **2019,** 1–17.

Somogyi, A.; Rosta, K.; Pusztai, P.; Tulassay, Z.; Nagy, G. Antioxidant Measurements. *Physiol. Meas.* **2007,** *28*, R41.

Stolarzewicz, I. A.; Ciekot, J.; Fabiszewska, A. U.; Białecka-Florjańczyk, E. Plant and Microbial Sources of Antioxidants. *Postepy Hig. Med. Dosw.* **2013,** *67*, 1359–1373.

Sundaram Sanjay, S.; Shukla, A. K. Free Radicals Versus Antioxidants. In *Potential Therapeutic Applications of Nano-Antioxidants*; Springer, 2021; pp 1–17.

Tekwani, B. L. Editorial [Infectious Disorders Drug Targets-An Arsenal of Knowledge on Pathogen Targets]. *Infect. Disord. Drug Targets* **2008,** *8*, 46–47.

Thomas, M. J. The Role of Free Radicals and Antioxidants: How do we know that they are Working? *Crit. Rev. Food Sci. Nutr.* **1995,** *35*, 21–39.

Travaglione, S.; Fabbri, A.; Fiorentini, C. The Rho-activating CNF1 Toxin from Pathogenic E. coli: A Risk Factor for Human Cancer Development? *Infect. Agents Cancer* **2008,** *3*, 1–9.

Valenzuela, A.; Sanhueza, J.; Nieto, S. Cholesterol Oxidation: Health Hazard and the Role of Antioxidants in Prevention. *Biol. Res.* **2003,** *36*, 291–302.

Valko, M.; Leibfritz, D.; Moncol, J.; Cronin, M. T. D.; Mazur, M.; Telser, J. Free Radicals and Antioxidants in Normal Physiological Functions and Human Disease. *Int. J. Biochem. Cell Biol.* **2007,** *39*, 44–84.

van den Berg, R.; Haenen, G. R. M. M.; van den Berg, H.; Bast, A. Applicability of an Improved Trolox Equivalent Antioxidant Capacity (TEAC) Assay for Evaluation of Antioxidant Capacity Measurements of Mixtures. *Food Chem.* **1999,** *66*, 511–517.

Wang, N.; Tan, H. Y.; Li, L.; Yuen, M. F.; Feng, Y. Berberine and Coptidis Rhizoma as Potential Anticancer Agents: Recent Updates and Future Perspectives. *J. Ethnopharmacol.* **2015,** *176*, 35–48.

Wipf, P.; Reeves, J. T.; Day, B. W. Chemistry and Biology of Curacin A. *Curr. Pharm. Design* **2004,** *10*, 1417–1437.

Wu, D.; Cederbaum, A. I. Alcohol, Oxidative Stress, and Free Radical Damage. *Alcohol Res. Health* **2003,** *27*, 277.

Žebeljan, A.; Vico, I.; Duduk, N.; Žiberna, B.; Krajnc, A. U. Profiling Changes in Primary Metabolites and Antioxidants During Apple Fruit Decay Caused by Penicillium crustosum. *Physiol. Mol. Plant Pathol.* **2021,** *113*, 101586.

Zhang, Y.; Lin, H.; Liu, C.; Huang, J.; Liu, Z. A Review for Physiological Activities of EGCG and the Role in Improving Fertility in Humans/Mammals. *Biomed. Pharmacother.* **2020,** *127*, 110186.

Zhang, D.; Xu, H.; Wang, L.; Li, Y.; Sun, P.; Wu, X.; Wang, G.; Chen, W.; Ye, W. Betulinic Acid and its Derivatives as Potential Antitumor Agents. *Med. Res. Rev.* **2015,** *35*, 1127–1155.

Zhou, H. Y.; Zhu, H.; Yao, X. M.; Qian, J. P.; Yang, J.; Pan, X. D.; Chen, X. D. Metformin Regulates Tight Junction of Intestinal Epithelial Cells via MLCK-MLC Signaling Pathway. *Eur. Rev. Med. Pharmacol. Sci.* **2017,** *21*, 5239–5246.

INDEX

A

Acute stress disorder (ASD), 284
Allium sativum (Lasun), 106
Antioxidants, 40, 305
  anticancer activity
    berberin and coptis, 319–320
  anti-inflammatory activities, 308
  aplidine, 328
  betulinic acid, 321
  butylated hydroxy toluene (BHT), 311
  butylated hydroxyl anisole (BHA), 311
  capsaicin, 322
  catechin, 322
  characteristics, 316
  classification, 309
    endogenous antioxidants, 309–310
    exogenous antioxidants, 310–311
  Curacin A, 329
  dichlorofluorescein (DCF), 316
  dichlorofluorescein diacetate (DCFDA), 316
  didemnin B, 328
  2,4-dinitrophenylhydrazine (DNPH), 315
  dolastatin, 328
  ecteinascid-743, 328–329
  effects, 317–318
  epicatechin, 322–323
  exogenous antioxidants
    natural antioxidants, 310–311
    synthetic antioxidants, 311
  ferrous oxidation-xylenol orange (FOX), 315
  folin ciocalteu (FC), 313
  lanthanides as anticancer agents, 318
  lycopene as potential anticancer agent, 318
  malondialdehyde (MDA), 315
  marine-derived anticancer molecules, 325–327
  mechanism(s) of anticancer activity, 327
  metal chelating agent (EDTA), 311
  nordihydroguaiaretic acid (NDGA), 311
  origin, 307–309
  our body, antioxidants system, 316–317
  oxygen radical absorption capacity (ORAC), 313
  podophyllotoxin, 321
  polyunsaturated fatty acid (PUFA), 310
  propyl gallate (PG), 311
  psammaplin-A, 327
  quercetin, 323–325
  reactive oxygen species (ROS), 319
  red blood cells
    significance, 329–330
  rich food sources, 265, 266–268
    agriculture, 268–269
    Alzheimer's disease, 271
    antioxidants, 269–270
    brain, 274
    brain function, 274–275
    breast cancer, 273
    cardiovascular disease, 272
    dietary sufficiency, 274
    elderly individuals, 266
    feeding the elderly, 273–274
    food, 268–269
    food color, 274
    food flavor, 274–275
    fragrant herbs, 270–271
    general, 275
    health, 266
    health promotion, 276
    nutrition, 268
    nutritional antioxidants, 272
    prevention of neurodegeneration, 275
    reno-protective dietary antioxidants, 272
    spices, 270–271
  selenium derivatives as cancer-preventive agents, 319
  sources, 307–309
  superoxide dismutase (SOD), 316
  techniques for measurement, 313
    biochemical assays, 315

chemical assays, 313
DPPH assay (1,1-diphenyl-2-picrylhydrazyl), 314
ferric-reducing antioxidant power, 314
FOX, 315
oxygen radical absorption capacity, 313
protein carbonyl, 315
ROS, 316
SOD, 315
TBARS, 315
total phenolic content (TPC), 313–314
total reducing power (TRP), 314
trolox equivalent, 314
tertiary butyl hydroquinone (TBHQ), 311
therapeutic properties, 330
thiobarbituric acid (TBA), 315
types, 311
ascorbic acid, 311
glutathione, 312
melatonin, 312
tocopherols, 312–313
tocotrienols, 312–313
Anti-stress functional foods, 283
acetylcholine (ACh), 290
acute stress disorder (ASD), 284
symptoms, 285
adaptogenic, 297–298
beans, 296
berries, 292–293
blueberries, 293
brain function complications, 286–287
destructive effects of stress CNS function, 287
learning, 288
stress affects cognition, 288
cardiovascular system, 289
chronic obstructive pulmonary disease (COPD), 289
chronic stress
impacts on the human body, 286
corticotropin-releasing hormone 2 (CRH-2), 288
dietary neurotransmitters, 291
dry volume (DV), 296
fruits, 291–292
gamma-aminobutyric acid (GABA), 290
gastrointestinal system, 288–289
linolenic acid (LNA), 296
megadosages stress therapy, 298–299
neurotransmitters (NTs), 290
nootropic, 297–298
oranges, 294
phytoconstituents, 292
plums, 294–295
pomegranates, 296
post-traumatic stress disorder (PTSD), 284
probiotics, 297
prunes, 295
recommended dietary allowance (RDA), 298
red grapes, 295–296
red wine, 298
reproductive system, 289–290
respiratory system, 289
resveratrol, 298
seeds, 296–297
strawberries, 293–294
stress, 284
acute stress, 284
chronic stress, 286
dietary neurotransmitters, 290–291
World Health Organization (WHO), 284
2, 2-Azino-bis (3-ethyl benzothiazoline-6 sulfonic acid) diammonium salt) ABTS method, 23

B

Bacillus Calmette–Guérin (BCG), 108
Bilateral common carotid artery occlusion (BCCAO), 209
Brain-derived neurotrophic factor (BDNF), 207
Butylated hydroxy toluene (BHT), 311
Butylated hydroxyl anisole (BHA), 311

C

Camella sinensis L. *(Theaceae),* 107
Cardiovascular diseases (CVDs), 128
antioxidant defense mechanism
catalase (CAT), 135
glutathione peroxidase (GPx), 135
superoxide dismutase (SOD), 135
nutraceuticals used in
coenzyme Q10, 148–149
flavonoids, 146–148
human heart, 137–140
lycopene, 144–146

selenium (Se), 136–137
vitamin C, 143–144
vitamin E, 140–142
reactive oxygen species (ROS), 129
atherosclerosis, 133–135
hypertension, 132–133
production in cytosol, 130
production in mitochondria, 130–132
Catalase (CAT), 135
Cerebrospinal fluid (CSF), 210
Chronic inflammatory diseases, 157
adenosine triphosphate (ATP), 167
asthma, 175–176
cancer, 172–173
cardiovascular disease (CVD), 173
central nervous system (CNS), 176
chronic liver disease (CLD), 159
chronic obstructive pulmonary disease (COPD), 175
classification of inflammation, 158
acute inflammation, 158–159
chronic inflammation, 159–160
CNS related diseases, 176
C-reactive protein (CRP), 173
cyclooxygenase (COX), 162
depression, 176
diabetes, 173
different biological activities, 180–181
diseases, 172
electron spin resonance (ESR), 160
free radicals, 177–178
history, 160
principles, 161
types, 161
inflammatory bowel disease (IBD), 175
mechanistic insight of oxidative stress, 169–171
myocardial infarction (MI), 173
natural compounds, 178–181
nucleic acid phosphatase (NCP), 178
obesity, 173–174
osteoporosis, 174
oxidative damage, targets, 163
DNA, 165
lipids, 163–164
proteins, 164
oxidative stress (OS), 171
Parkinson's disease, 176–177
reactive nitrogen species (RNS), 160
reactive oxygen species (ROS), 160, 165
DNA oxidation, 168–169
ion channels, 167
lipid peroxidation, 167–168
protein modifications, 168
redox-sensitive transcript factors, 165–166
triggering of protein kinases, 166
rheumatoid arthritis (RA), 174–175
stress-activated protein kinase C-JUN N-terminal kinase (SAPK-JNK), 166
Substantia Nigra Pars Compacta (SNPC), 176
suppressors of cytokine signaling (SOCS), 171
tumor microenvironment (TME), 170
types
hydrogen peroxide, 163
peroxyl radical (ROO), 163
reactive oxygen species (ROS), 161–162
superoxide, 162–163
unfolded protein response (UPR), 167
Chronic obstructive pulmonary disease (COPD), 289
Corticotropin-releasing hormone 2 (CRH-2), 288
Cyclooxygenase (COX), 106

D

Diabetes mellitus (DM), 26, 230
anthocyanins, 244
chromium, 233–234
curcuma longa, 232–233
flavanones, 241
flavones, 243
flavonol, 240
lipoic acid, 234–235
magnesium, 234
resveratrol, 245–246
selenium, 235
vitamin E, 236–237
zinc, 230–232
Dichlorofluorescein (DCF), 316
Dichlorofluorescein diacetate (DCFDA), 316
2,4-Dinitrophenylhydrazine (DNPH), 315
1, 1 Diphenyl-2-picrylhydrazyl (DPPH) method, 22
DMPD (N, N-dimethyl-P-phenylenediamine dihydrochloride) method, 24

DPPH assay (1,1-diphenyl-2-picrylhydrazyl), 314
Dry volume (DV), 296

E

Epigallocatechin gallate (EGCG)
  green tea bioactives, 69
    absorption and distribution, 70
    cardiovascular diseases, 75–76
    excretion, 71–72
    health and wellness, 72
    hematologic diseases, 73–75
    metabolism, 71
    mutagenicity and carcinogenicity, 77–78
    neurological diseases, 76–77
  polyphenol oxidase (PPO), 68
  therapeutic potential
    gold nanocarriers, 84–85
    lipid nanoparticles, 79, 81–82
    liposomes, 82–83
    nanocarriers, 78–79
    polymeric nanocarriers, 83–84

F

Ferrous oxidation-xylenol orange (FOX), 315
Folin ciocalteu (FC), 313
Food and nutrition board (FNB), 236

G

Gamma-aminobutyric acid (GABA), 290
Glial fibrillary acidic protein (GFAP), 209
Glutathione peroxidase (GPx), 12, 135
Glutathione reductase (GR), 12
Glutathione-S-transferases (GST), 12–13
Green tea bioactives, 69
  absorption and distribution, 70
  cardiovascular diseases, 75–76
  excretion, 71–72
  health and wellness, 72
  hematologic diseases, 73–75
  metabolism, 71
  mutagenicity and carcinogenicity, 77–78
  neurological diseases, 76–77

H

Huntington's disease (HD), 196

I

Immunomodulators
  antioxidants
    Allium sativum (Lasun), 106
    applications of, 103
    Bacillus Calmette–Guérin (BCG), 108
    Camella sinensis L. *(Theaceae),* 107
    challenges and, 115–116
    curcumin crude extract, 105
    cyclooxygenase (COX), 106
    and defense, 100–102
    lipoxygenase (LOX), 106
    NALP3 inflammasome, 109
    NRLP3 inflammasome, 110
    peripheral blood mononuclear cells (PBMCs), 109
    plant-derived antioxidants, 111–114
    Quillaja saponaria, 108
    Stephania tetrandra S., 108
    vitamin C (ascorbic acid), 104
  free radicals, 96
  immune system, 97–98
  immunomodulating agents, 98–99
  need for, 99–100

L

Linolenic acid (LNA), 296
Lipoxygenase (LOX), 106

M

Macrophage-derived chemokine (MDC), 206
Malondialdehyde (MDA), 315
Megadosages stress therapy, 298–299
Mitogen-activated protein kinase (MAPK), 209

N

Natural antioxidants
  antioxidants, 7
    1, 1 diphenyl-2-picrylhydrazyl (DPPH) method, 22
    2, 2-azino-bis (3-ethyl benzothiazoline-6 sulfonic acid) diammonium salt ABTS method, 23
    capsicum annuum, 20
    carotenoid linoleate model, 24
    chain breaking, 8

conjugated diene assay, 22
curcumin, 20
DMPD (N, N-dimethyl-P-phenylenediamine dihydrochloride) method, 24
estimation of, 22
eugenia caryophyllus, 20
flavonoids, 16–17
fruits and vegetables, 15–16
garlic *(Allium sativum),* 19–20
geranium sanguineum, 21
hydroxyl radical scavenging activity, 23
Leea indica, 21–22
marine sources, 18–19
mechanism of action, 8–9
medicinal plants and spices, 19–22
mushrooms, 19
nitric oxide radical inhibition activity, 23
nitro blue tetrazolium (NBT), 22
oxygen radical absorbance capacity (ORAC), 24
peroxynitrite radical scavenging activity, 23
phosphomolybdenum method, 23
pistacia lentiscus, 21
Polyalthia cerasoides, 22
polyphenols, 16
polyunsaturated fatty acid (PUFA), 22
prevention of oxidation, 8
recycle waste, 17–18
salvia officinalis, 21
superoxide radical scavenge activity, 22
total radical trapping antioxidant potential (TRAP) technique, 24
Trolox equivalent (TE) equivalent, 24
uncaria tomentosa, 21
classification, 10
catalase (CAT), 12
enzyme-based antioxidants, 11
glutathione, 13
glutathione peroxidase (GPx), 12
glutathione reductase (GR), 12
glutathione-S-transferases (GST), 12–13
superoxide dismutase (SOD), 11–12
health benefits and potential role, 24
cancer, 26–27
cardiovascular diseases, 26
diabetes mellitus (DM), 26
neurodegenerative disorders, 25
natural antioxidants, 9–10
non-enzymatic antioxidants
carotenoids (β-Carotene), 15
ceruloplasmin, 14
lactoferrin, 14
selenium (Se), 13–14
transferrin, 14
vitamin A, 14
vitamin C, 14
vitamin E, 14–15
nutraccuticals, 5
oxidation process, 6–7
Neurodegenerative disorders (NDs), 195, 201
Alzheimer's disease (AD), 201–202
amyotrophic lateral sclerosis (ALS), 203
Huntington disease (HD), 202–203
Parkinson's disease (PD), 202
spinal muscular atrophy (SMA), 204
spinocerebellar ataxia (SCA), 204
Neurotransmitters (NTs), 290
Nitro blue tetrazolium (NBT), 22
Non-enzymatic antioxidants
carotenoids (β-Carotene), 15
ceruloplasmin, 14
lactoferrin, 14
selenium (Se), 13–14
transferrin, 14
vitamin A, 14
vitamin C, 14
vitamin E, 14–15
Nordihydroguaiaretic acid (NDGA), 311
Nutraceutical antioxidants, 225
anthocyanins
cyanidin, 244–245
delphinidin, 245
pelargonidin, 245
diabetes mellitus, 226
oxidative stress, 228–229
pathophysiology of diabetes, 226–227
vitamin D, 246
diabetes mellitus (DM), 230
anthocyanins, 244
chromium, 233–234
curcuma longa, 232–233
flavanones, 241
flavones, 243
flavonol, 240
lipoic acid, 234–235

magnesium, 234
resveratrol, 245–246
selenium, 235
vitamin E, 236–237
zinc, 230–232
flavanones
hesperidin, 241–242
naringenin, 242–243
flavones
apigenin, 243
wogonin, 243–244
flavonol
kaempferol, 240–241
food and nutrition board (FNB), 236
glutathione peroxidase (GPx), 249
glutathione reductase (GR), 249
nitric oxide (NO), 249
nutraceuticals, 229–230, 231
reactive oxygen species (ROS), 228
role
diabetes retinopathy, 237–238
diabetic nephropathy, 237
selenium (Se)
insulin resistance, role of selenium, 235–236
types of diabetes, 228
vitamin D
diabetic peripheral neuropathy, 248
effect on diabetic nephropathy, 249
effect on diabetic retinopathy, 249–250
impact on glycemic control, 246–248
vitamin E
protective action, 240
role, 237
role of vitamin as endogenous antioxidant defenses, 239
Nutraceuticals, 3

O

Oxygen radical absorbance capacity (ORAC), 24, 313

P

Peroxyl radical (ROO), 163
Phytochemical antioxidants
carotenoids, 49
β-carotene, 50–51
β-cryptoxanthin, 52–53
curcumin, 51–52
lutein, 52
lycopene, 51
non-protein
bilirubin, 56–57
ubiquinone, 57–58
uric acid, 58–59
polyphenolic acid
ferulic acid, 48–49
hydroxycinnamic acid, 48
polyphenols, 46–47
ginger, 48
proteins
albumin, 53–54
ceruloplasmin, 54
haptoglobin, 54–55
lactoferrin, 55–56
transferrin, 56
vitamin A, 41–42
vitamin B, 42
vitamin cofactors and minerals
coenzyme Q 10 (CoQ-10), 43
copper, 45
iodine, 46
manganese, 44
selenium, 44–45
zinc, 45–46
vitamin E, 42
Phytochemicals, 39
Plant-derived antioxidant nutraceuticals, 195
Alzheimer's disease (AD), 195
amyloid precursor protein (APP), 206
amyotrophic lateral sclerosis (ALS), 196
bilateral common carotid artery occlusion (BCCAO), 209
brain-derived neurotrophic factor (BDNF), 207
central nervous system (CNS), 196
cerebrospinal fluid (CSF), 210
glial fibrillary acidic protein (GFAP), 209
Huntington's disease (HD), 196
macrophage-derived chemokine (MDC), 206
mitogen-activated protein kinase (MAPK), 209
neurodegenerative disorders (NDs), 195, 201

Alzheimer's disease (AD), 201–202
amyotrophic lateral sclerosis (ALS), 203
Huntington disease (HD), 202–203
Parkinson's disease (PD), 202
spinal muscular atrophy (SMA), 204
spinocerebellar ataxia (SCA), 204
neuropharmacological perspective, 204–205
curcumin, 209–210
ginkgo biloba, 210
grape seed extract, 211–212
green tea polyphenols, 212
guarana seed extract, 214–215
lycopene, 207–209
magnolol, 211
pycnogenol, 212–213
resveratrol, 205–206
vitamin C (ascorbic acid), 210–211
vitamin E, 213–214
xanthorrhizol, 213
nitric oxide (NO), 209
Parkinson's disease (PD), 195
spinal muscular atrophy (SMA), 196
spinocerebellar ataxia (SCA), 196
superoxide dismutase (SOD), 209
thiobarbituric acid reactive substances (TBARS), 207
tocotrienol-rich fraction (TRF), 214
total cholesterol (TC), 208
treatment of NDs, 198–199
Polyalthia cerasoides, 22
Polyphenol oxidase (PPO), 68
Polyunsaturated fatty acid (PUFA), 22, 310
Post-traumatic stress disorder (PTSD), 284
Propyl gallate (PG), 311
Psammaplin-A, 327

Q

Quercetin, 323–325
Quillaja saponaria, 108

R

Reactive oxygen species (ROS), 4, 129, 165, 319
atherosclerosis, 133–135
DNA oxidation, 168–169
hypertension, 132–133
ion channels, 167
lipid peroxidation, 167–168
production in cytosol, 130
production in mitochondria, 130–132
protein modifications, 168
redox-sensitive transcript factors, 165–166
triggering of protein kinases, 166
Recommended dietary allowance (RDA), 298
Rheumatoid arthritis (RA), 174–175

S

Selenium (Se), 136–137
derivatives as cancer-preventive agents, 319
insulin resistance, role of selenium, 235–236
Spinal muscular atrophy (SMA), 204
Spinocerebellar ataxia (SCA), 204
Stephania tetrandra S., 108
Stress, 284
acute stress, 284
chronic stress, 286
dietary neurotransmitters, 290–291
Stress-activated protein kinase c-jun N-terminal kinase (SAPK-JNK), 166
Substantia nigra pars compacta (SNPC), 176
Superoxide dismutase (SOD), 11–12, 135, 316
Suppressors of cytokine signaling (SOCS), 171

T

Tertiary butyl hydroquinone (TBHQ), 311
Thiobarbituric acid (TBA), 315
Thiobarbituric acid reactive substances (TBARS), 207
Total phenolic content (TPC), 313–314
Total reducing power (TRP), 314
Trolox equivalent, 314
Trolox equivalent (TE) equivalent, 24
Tumor microenvironment (TME), 170

U

Uncaria tomentosa, 21
Unfolded protein response (UPR), 167

W

Wogonin, 243–244
World Health Organization (WHO), 284